FORREST GENERAL MEDICAL

ADVANCED MEDICAL TRANSCRIPTION COURSE

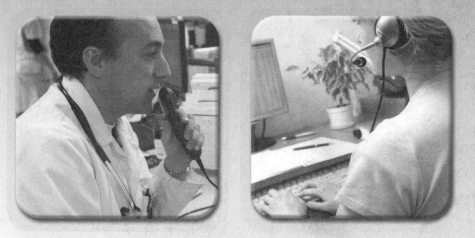

ADVANCED HEALTHCARE DOCUMENTATION SPECIALTY COURSE

FOURTH EDITION

FORREST GENERAL MEDICAL CENTER

ADVANCED MEDICAL TRANSCRIPTION COURSE

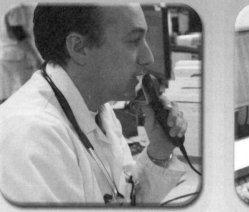
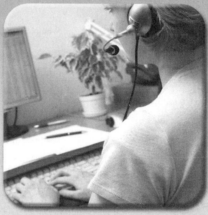

ADVANCED HEALTHCARE DOCUMENTATION SPECIALTY COURSE

FOURTH EDITION

DONNA L. CONERLY-STEWART, Ed.D.
Professor Emeritus
Business Technology Education
The University of Southern Mississippi
Hattiesburg, MS

PATRICIA A. IRELAND, CMT, AHDI-F
Multispecialty Medical Transcriptionist,
Instructor, Medical/Technical Author and Editor
San Antonio, TX

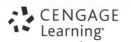
CENGAGE
Learning·

Australia • Brazil • Mexico • Singapore • United Kingdom • United States

Forrest General Medical Center: Advanced Medical Transcription Course, Fourth Edition
Donna L. Conerly-Stewart, Patricia A. Ireland

Product Director: Steve Helba

Associate Product Manager: Christina Gifford

Senior Director, Development: Marah Bellegarde

Product Development Manager: Juliet Steiner

Senior Content Developer: Natalie Pashoukos

Content Developer: Lauren Whalen

Editorial Assistant: Cassie Cloutier

Vice President, Marketing: Jennifer Ann Baker

Marketing Director: Wendy Mapstone

Production Director: Wendy A. Troeger

Production Manager: Andrew Crouth

Senior Content Project Manager: Kathryn B. Kucharek

Senior Art Director: David Arsenault

Media Developer: Deborah Bordeaux

Copyeditor: Kristin Wall

Cover image(s): background art/texture: © VikaSuh/www.Shutterstock.com; physician doing dictation: © Reza Estakhrian/Stone/Getty Images; woman with computer and headset: © pryzmat/www.Shutterstock.com

For product information and technology assistance, contact us at
Cengage Learning Customer & Sales Support, 1-800-354-9706
For permission to use material from this text or product,
submit all requests online at **www.cengage.com/permissions.**
Further permissions questions can be e-mailed to
permissionrequest@cengage.com

Library of Congress Control Number: 2013948995

ISBN-13: 978-1-111-53984-9

Cengage Learning
200 First Stamford Place, 4th Floor
Stamford, CT 06902
USA

Cengage Learning is a leading provider of customized learning solutions with office locations around the globe, including Singapore, the United Kingdom, Australia, Mexico, Brazil, and Japan. Locate your local office at: **www.cengage.com/global**

Cengage Learning products are represented in Canada by Nelson Education, Ltd.

To learn more about Cengage Learning, visit **www.cengage.com**

Purchase any of our products at your local college store or at our preferred online store **www.cengagebrain.com**

Notice to the Reader

Printed in the United States of America
1 2 3 4 5 6 7 18 17 16 15 14

DEDICATION

This textbook is dedicated to the memory of
Janet Clark Broom and James C. "Shrimp" Thompson,
whose families provided many of the authentic patient
records used for our students' edification.

Also, in loving gratitude to my dear husband, Vic Stewart, for his
patience and understanding—without which this revision could not
have been brought to fruition.

"It is better to know some of the questions than all of the answers."

–James Thurber

CONTENTS

PREFACE

Forrest General Medical Center: Advanced Healthcare Documentation Specialty Course, 4th edition, has been completely revised and updated. This comprehensive text is designed primarily for the advanced healthcare documentation specialist (HDS) student at the postsecondary level—community colleges, proprietary institutions, and four-year colleges or universities. One should possess a good foundation in English grammar and punctuation, keyboarding, medical terminology, and anatomy/physiology before beginning the study of these materials. Having completed a beginning healthcare documentation course would be a plus.

This text is designed to be used in a traditional classroom setting, in online courses, and in hospital in-service education departments. Either the newly employed or those being cross-trained or retrained would find it useful. The text could also be used in the training/retraining of veterans and their spouses, the disabled and their caregivers, and retirees who are looking for a new career. These materials could also prove useful in transitioning from a traditional transcription setting to voice/speech recognition and medical editing.

Conceptual Development of Text

The authors developed this revision of *Forrest General Medical Center* because the Healthcare Documentation Specialty field has changed and grown over the past several years. New issues have become important to the practitioners—for example, voice/speech recognition and medical editing, robotic surgery, new drugs, and new medical terms. We also wanted to address correspondence and provide tips on job searching.

Market needs at this time are for full-time employees; in that regard, we have tried to lay out the necessary learning materials for students in today's world to work at becoming full-time employees.

Organization and Design

The 4th edition contains 20 chapters organized into an introductory chapter, 17 medical specialty chapters, a chapter containing correctly formatted sample correspondence pieces, and proofreading exercises. The final chapter addresses professionalism and ethics within the profession. The organization of the material is intended to prepare students to enter and pursue a successful career in the healthcare documentation specialty field. The design of the material is intended to provide ease in learning.

Chapter 1 includes

- Helpful references and pointers
- CMTips with healthcare documentation specialty rules
- Report formatting
- Major types of medical reports, including the "basic four," and 15 model report forms

Chapters 2–18 include

- Introduction to each specific medical specialty
- Critical thinking exercises
- Lists of abbreviations with meanings
- Anatomic illustrations
- Lists of terminology specific to each specialty (with phonetic pronunciations)
- Transcription tips for each specialty
- Supportive web sites for each specialty
- Index listing each patient with name and type of report/procedure

Chapter 19 includes

- Examples of letters and memos
- Critical thinking exercise
- Twelve proofreading exercises with an index listing each patient

Chapter 20 includes

- Introduction and critical thinking exercise
- Tips on job searching, interviewing, résumé creation
- In-depth discussion of the healthcare documentation specialty career field

New and Updated Features

New features include three new chapters: Endocrinology, Arthritis/Rheumatology, and Podiatry.

All new transcription exercises, including clinic notes, HPIP notes, and SOAP notes. Other new elements include:

- New illustrations in most chapters,
- Information on quality assurance, scribes in the medical profession, speech recognition, medical editing, and text expanders,
- Material on an effective job search, which includes samples of employment documents and interviewing tips
- CMTips, computer safety, report formatting, and a discussion of the "basic four,"
- A list of the healthcare professional names that appear in the dictated reports along with their specialties; accents are included for each one who dictates,
- "Do not use" list from The Joint Commission,
- Two-state postal codes from United States Postal Service, and
- Proofreading marks on inside back cover of text.

Updated features include an updated chapter on Infectious Diseases, which is a stand-alone chapter in the 4th ed. Other updated elements include:

- New critical thinking exercises,
- Expanded abbreviations, terms, and laboratory/ diagnostic testing lists,
- Updated lists of reference materials, and
- Updated/expanded web site sections in each chapter.

Other Key Features

The basic educational features of *Forrest General Medical Center* have remained the same. They are:

- Realistic dictation with background noise in 17 specialties by professionals from various ethnic groups,
- Comprehensive lists of terms specific to each specialty,
- Realistic anatomic visuals,
- Comprehensive appendix to include confusing words, types of sutures and suture materials, dressings, medical instruments, anesthetic agents, surgical incisions, operative positions, and related web sites, and
- Selected resources recommended by authors.

List of Names, Addresses, and Phone Numbers for Forrest General Medical Center and its Feeder Clinics

Forrest General Medical Center
1038 Superior Street NW
Nashville, TN 37189
Phone 615.555.5000

Merwin B. Moore Memorial Clinic
6249 Broad Street
Lebanon, TN 37106
Phone 615.555.2500

James C. Thompson Memorial Clinic
#1 Lincoln Circle
Paris, TN 37904
Phone 731.555.3700

Carl E. Loftin Memorial Clinic
9465 Enterprise Circle
Cookeville, TN 37269
Phone 931.555.4900

Greater Nashville Gastroenterology Associates, P.A.
1200 Superior Street NW
Nashville, TN 37189
Phone 615.555.2600

The Nashville Diagnostic Clinic
12221 N. Cleary Expressway
Nashville, TN 37758
Phone 615.901.1111

The Nashville Eye Clinic
Cataract & Lasik Surgery Center
7790 Iris Lane Suite 300
Nashville, TN 37758
Phone 615.801.8111

Pebble Hill Podiatry
3026 Hillcrest Drive Suite 100
Nashville, TN 37758
Phone 615.555.7111

ACKNOWLEDGMENTS

We appreciate the assistance of all who helped in the production of this 4th edition. Our particular thanks go to the following professionals for their advice and review:

Ruth Bass, Neurology, Hattiesburg, MS
Jerrie Bolton, Medical Transcriptionist, Galveston, TX
Terisa Carter MT (ASCP), Reno, NV
B. Craig Chancellor, ACNP, Cardiology/Cardiovascular Surgery, Hattiesburg, MS
Carol Crumrine, Medical Transcriptionist, Columbia, NJ
India Dunaway, Supervisor, Pathology, Hattiesburg, MS
Linda Galbraith, Medical Transcriptionist, Foley, AL
Pam Hall, CMT, Clayton, NC
Holly Hammett, JD, PHR, Hattiesburg, MS
James R. Lantis Jr, MHA, MS, RHIA, HIM Director, University of Alabama Hospital, Birmingham, AL
Judy Matos, Medical Transcriptionist, Sandy Hook, CT
Deanna Aileen Martin, Medical Transcriptionist, San Antonio, TX
Cheryl L. Mauzy, MSN, RNC, NNP, Neonatology, Hattiesburg, MS
Jerry Morris, Medical Physics, Radiology/Diagnostic Imaging, Hattiesburg, MS
Shelia Morse, RN, BSN, Plastic/Reconstructive Surgery, Hattiesburg, MS
Stacey L. McFarlin, Consolidated Computing Solutions, www.ccs.satx.com
Julie Naimi, Medical Transcriptionist, Ft. Lauderdale, FL
Marge Parker, Medical Transcriptionist, Hayes, VA

And for providing or reviewing material, we are deeply grateful to each of the following:

Richard C. Adam, DPM, FACFAS, San Antonio, TX
Louis W. Benton, MD, OB/GYN, Hattiesburg, MS
Jeff Bullock, MD, Gastroenterology, San Antonio, TX
Mark M. Casillas, MD, Orthopedics, San Antonio, TX
Gary C. David, PhD, Assoc. Professor of Sociology, Bentley College, Waltham, MA
Robert E. DeCoux, MD, Gastroenterology, Hattiesburg, MS
Endwell Family Physicians, Endwell, NY
Gardner L. Fletcher, MD, Respiratory/Pulmonary Medicine, Hattiesburg, MS
Portia Harris, MD, Arthritis, Hattiesburg, MS
J. Michael Herrington, MD, Hematology/Oncology, Hattiesburg, MS
James M. Hodges, MD, ENT/Oral Surgery, Hattiesburg, MS
Ralph C. Kahler, MD, Infectious Diseases, Hattiesburg, MS
John H. Kosko, MD, Orthopedics/Podiatry, Hattiesburg, MS

Joshua A. Maksi, MD, Neurology, Hattiesburg, MS
Beth W. Nauert, MD, Pediatrician, Austin, TX
Richard A. Pecunia, MD, Plastic/Reconstructive Surgery, Hattiesburg, MS
J. Gregory Powell, MD, Endocrinology, Hattiesburg, MS
Thomas Puckett, MD, Pathology, Hattiesburg, MS
David C. Stout, MD, Urology/Nephrology, Hattiesburg, MS
Z. Michael Taweh, MD, Family Medicine/Geriatrics, Danbury, CT
Joseph K. Young, Doctor of Optometry, Newtown, CT

CHAPTER 1
INTRODUCTION

This chapter reviews what each student will need in order to successfully complete the healthcare documentation specialty (HDS) activities presented. In order to produce quality work with efficiency, carefully study the information presented here before beginning the HDS activities.

Chapter 1 contains information on the following topics:

- Helpful References
    - Selected healthcare documentation specialist guides
    - Selected office reference manuals
- Helpful Pointers
- CMTips™
- Healthcare Documentation Specialty Rules
- Computer Safety
- Typical Formats for Reports
- AHDI Report Formatting Guidelines
- Major Types of Medical Reports
- Model Report Forms

The information in this chapter will be indispensable as you complete the HDS exercises in Chapters 2 through 19.

Helpful References

To work efficiently and accurately, English, medical, as well as Internet web site references will support your HDS activities. Select an English grammar and punctuation guide, such as *The Book of Style for Medical Transcription, 3rd Edition* (further referred to as the AHDI *Book of Style* in this text), and follow it consistently. If your employer/client has a style preference, use their guide of choice for their work.

The following publications are examples of selected HDS guides:

Sims LM. *The Book of Style for Medical Transcription*. 3rd ed. Modesto, CA: Association for Healthcare Documentation Integrity; 2008.

Blake RS. *The Medical Transcriptionist's Handbook*. 2nd ed. Clifton Park, NY: Delmar Publishers; 1998.

Pfeiffer M, ed. *Medical Transcription Do's and Don'ts*. Philadelphia: WB Saunders Company; 1999.

Pugh MB, ed. *American Medical Association Manual of Style*. 9th ed. Philadelphia: Lippincott Williams & Wilkins; 1998.

Selected references to assist with grammar and punctuation rules and other transcription trouble spots include:

Clark JL, Clark LR. *How 13: A Handbook for Office Professionals*. 13th ed. Albany: Cengage Learning; 2014.

Jaderstrom S, Kruk L, Miller J. *Complete Office Handbook*. 3rd ed. New York, NY: Random House; 2002.

Sabin W. *Gregg Reference Manual*. 10th ed. Blacklick, OH: Glencoe McGraw-Hill; 2005.

For a more extensive list of suggested references, see the Appendix.

■ Helpful Pointers

The Healthcare Documentation Specialist (HDS) is a very important member of the patient care team. The HDS is charged with the responsibility of assuring that the physician's words are recorded promptly and accurately. This involves excellent listening, proofreading, and editing skills in addition to critical-thinking skills.

Technology has benefitted the medical field, giving us speech recognition and voice recognition systems, electronic healthcare records, electronic signatures, and many other benefits that directly affect the career of the HDS.

When speech or voice recognition is the primary means of obtaining physician dictation, the HDS becomes a medical editor. The production rate accelerates, keying errors are reduced, and carpel tunnel injuries are greatly minimized.

Additionally, more and more facilities are turning to *electronic (computer-based) patient records* rather than paper-based patient records to make the clinical decision-making process more efficient. The electronic patient record stores comprehensive patient information from a variety of sources—clinic, laboratory, and pharmacy. Clinical examination results can be entered by clinicians at or near the point of care (POC). Automatic date and time stamping of entries facilitates documentation and tracking of patient care and outcomes over time.

An electronic record also makes it easier for the primary care physician and consultants to quickly locate and readily identify accurate, usable information about the patient at the POC. If necessary, the physician and other authorized personnel can view a document as soon as it is transcribed, even before it is edited or signed. However, the record must still be authenticated by the physician, as indicated by insertion of the physician's signature, to be considered legal.

Today many physicians use *electronic signatures* rather than taking the time to personally sign each document.

The words "electronically signed by [physician's name]" together with the date and time will be found on the document above the sign-off block.

At the end of this chapter, the model reports give examples of how dictated and documented information is styled according to the AHDI *Book of Style*. AHDI guidelines represent a standard for medical reports. Formatting guidelines begin on page 3.

On the model reports, notice the signature block at the end of each report. The name of the physician followed by the title is keyed below the signature line. Next, the reference initials, the date the report was dictated, and the date it was transcribed are recorded—this is called the sign-off block. These dates are critical and must be accurate. Different styles are used by different employers/clients, and sometimes they are added automatically. *NB*: In this textbook, we are using ---- (four hyphens) to indicate the year. A four-digit year is the trend today.

Model Report #5 illustrates an electronic signature. Note that the time and date when the signature was affixed are included. In the reference lines, the physician's complete name is typed, followed by the HDS's initials. The time the document was dictated and transcribed, together with the document number, are also included. This practice allows the facility to improve the audit trail.

Although we have made an attempt to be consistent in these reports, several correct ways exist to document medical dictation. For example, if a physician dictates "one 0 nylon suture," it may be transcribed as either "1-0 nylon suture" or "0 nylon suture." However, "2-0" should be keyed as "2-0," not "00," and "4-0" as "4-0," not "0000." Be guided by the preference of each employer/client plus the AHDI *Book of Style*. As an HDS, flexibility is an important attribute. Before beginning "work" at Forrest General Medical Center, review the following:

1. Prefixes, suffixes, word roots, and/or combining forms
2. Types of medical reports (see page 10 and the model report forms on pages 12 through 38)
3. Proper healthcare documentation and/or grammar rules (beginning on page 4)
4. Confusing words (Appendix, page 309)
5. Types of sutures, anesthesia, dressings, incisions, operative positions, frequently used drugs, instruments, and laboratory tests (Appendix, page 316)
6. Components of the major types of medical reports, including the "basic four" (page 10)

An HDS should be concerned with accuracy in grammar, punctuation, style, and format. The following sections review grammar, punctuation, style, and formatting guidelines.

CMTips™

Nonmetric Units of Measure

Do not abbreviate nonmetric units of measure (unless in a table).

6 feet 2 inches	*NOT: 6' 2" or 6 ft. 2 in*
7 pounds	*NOT: 7 lbs or 7#*

The patient is 4 feet 10 inches tall. (*NB*: no comma between the measurements)

The infant weighed 5 pounds 9 ounces.

Mom gave the child 2 tablespoons of Motrin.

It was a long leg cast, probably 3 feet or 3-1/2 feet long.

Time

Acceptable abbreviations for ante meridiem (before noon) and post meridiem (after noon) are written as AM or a.m., PM or p.m., with the lowercase being preferred. Use periods with a.m. and p.m. so that a.m. is not misread as "am." Do not use periods with uppercase AM and PM. Insert a space between numerals and the abbreviation.

8:30 a.m. or 8:30 AM	*NOT* 8:30 am
	NOT 8:30a.m.
	NOT 8:30AM

Do not use these abbreviations with a phrase such as "in the morning," "in the evening," "tonight," or "o'clock":

8:30 a.m.	*NOT 8:30 a.m. o'clock*
9:30 PM	*NOT 9:30 PM in the evening*

Military time identifies the day's 24 hours by numerals 0100 through 2400. Transcribe military time with four digits <u>without</u> a space or colon. You may add the word "hours" for clarity if dictated, but this is not absolutely necessary.

Noon = 1200 hours   Midnight = 2400 hours

The patient arrived at 1300 hours. (1 p.m.)

The woman fell at 1430 the day prior to admission. (2:30 p.m.)

No one was admitted before 0445 due to security issues. (4:45 a.m.)

Time Zones

In the United States, the latest time is always Eastern Standard Time (EST), next is Central Standard Time (CST), then Mountain Standard Time (MST), and finally the earliest is Pacific Standard Time (PST).

It goes like this: EST --> CST --> MST --> PST

Every time you move from left to right (the direction of the arrows), you subtract an hour. When going against the arrow, add an hour each time you cross an arrow.

The time would therefore be 4 p.m. EST, 3 p.m. CST, 2 p.m. MST, 1 p.m. PST.

Exceptions: Daylight savings time—Arizona and Hawaii do not recognize daylight savings time. For those states that do recognize it, during the time it is in effect, subtract one hour for Daylight savings time. (Remember, Fall back and Spring ahead.)

Proofread

Each sentence must make sense. It is easy to accidently use the wrong form of a word, making your sentence sound off. Type a few lines. Stop. Go back and read aloud without audio. Enunciate each syllable of each word. You should spot any errors. <u>Remember</u>: If it sounds weird or if it makes no sense, it could be wrong. Listen to that spot in the audio again and edit any mistake. After all, physicians can dictate errors in their work; also, it is easy to add a stray letter, transpose letters or numbers, and/or leave out punctuation when typing fast. (*NB*: We offer proofreading exercises to help students learn this process.)

Examples:

- The patient take here medications first thing in the mornings and again after dinner.
  Edited: The patient takes her medications first thing in the morning and again after dinner.

- Patients past history is noncontributory.
  Edited: Patient's past history is noncontributory.

- On exam, vital sings are WNL; BP 120/80, afebrile, weight 175 lbs.
  Edited: On exam, vital signs are WNL; BP 120/80, afebrile, weight 175 pounds.

Graves disease: The term *Graves* disease does not contain an apostrophe. It is not *Grave's* disease or *Graves'* disease, as is often mistakenly transcribed. It can even be listed incorrectly in spell-check. The same is true with *Wilms* tumor and *Perthes* disease.

Remember: *Labia minora* is a plural term in the female anatomy. If the dictation concerns one side—left or right—you must transcribe the following, a singular term, whether it has been dictated or not: *labium minus*.

As such, *labia majora* is a plural term in the female anatomy. When the dictation regards one side, transcribe the following singular term, whether or not it was dictated: *labium majus*.

Regimen, Regime, Regiment

These soundalike words are often confused by both the HDS and the dictator.

A *regimen* is a treatment plan.

A *regime is a government authority.*

A *regiment* is an army unit.

Therefore, in medicine, you would use the word *regimen* to describe a treatment plan, even if the wrong soundalike word is dictated by the physician.

Healthcare Documentation Specialty Rules

The following selected rules adhere to the AHDI *Book of Style.* Consult that style guide for situations that are not addressed in the information that follows.

Capitalization

General Rules

1. Capitalize the trade names of drugs and brand names of manufactured products and equipment. **Do not** capitalize the generic names of drugs or products.

Advil	ibuprofen
Pepcid AC	famotidine
DepoDur	morphine
Humulin N	insulin
Kleenex	tissue

2. Capitalize eponyms but not the word(s) that accompany or modify them. An apostrophe occurs in some eponyms. The AHDI *Book of Style* recommends that the apostrophe be dropped; other references retain the apostrophe. Words derived from eponyms (such as adjectival forms) are not capitalized.

Parkinson disease	parkinsonism
Banks graft	Knowles hip pin
Down syndrome	Henry master knot
Deaver skin incision	Nesbit tuck procedure

3. When the full genus and species names are used, the genus takes an initial capital letter. When the genus is referred to as a single letter, that letter is uppercased. Species names should not be capitalized, nor should adjectival forms.

Streptococcus	streptococcal
	strep throat
Rickettsia japonica	R japonica
Pseudomonas	P aeruginosa
methicillin-resistant	MRSA
Staphylococcus aureus	

Escherichia coli	E coli
	E coli pneumonia
Giardia	giardiasis dysentery

   NB: Some reference books suggest italicizing the singular form of a genus and species name in formal publication.

4. Do not capitalize general references to departments or rooms in a medical facility. For example, *emergency room* and *recovery room* are lowercased, as generic terms. Specially designated rooms, however, should be capitalized; for example, the Crystal Dining Room.

5. When indicating positive allergy information, use a format that will draw attention to the data—either upper case or bold. The allergy's results should be included, whenever known, but it is unnecessary to upper case or bold that part of the sentence. Refer to your employer/client for preference in style. Acceptable formats include:

   ALLERGIES
   1. CODEINE, which causes a generalized rash.
   2. PENICILLIN, which causes anaphylactic shock.

   ALLERGIES
   1. **Codeine,** which causes a generalized rash.
   2. **Penicillin,** which causes anaphylactic shock.

6. Capitalize acronyms but not the words from which the acronym is obtained, unless it involves an eponym. When an acronym is dictated, spell out the phrase at first use, placing the acronym in parentheses. Then the acronym can be used throughout the report.

OAG	open-angle glaucoma
LD	Lyme disease
FOBT	fecal occult blood test
AICD	automatic implantable cardioverter-defibrillator

7. Regarding numbers in cancer grades and stages for classifications—check appropriate references. Diastolic and systolic murmurs use lowercase grade with arabic numerals. The stages of labor use lowercase stage and arabic numerals.

stage 1 (early/active labor)	grade 1 murmur (barely heard)
stage 2 (pushing/ delivering baby)	grade 2 murmur (clearly heard)
stage 3 (delivering placenta)	grade 3 murmur (loudly heard)

8. Do not capitalize disease names except for eponyms that may form part of the name.

Alzheimer disease   dementia
celiac disease   Crohn disease
black lung disease   mu heavy chain disease

9. Capitalize all major section headings in medical reports, e.g.,
   CHIEF COMPLAINT, ADMITTING DIAGNOSIS, PREOPERATIVE DIAGNOSIS, POSTOPERATIVE DIAGNOSIS, SUBJECTIVE, PHYSICAL EXAMINATION, OBJECTIVE, LABORATORY DATA, ASSESSMENT, IMPRESSION, PLAN, PROGNOSIS
   For subsection headings within a paragraph, use initial caps only, e.g.,
   PHYSICAL EXAMINATION: Vital Signs, HEENT, Neck, Lymph Nodes, Chest, Heart, Lungs, Abdomen, Extremities, Neurologic/ Psychiatric
   These subsections may be transcribed in paragraph style or flush left—both styles are equally correct.

10. Medical specialties, such as orthopedics, pediatrics, or internal medicine, are common nouns and, as such, are lowercase. Reference to a specialist, as an orthopedist, a pediatrician, or an internist should also be lowercase. In the signature block, however, transcribe the full name with title in initial caps, thus:

Robert J. Allen, MD, Internal Medicine

Gene Patrick, MD, PhD, Orthopedic Surgery

NB: When the name of a department is considered part of an organizational entity, the word should be in initial caps. See examples below.

The patient was referred to Endocrinology for diabetic studies.

Specimen sent to Pathology for gross and microscopic examination.

11. Brand names for items such as dressings, sutures, instruments, and drugs are uppercased; however, generic names or the adjectival forms that accompany the brand name are lowercased.

Emmett tenaculum   Adaptic gauze dressing
milk of magnesia   solid-state silk sutures
Gemini clamp   Stahl lens gauge
Ace   elastic bandage

Numbers

In this text we are following the AHDI *Book of Style* in the expression of numbers. Because figures (arabic numerals) are more distinguishable from surrounding text than are spelled-out numbers, AHDI recommends the use of figures in most instances. Specific guidelines follow.

General Rules

1. Use arabic numerals when typing units of measure, ages, and other vital statistics, including laboratory values.

3-year-old male   1.5 cm wound   26 mcg
5 feet 6 inches tall 42 years old   WBC 18.5
hemoglobin 14.7   9 eosinophils   2.7 mL

2. Use ordinal numbers (1st, 2nd, 3rd, …) to express position in a series or order.

Ms. Davis is in her 3rd month of pregnancy.

The 5th lumbar vertebra is involved.

Look at the 7th entry on the form.

Patient is to return in followup on the 11th and 24th of next month.

3. Follow the standard rules concerning the expression of dates. If the day precedes the month, use ordinal numbers; if it follows the month, use figures. Note the correct use of the comma when the year appears with the day and month and the correct format when only the year appears with the month.

On the 13th of January the patient took a turn for the worse.

The report is due October 23.

On April 4, 2014, Mary is to return. Her husband is to return in January 2014.

This surgery is scheduled 5 Dec 2014.

Use numbers with virgules (forward slashes) in the sign-off block with no spaces in the date. *NB*: In this text, we are using ---- to indicate a four-digit year.

D: 6/17/----

T: 6/18/----

4. Spell out numbers that begin a sentence or rewrite the sentence to place the number elsewhere. Keep numbers that relate to specific terms or measurements on the same line. A hard space or a hard hyphen will keep phrases together, unseparated, at the end of a line.

5. No comma is used in four-digit numbers, but use a comma in numbers with five or more digits.

White count was 6600.   Platelet count was 304,000.

The price was high at $7500.   There are more than 1,000,000 stars.

6. Preceding/trailing zeros: When a quantity of less than one is dictated, place a zero before the decimal point. However, no preceding zero is used in bullet calibers.

0.4 mg   *BUT*   .22 caliber rifle

When a whole number is dictated, do not add a decimal with a trailing zero, especially with drug references—this is considered dangerous. (See *Joint Commission Standards* in *The Book of Style for Medical Transcription*, 3rd ed., Section 9.3.1.)

7. Roman numerals are used for certain, specific classification systems; for example, the axis designations for psychiatric diagnoses, blood factors, cancer stages, Clark levels for malignant melanoma, decubitus ulcers, EKG standard bipolar leads, and several other instances. Check a reputable dictionary or other medical reference material for exact usage of roman numerals.

Punctuation

Commas

General Rules

1. In this text we are following the AHDI *Book of Style* for punctuation. Commas are used to improve clarity, enhance readability, and to avoid confusion or misunderstanding.

2. Use a comma between coordinate adjectives— adjectives that modify the same noun. Use a comma before "and" or "or" in a series.

   Physical examination revealed a tall, emaciated, underweight man.

   (*NB*: No comma is placed between the last adjective and the noun.)

   Patient's chief complaint included pain in the neck, shoulders, thumbs, hips, and knees.

3. If an adjective or adjectival phrase follows the noun it modifies, set it off with commas.

   She has tendinitis, right shoulder, with much discomfort.

4. Use commas between independent clauses that do not contain internal commas. If either (or both) contains internal commas, use a semicolon to separate the clauses. Remember, a *phrase* is a group of words that contains no subject and verb; a *clause* is a group of words that does contain a subject and a verb.

   The patient was begun on Ativan, and her symptoms subsided.

   (Independent clauses with no internal commas and are joined by a conjunction.)

   The patient, who was brought in by his mother, was begun on Ativan; and after about 2 hours, his symptoms subsided.

   (Independent clauses that do contain internal commas and are joined by a conjunction.)

5. Use commas to set off dependent nonrestrictive (or nonessential) clauses. Remember, a dependent clause is a group of words that "depends" on the rest of the sentence to make sense. It cannot stand alone as a sentence.

   The patient, who was brought in by his mother, was bleeding from the ear.

   NB: "who was brought in by his mother" is a dependent clause.

6. Do not set off dependent restrictive (essential) clauses with commas.

   The cut that was from the shoulder to the elbow was bleeding profusely.

   NB: "that was from the shoulder to the elbow" is restrictive; it tells which cut; therefore, it is necessary for clarity of the sentence and does not require commas.

7. When typing information concerning weights, spell out *pounds* and *ounces*. Do not separate with a comma.

   The newborn weighed 6 pounds 10 ounces.

Periods

1. Use periods with lowercased abbreviations and acronyms, whether English or Latin. If a sentence ends with an abbreviation that uses periods, no further period is needed to end the sentence.

etc. (and other things, and so forth)	p.r.n. (pro re nata)
a.m. (morning)	t.i.d. (ter in die)
et al. (and other people)	n.p.o. (nil per os)
pp. (pages)	a.c. (before food)
q.6 h. (every 6 hours)	p.c. (after food)

2. For plural forms of capitalized abbreviations, use a lowercase *s*.

   EOMs   PVCs   RBCs

3. To form the plural of lowercased abbreviations, use *'s*.

   wbc's   cbc's
   kcal's   serial 7's

4. See The Joint Commission's "Do Not Use" list (Appendix) for dangerous abbreviations. Also, make a good abbreviation book part of your medical reference material.

Semicolons

1. Use a semicolon to separate two independent clauses not joined by a conjunction.

   > Mrs. Davis has emphysema; her quality of life is very poor.

   > Mr. Clark was taken to a private room; his wife was taken to surgery.

2. A semicolon is used to join independent clauses, one or both of which contain internal commas.

   > Jesse, who is Jane's brother, was injured seriously in the accident; Jane was not injured.

   > There was some spasm in the sigmoid colon; otherwise, there were no mucosal lesions, mass lesions, friability, or ulceration seen throughout the colon.

3. Use a semicolon to separate two independent clauses joined by an adverbial connective (conjunctive adverb).

   > The patient was considered to be terminally ill; therefore, a DNR was to be signed and notarized.

Colons

1. The primary function of a colon is to introduce a list, series or enumeration, and in expressions of time. ***NB***: Military time takes no punctuation.
   Unless your employer/client prefers otherwise, use one space after a colon. Capitalize the word immediately following the colon, even if it is normally a lowercase word. Do not capitalize the first word after a colon if the material that follows is subordinate and cannot stand alone as a sentence. If the material that follows the colon forms an independent clause, however, do capitalize the first word to express special emphasis.

   > Medications include the following: glucophage and Mylanta.

   > Heart: Regular rate and rhythm. Lungs: Clear to A&P.

> Surgery was begun at 9:30 a.m. and was completed at 2 p.m.

> 1615 hours is 4:15 p.m.   2400 hours is midnight

2. Use a colon to express a ratio but not a range.

   ratio of 1:100,000   from 70 to 150 *NOT* 70:150

Hyphens

1. Use a hyphen to join compound modifiers occurring before a noun.

   > The well-developed, well-nourished young man was admitted for observation.

   When compound modifiers occur after the noun, the hyphens are omitted except when listed in the dictionary with hyphens. Compound adjectives shown in the dictionary with hyphens are considered permanently hyphenated. Regardless of whether the compound appears before or after a noun, the phrase retains the hyphen. Examples of some of these permanently hyphenated compounds include:

first-class	short-term
up-to-date	well-known
old-fashioned	well-rounded
cul-de-sac	SSN 000-00-0000

   When the parts of compound adjectives are separated (or suspended), hyphenate each part.

   > The 6-, 7-, and 8-year-old patients are to be moved from the pediatric floor to the emergency room until the windows are repaired.

   Adjective/adverb combinations should not be hyphenated.

   > This terminally ill young man is in desperate need of financial help.

2. When hyphenated compound words become well established, many times the hyphen is dropped and the words are joined to form one word—such as weightbearing, which has evolved into one word. When such words can be used as nouns, verbs, or adjectives, the noun/adjective forms are joined without a hyphen. When the compound word is used as a verb and one of the words is a preposition, the compound remains as two separate words.

VERB	NOUN, ADJECTIVE
follow up	followup
follow through	followthrough
check up	checkup
work up	workup

Abbreviations and Symbols

1. Abbreviate metric units of measurement when a numeric quantity precedes the unit of measure. Do not use a period after the abbreviation (for example, 50 cm or 4 g).
2. Write out abbreviations that are dictated in full except for metric units of measurement. A sentence may begin with a dictated abbreviation, acronym, or brief form; however, the sentence may also be recast.
3. Spell in full any abbreviation that is used in the admission, discharge, preoperative, or postoperative diagnosis lines. Also, a conclusion in a consultation plus information in the title of an operation should be written out, not abbreviated.

Use of Dates Within Medical Reports

1. Spell out the month within the context of a report. Use numerals to represent the day of the month.

    The patient was brought to the hospital via ambulance on September 12, ----.

    On May 29, ----, patient was involved in a car accident; he expired on June 26.

    (Note the use of commas to set off the year in the date above.)

    Mr. Jonathan P. Andrews was named CEO of the hospital in October 2003.

2. Use one space after D and T in the sign-off block, which is transcribed two lines under the signature line.

    (D = date dictated; T = date transcribed)

    Grace Mosel, MD

    GM:pai
    D: 5/20/----
    T: 5/21/----

3. When typing dates, keep the month and day on the same line; the year can go onto the next line, if necessary. A hard space will keep this information together on the same line.

    NOT . . . . October
    24, ---- *BUT* . . . . October 24, ----.

Miscellaneous Rules

1. For words that require accent marks, the trend is to omit the accent in transcribed medical reports because of equipment limitations and the possibility of making errors in placement. Never place them in handwritten form.

2. When an acronym is dictated, transcribe the words in full at first use; then, you may use the short form throughout the report except in the admitting or discharge diagnosis lines, preoperative or postoperative lines, or diagnosis lines.

3. Use of the ampersand (&) should be limited to certain single-letter abbreviations (i.e., D&C, I&A, C&S, T&A). No space should precede or follow the ampersand. Do not use in operative titles or diagnosis lines.

4. Limit use of the degree sign to information in tables except when giving temperature. Write out *degrees* in text when expressing angles.

    The knee was bent to 30 degrees' flexion.

    Temperature was 48 degrees F. *OR* 48 °C (if degree symbol is available)

5. When transcribing measurements, use a lowercase *x* or the multiplication symbol with one space before and after it.

    The wound measured 4 x 6 inches.

    Specimen measuring $0.5 \times 1.2 \times 2.0$ cm was removed and sent to Pathology.

Decimals

When metric measures are dictated, always use the decimal form of the number.

The incision was 4.5 cm long. *NOT* 4-1/2 cm long.

Percent

When "percent" is dictated, transcribe % or *percent* within the report. Do not use the abbreviation "*pct.*" for *percent* except in tables. Use % with no space after a number; use *percent* when the number is written in full. Remember, percent is one word.

40% or 40 percent   Twenty percent   15% or 15 percent

Punctuation with Quotation Marks

1. Periods and commas always go <u>inside</u> the final quotation marks. Colons and semicolons always go <u>outside</u>. Placement of the question mark and exclamation mark depends on the wording of the sentence.

    The physician said, "Mrs. Anderson should be taken to an extended-care facility."

2. If the quotation is asking the question, place the question mark inside the quotation marks.

If, however, the sentence is stated in the form of a question but the quotation is not, place the mark outside the quotation marks.

> The social worker asked, "Is he to be admitted to rehab?"

> Did the social worker say, "We cannot accept his admission"?

Drug Information

1. Transcribe information relating to drug dosages as dictated. It is acceptable to abbreviate units of time if that is the preference of the employer/client. Examples as follows:

   > Dictated: penicillin four milligrams three times a day

   > Transcribe: penicillin 4 mg 3 times a day OR penicillin 4 mg t.i.d.

   > Dictated: Keflex two hundred fifty milligrams every four hours

   > Transcribe: Keflex 250 mg every 4 hours OR Keflex 250 mg q.4 h.

2. Do not use commas to separate drug names from instructions and doses. The commas go between the drug and all its dosage information, as follows:

   > The patient was instructed to take erythromycin 250 mg q.i.d., Keflex 500 mg q.6 h., and Reglan 10 mg at bedtime; she is to hold off on NSAIDs for now.

NB: If more than three medications are listed, it is helpful to transcribe them in list form—this makes the report easier to read and code.

Computer Safety

Your computer is your lifeline in healthcare documentation.

1. Change your password often—some say every three months—and use a complicated password.
2. Save your work early and often—do not take a chance on losing even one report.
3. Backup your files every day—to a thumb drive or an external hard drive or both. Companies often have their files backed up and stored off site; however, if you are an independent contractor, backup is your responsibility.
4. Use basic preventive maintenance to keep your computer running smoothly. Have current antivirus and firewall software installed and running at all times. This is **not** optional. There are free programs to download as well as ones that cost money. Examples include Advanced System Care, AVG, www.webroot.com, and others.
5. Employ "professional computer repair" for problems that are not routine.

Remember: Your computer is your means of communication and your means of making a living. Keep it clean, safe, in good repair, and away from children and pets.

Typical Formats for Reports

The formatting of each medical report can differ from one facility to another; therefore, the HDS or the medical editor should be prepared to demonstrate flexibility in transcribing or editing reports.

In some facilities, medical records are printed on plain paper (sometimes colored to identify specific reports); other facilities have a prepared form onto which dictation is transcribed. Some prepared forms include a line at the bottom of the page for the signature of the dictating healthcare professional. When this is the case, you should type the dictator's name and title directly under the line; otherwise, the HDS creates a line. The sign-off block is transcribed flush left and double spaced below the signature line; it includes dictator initials, HDS initials, date dictated, and date transcribed. It can include the exact time of dictation and transcription as well—sometimes this information is automated. The dictating healthcare professional will sign above the typed signature line.

Many medical facilities provide equipment that allows the HDS to download patient information and demographics directly from the mainframe. This information can be placed at the top or at the bottom of the first page of each report, depending upon the employer's/client's preference. The HDS selects account information on the patient and copies all relevant data automatically into the document. Then the HDS begins keying pertinent dictation into the body of the report, never having to manually enter patient data.

If a procedure is considered normal, many facilities have prerecorded "normal" templates. The HDS is instructed to retrieve a "normal 1" or a "normal 2," for example. When a "normal" template is to be used, the HDS starts a new document and inserts the "normal" text, which saves time and the possibility of introducing errors for both the HDS and/or the originator.

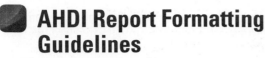

AHDI Report Formatting Guidelines

Adhering to the following guidelines and studying the model reports will aid in formatting reports correctly. Although AHDI guidelines are the "standard," a facility may (1) prefer or require the use of a different style guide or even (2) require "verbatim" documentation.

1. Use block format for all reports with left justification.
2. Leave 1/2- to 1-inch top, bottom, left, and right margins.
3. Hyphenate words at the end of lines only when typing words with preexisting hyphens. Use a hard hyphen to keep words together on the same line.
4. Begin a new paragraph where the dictator indicates except when paragraph use is excessive. If no paragraphs are dictated, paragraph when appropriate or when the subject changes.
5. Type major headings in all capitals, as dictated, flush left.
6. Rekey the diagnosis if the dictator uses "same" for the postoperative diagnosis (meaning it is the same as the preoperative diagnosis). Do not type "same," even if you have a "verbatim" employer/client.
7. Enumerate items as dictated. If some are numbered and some are not, keep your work consistent. Rule of thumb: If there are more than three, use a numbered list.
8. Double space between major sections of reports but single space between subheadings that are listed vertically.
9. Avoid abbreviating headings, even if dictated, except for widely used and readily recognizable abbreviations, such as HEENT.
10. Use a colon followed by one space if information follows a heading on the same line.
11. Omit the colon after the heading if the information begins on the next line at the left margin.
12. Enter the signature block at the left margin four spaces after the last line of type. Type the originator's full name and title. If necessary, a long title can be typed directly beneath the name.
13. Identify each report by the originator and the HDS's initials, date of dictation, and date of transcription, called the "sign-off block," typed flush left and entered two lines below the originator's name and title. Employers/clients will have their own style for this information. The only punctuation would be a colon or a virgule, as shown.

DS:pai	OR	ds:pai
DS/pai	OR	ds/pai
D: 05/03/----	OR	D: 5/3/----
T: 05/04/----	OR	T: 5/4/----

14. Continue a report onto a second or succeeding page by keying "continued" at the bottom of each page and inserting a heading at the top of each succeeding page. See the model reports for examples.
15. Use the "widow/orphan" feature of your word processor to avoid having a single line of type appear as the last line on the page or the first line of a new page. Each page of a report must contain at least two lines of text. Never leave only a signature block and sign-off block alone on a page.
16. Type a copy line two spaces underneath the sign-off block, flush left. Use a colon after the "c," or "cc" (courtesy copy) or "bc" (blind copy). A tab is often used after the colon so that the names align and for better readability; however, one space after the colon is also acceptable.

    c: Carole J. Downey, MD, OB/GYN

    bc: Patricia Maloney, JD, PhD

Major Types of Medical Reports

The "basic four" includes the *history and physical exam, operative report, consultation,* and *discharge summary.* Radiology and pathology reports are not included in the basic four.

Becoming familiar with the following information about the "basic four" plus radiology and pathology reports will help you understand the components of each.

1. History and physical examination—Often dictated by the admitting physician or resident; however, "hospitalists" are physicians who deal only with hospitalized patients. The hospitalist often will take care of the H&P for clinicians and surgeons. The "history" includes the chief complaint, history of present illness, and information about the patient's past, social, and family histories that contributed to the present illness. In addition, a review of systems and physical findings are part of this report. The review of systems is subjective (what the patient tells the doctor), but the physical is objective information—what is seen and felt on physical evaluation of the patient at the time of admission. Vital signs are included in the physical exam section. (See Model Report #1, p. 12)
2. Consultation—When a second opinion about a patient's condition or diagnosis is required, a consulting physician evaluates the patient. This report is dictated by the consultant, addressed to

the attending physician, and generally includes the date of and reason for the consultation, the physical exam, and laboratory data, and the consultant's impression and recommendations. A note of appreciation for the consultation may also be included. (See Model Report #2, p. 15)

3. Operative report—Dictated by the surgeon or PA (physician's assistant), this includes specific information regarding an operative procedure. Preoperative and postoperative diagnoses, surgeon name(s), anesthesiologist name(s), type of anesthesia, operative findings, and a detailed description of the procedure are typical parts of this report. A prognosis may be included. (See Model Report #3, p. 17)

4. Discharge summary (DS)—Often dictated by the admitting physician or resident when the patient is dismissed from the hospital. Again, if a hospitalist has been used for the patient, he would dictate the discharge summary. The DS includes a review of why the patient was admitted and a history of the hospital stay. It can also include information on laboratory data, followup instructions, discharge medications, condition of the patient on discharge, and the prognosis. The primary focus of the discharge summary is a summary of events that occurred while the patient was in the hospital plus discharge diagnoses. (See Model Report #5, p. 24)

5. Radiology report—Dictated upon completion of a diagnostic procedure, this includes the impression and findings. Examples include CT scans, MRI scans, therapeutic x-rays, nuclear medicine scans, mammograms, and fluoroscopic examinations. (See Model Report #6, p. 27)

6. Pathology report—Includes gross description and microscopic diagnosis of tissue removed at surgery. This is done in anatomic pathology and does not include clinical laboratory information. It contains detailed information on the tissue, both as seen by the naked eye (gross) and as seen under the microscope. (See Model Reports 4a and 4b, pp. 20 and 22)

Some practitioners dictate the *problem-oriented record (POR)* so that specific problems are defined, numbered, and referred to by number throughout the record. Components of the POR may vary according to the particular setting in which the system is used. However, every system includes the following:

1. The *initial data base,* which consists of the patient's comprehensive health history, a complete physical exam, and available laboratory data.

2. The *problem list.*

3. *Progress notes, chart notes,* and *followup notes* may be organized in different formats—SOAP or HPIP are two popular formats. The note begins with the problem and continues as follows:

H = History   S = Subjective examination
P = Physical   O = Objective examination
I = Impression   A = Assessment
P = Plan   P = Plan

Model Report Forms

Model Report No. 1: History and Physical Examination

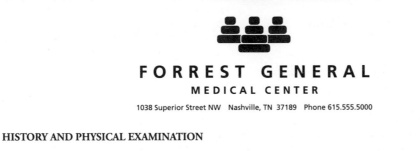

FORREST GENERAL
MEDICAL CENTER
1038 Superior Street NW   Nashville, TN 37189   Phone 615.555.5000

HISTORY AND PHYSICAL EXAMINATION

Patient Name: AULTMAN, Johnny   **Admitting Physician**: A. Phipps, MD
Patient ID: 3798670   **Sex/Age**: M/76   **DOB**: May 2, ----
Date of Admission: March 14, ----

CHIEF COMPLAINT
Black, tarry stools.

PRESENT ILLNESS
This 76-year-old white male presented to the ER because of black, tarry stools. He had been having these for a short period of time, has had only 2 stools over the past month, has had no indigestion or heartburn. Has a history of peptic ulcer disease with bleeding x2. Each of those times he had no pain or indigestion, no nausea or vomiting.

PAST HISTORY
In relatively good health, he has had hypertension for about 6 years. No history of thyroid disease, asthma, TB, or pneumonia. A borderline diabetic for 5 years with no previous surgery.

FAMILY HISTORY
Father died of a CVA. A brother has prostate CA and a sister has CA of the spleen.

SOCIAL HISTORY
He smoked about 2 packs a day for 25 years but stopped about 16 years ago. He does not drink. He is a widower with 2 grown children who are L&W.

CURRENT MEDICATIONS
Dyazide, 1 daily; a 1500-calorie ADA diet, takes aspirin occasionally.

ALLERGIES
He has no known drug allergies.

REVIEW OF SYSTEMS
HEENT: Has a cataract on the right eye with decreased vision in that eye.
PULMONARY: Some chronic productive cough with some shortness of breath on exertion. There is no hemoptysis, no PND, no orthopnea.
CARDIOVASCULAR: No chest pains, palpitations, or fluttering.
GASTROINTESTINAL: See PRESENT ILLNESS.
GENITOURINARY: No dysuria, hematuria, frequency, or urgency. Some decrease in size and force of his stream at times. He also has some terminal dribbling. Nocturia 1 to 2 times per night.

(Continued)

HISTORY AND PHYSICAL EXAMINATION
Patient Name: AULTMAN, Johnny
Date of Admission: March 14, ----

NEUROMUSCULAR: Stiffness in his left shoulder and right shoulder pain at times.

PHYSICAL EXAMINATION
GENERAL: Well-developed, well-nourished white male in no acute distress.
VITAL SIGNS: Blood pressure 142/70, respirations 18, pulse 100, and temperature 97.5 °F.
HEENT: Pupils are equal, round, and reactive to light and accommodation. He has a right cataract. Fundi are normal. He has dentures.
NECK: No carotid bruits. Some fullness over the thyroid but no palpable gland.
HEART: Regular rate without murmur, rub, or gallop.
LUNGS: Clear to auscultation and percussion.
ABDOMEN: Soft and nontender. No masses palpable, no bruits, no palpable organomegaly.
RECTAL: He has some black, tarry stool in the rectal vault that is Hemoccult positive. His prostate is 1+ to 2+ enlarged, but there are no hard nodules.
NEUROLOGICAL: Affect is WNL. Extremities move well. Sensory and motor function normal. DTRs are symmetrical.
EXTREMITIES: No clubbing, cyanosis, or edema.

IMPRESSION
Melena; rule out bleeding peptic ulcer disease. Patient is to discontinue aspirin at this time.

_____

Doris Robertson, MD, Gastroenterology

DR:ds
D: 3/14/----
T: 3/14/----

C: Anderson Phipps, MD, Family Medicine/Geriatrics

Model Report No. 2: Consultation

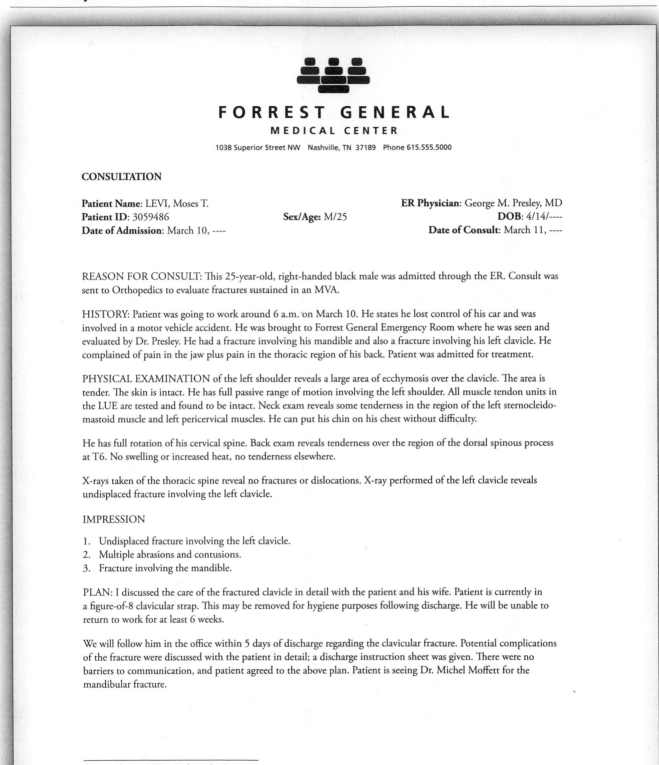

FORREST GENERAL
MEDICAL CENTER
1038 Superior Street NW   Nashville, TN 37189   Phone 615.555.5000

CONSULTATION

Patient Name: LEVI, Moses T.
Patient ID: 3059486   **Sex/Age:** M/25
Date of Admission: March 10, ----

ER Physician: George M. Presley, MD
DOB: 4/14/----
Date of Consult: March 11, ----

REASON FOR CONSULT: This 25-year-old, right-handed black male was admitted through the ER. Consult was sent to Orthopedics to evaluate fractures sustained in an MVA.

HISTORY: Patient was going to work around 6 a.m. on March 10. He states he lost control of his car and was involved in a motor vehicle accident. He was brought to Forrest General Emergency Room where he was seen and evaluated by Dr. Presley. He had a fracture involving his mandible and also a fracture involving his left clavicle. He complained of pain in the jaw plus pain in the thoracic region of his back. Patient was admitted for treatment.

PHYSICAL EXAMINATION of the left shoulder reveals a large area of ecchymosis over the clavicle. The area is tender. The skin is intact. He has full passive range of motion involving the left shoulder. All muscle tendon units in the LUE are tested and found to be intact. Neck exam reveals some tenderness in the region of the left sternocleido-mastoid muscle and left pericervical muscles. He can put his chin on his chest without difficulty.

He has full rotation of his cervical spine. Back exam reveals tenderness over the region of the dorsal spinous process at T6. No swelling or increased heat, no tenderness elsewhere.

X-rays taken of the thoracic spine reveal no fractures or dislocations. X-ray performed of the left clavicle reveals undisplaced fracture involving the left clavicle.

IMPRESSION

1. Undisplaced fracture involving the left clavicle.
2. Multiple abrasions and contusions.
3. Fracture involving the mandible.

PLAN: I discussed the care of the fractured clavicle in detail with the patient and his wife. Patient is currently in a figure-of-8 clavicular strap. This may be removed for hygiene purposes following discharge. He will be unable to return to work for at least 6 weeks.

We will follow him in the office within 5 days of discharge regarding the clavicular fracture. Potential complications of the fracture were discussed with the patient in detail; a discharge instruction sheet was given. There were no barriers to communication, and patient agreed to the above plan. Patient is seeing Dr. Michel Moffett for the mandibular fracture.

_____
Olivia Glover, MD, Orthopedic Surgery

OG:ds
D: 3/11/----
T: 3/11/----

C: Michel Moffett, MD, ENT/Oral Surgery

Model Report No. 3: Operative Report

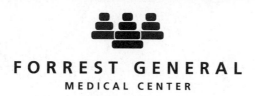

FORREST GENERAL
MEDICAL CENTER
1038 Superior Street NW   Nashville, TN 37189   Phone 615.555.5000

OPERATIVE REPORT

Patient Name: TOUPS, Wallis   **Admitting Physician**: Anderson Phipps, MD
Patient ID: 543-9207   **Sex/Age**: M/65   **DOB**: 6/18/----
Date of Admission: March 15, ----   **Surgeon**: Jeffrey Wolfe, MD

PREOPERATIVE DIAGNOSIS
Intermittent atrial flutter/fibrillation with severe ventricular bradycardia.

POSTOPERATIVE DIAGNOSIS
Intermittent atrial flutter/fibrillation with severe ventricular bradycardia.

PROCEDURE
Implantation of permanent transvenous cardiac pacemaker (Medtronic model 5985).

ANESTHESIA
Local 1% Xylocaine administered by Diane Davis, CRNA.

FINDINGS (including the condition of all organs examined)
Patient was admitted with episodes of atrial flutter/fibrillation with very slow ventricular response in low 40s. He was entirely uncooperative and combative during the course of the operation. It took 5 people to hold him on the cath table. Also, his heart rate was between 140 and 180. He had very small veins in the region of the deltopectoral groove.

All these problems led to great difficulty in putting this pacemaker in place. However, the electrode was finally positioned in the apex of the right ventricle, and I assumed that his threshold was satisfactory; but we could not be entirely sure of this because of his very fast ventricular rate of 140 to 160. It appeared that the threshold was an MA of 0.8, voltage of 0.5, with resistance of 610 ohms. R-wave sensitivity was 7.3.

PROCEDURE IN DETAIL
With the patient in the supine position, the right pectoral region was prepped and draped in the usual fashion. As mentioned above, the patient was entirely combative and uncooperative so that 5 people had to hold him down. After satisfactory local anesthesia and regional anesthesia were induced, a transverse incision was made and the deltopectoral groove was dissected. One vein appeared to be slightly larger than the rest of the very small venules in this area. It was cannulated with a cardiac electrode; with some difficulty, this was threaded into the apex of the right ventricle under fluoroscopic control.

As mentioned above, the patient's threshold appeared to be satisfactory, though this was not entirely certain. Electrode was ligated in place with heavy silk, after which it was attached to the Medtronic pacemaker model 5985. The unit was implanted into the subcutaneous pocket. It should be noted that the patient had practically no subcutaneous fat, so only a very thin layer of subcutaneous tissue and skin overlies the pacemaker.

(Continued)

OPERATIVE REPORT   Page 2
Patient Name: TOUPS, Wallis   Admitting Physician: Anderson Phipps, MD
Patient ID: 543-9207   Date of Admission: March 15, ----

The wound was closed in 2 layers. Sterile dressings were applied. Instrument count was correct x2. Blood loss was minimal. Patient was taken to SICU in stable condition, much calmer. He can be returned to his room after 24 hours in SICU.

NB: Patient must be monitored closely. I have informed the floor nurses and the SICU nurses that they are to contact me and/or my PA immediately should he become confused or uncooperative.

_____

Jeffrey Wolfe, MD
Cardiac Surgery

JW:pai
D: 3/15/----
T: 3/15/----

Model Report No. 4a: Pathology Report

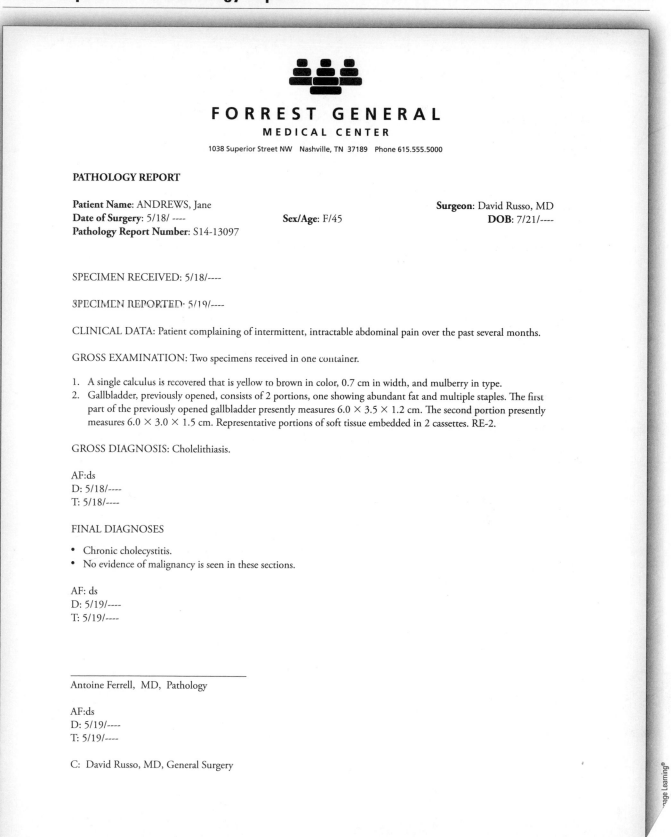

FORREST GENERAL
MEDICAL CENTER
1038 Superior Street NW   Nashville, TN 37189   Phone 615.555.5000

PATHOLOGY REPORT

Patient Name: ANDREWS, Jane   **Surgeon**: David Russo, MD
Date of Surgery: 5/18/ ----   **Sex/Age**: F/45   **DOB**: 7/21/----
Pathology Report Number: S14-13097

SPECIMEN RECEIVED: 5/18/----

SPECIMEN REPORTED: 5/19/----

CLINICAL DATA: Patient complaining of intermittent, intractable abdominal pain over the past several months.

GROSS EXAMINATION: Two specimens received in one container.

1. A single calculus is recovered that is yellow to brown in color, 0.7 cm in width, and mulberry in type.
2. Gallbladder, previously opened, consists of 2 portions, one showing abundant fat and multiple staples. The first part of the previously opened gallbladder presently measures 6.0 × 3.5 × 1.2 cm. The second portion presently measures 6.0 × 3.0 × 1.5 cm. Representative portions of soft tissue embedded in 2 cassettes. RE-2.

GROSS DIAGNOSIS: Cholelithiasis.

AF:ds
D: 5/18/----
T: 5/18/----

FINAL DIAGNOSES

- Chronic cholecystitis.
- No evidence of malignancy is seen in these sections.

AF: ds
D: 5/19/----
T: 5/19/----

_____

Antoine Ferrell, MD, Pathology

AF:ds
D: 5/19/----
T: 5/19/----

C: David Russo, MD, General Surgery

Model Report No. 4b: Pathology Report

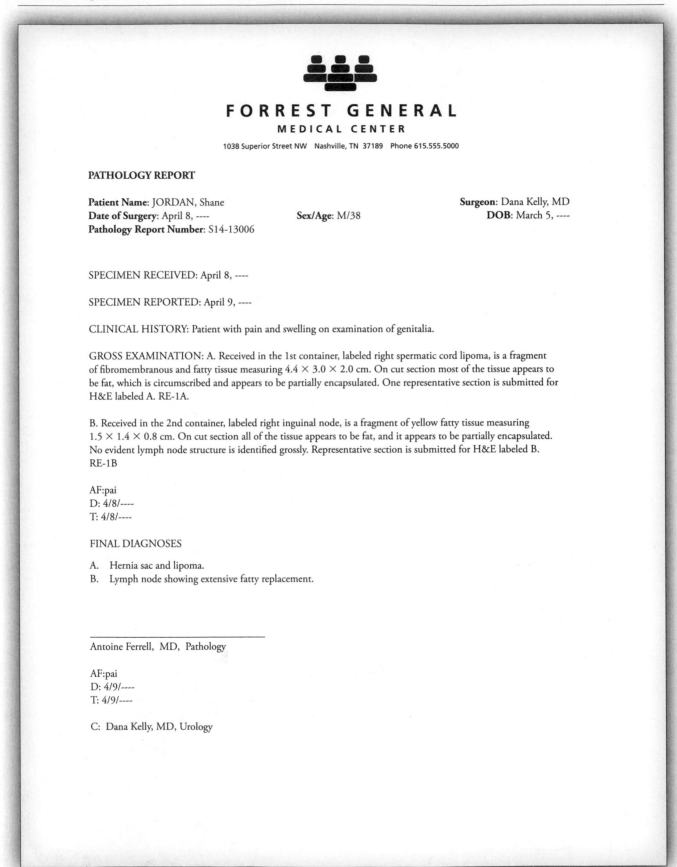

FORREST GENERAL
MEDICAL CENTER
1038 Superior Street NW   Nashville, TN 37189   Phone 615.555.5000

PATHOLOGY REPORT

Patient Name: JORDAN, Shane   **Surgeon**: Dana Kelly, MD
Date of Surgery: April 8, ----   **Sex/Age**: M/38   **DOB**: March 5, ----
Pathology Report Number: S14-13006

SPECIMEN RECEIVED: April 8, ----

SPECIMEN REPORTED: April 9, ----

CLINICAL HISTORY: Patient with pain and swelling on examination of genitalia.

GROSS EXAMINATION: A. Received in the 1st container, labeled right spermatic cord lipoma, is a fragment of fibromembranous and fatty tissue measuring 4.4 × 3.0 × 2.0 cm. On cut section most of the tissue appears to be fat, which is circumscribed and appears to be partially encapsulated. One representative section is submitted for H&E labeled A. RE-1A.

B. Received in the 2nd container, labeled right inguinal node, is a fragment of yellow fatty tissue measuring 1.5 × 1.4 × 0.8 cm. On cut section all of the tissue appears to be fat, and it appears to be partially encapsulated. No evident lymph node structure is identified grossly. Representative section is submitted for H&E labeled B. RE-1B

AF:pai
D: 4/8/----
T: 4/8/----

FINAL DIAGNOSES

A.   Hernia sac and lipoma.
B.   Lymph node showing extensive fatty replacement.

_____

Antoine Ferrell, MD, Pathology

AF:pai
D: 4/9/----
T: 4/9/----

C: Dana Kelly, MD, Urology

Model Report No. 5: Discharge Summary

FORREST GENERAL
MEDICAL CENTER
1038 Superior Street NW   Nashville, TN 37189   Phone 615.555.5000

DISCHARGE SUMMARY

Patient Name: DONALDSON, Gayle
Patient ID: 490-3982   **Sex/Age**: F/55
Date of Admission: June 10, ----

Admitting Physician: Doris Robertson, MD
DOB: April 4, ----
Date of Discharge: June 16, ----

ADMITTING DIAGNOSES

1. Atrophic gastritis.
2. Irritable bowel syndrome.
3. Heme-positive stool.

PROCEDURE PERFORMED
Esophagogastroduodenoscopy done 6/11/---- with no complications.

HISTORY AND PHYSICAL ON ADMISSION
This 55-year-old white female was admitted for evaluation of abdominal pain, nausea and vomiting, and reports
of coffee-grounds emesis. Several weeks ago she was evaluated at Forrest General Emergency Room for similar
symptoms and was told she had several ulcers in her distal esophagus. She was started on medications; however, she
was told that she might have to have surgery. She did fairly well after the initiation of medication, but over the 3 days
prior to admission, she had increasing left upper quadrant discomfort along with nausea, vomiting, and hematemesis.
She gives history of a 35-pound weight loss over the last 18 months. Two years ago patient underwent evaluation at
Greater Nashville Gastroenterology Associates and was found to have erosive gastritis with duodenitis as well as reflux
esophagitis. She also had some left upper quadrant pain at that time that was attributed to some post herpes zoster
neuritis. She previously had cholecystectomy and appendectomy.

PHYSICAL EXAM on admission (limited to the GI system) shows multiple well-healed abdominal scars. Abdomen
soft, no masses palpable. Some mild discomfort elicited on palpation of the left upper quadrant. Bowel sounds
WNL. Stool is Hemoccult positive.

LABORATORY DATA ON ADMISSION
Admission labs showed hemoglobin 13.8 with WBCs 8000. Urinalysis with 3+ protein with 1 to 3 RBCs/hpf.
SMAC was WNL except for slight elevation of BUN at 38.

HOSPITAL COURSE
The patient underwent EGD by Dr. Robertson on June 11 with findings of some mild erythema in the prepyloric
area, but it was otherwise unremarkable. CT scan of the abdomen was normal. Serum gastrin was slightly elevated
at 256. Gastric analysis was done and showed basal of 0.3 mEq/hr, which was quite low; maximal acid output 7.1,
which was also low; and peak acid output of 10 mEq/hr. Zantac was discontinued 24 hours prior to gastric analysis.
Lactose tolerance test was done, which showed normal curve. Barium enema was done, which was grossly normal.

(Continued)

DISCHARGE SUMMARY   Page 2
Patient Name: DONALDSON, Gayle   Admitting Physician: Doris Robertson, MD
Patient ID: 490-3982
Date of Admission: June 10, ----   Date of Discharge: June 16, ----

IMPRESSION on discharge is that patient has elements of atrophic gastritis. She was started on Reglan while in the hospital and has shown marked improvement with regard to her nausea and abdominal discomfort. I suspect that she has some element of irritable bowel syndrome.

DISCHARGE PLAN
We are instituting a high-fiber diet and continuing Reglan and Zantac. Patient has been instructed to continue a bland diet and to add additional foods, one at a time. She is to return to my office in 3 weeks for followup. We will repeat the Hemoccult test at that time.

MEDICATIONS AT TIME OF DISCHARGE

1. Zantac 150 mg p.o. b.i.d.
2. Reglan 10 mg p.o. a.c. and at bedtime
3. Restoril 30 mg at bedtime p.r.n. sleep.
4. Darvocet-N 100 1 q.4 h. p.r.n. pain.

Electronically signed by Doris Robertson, MD, Gastroenterology, 6/16/---- at 6:20 p.m.

DR:ds
DD: 6/16/----
DT: 6/17/----

Model Report No. 6: Radiology Report

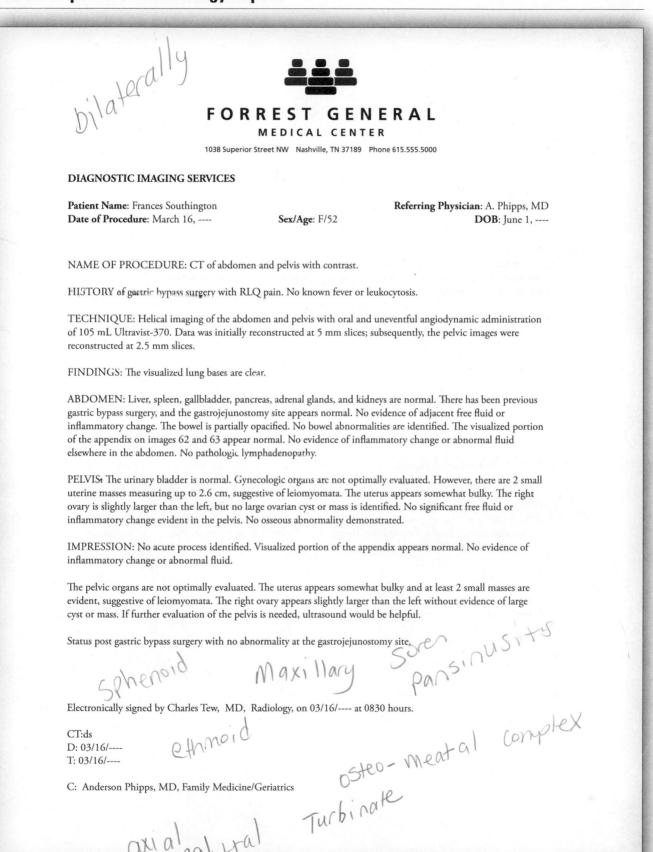

FORREST GENERAL
MEDICAL CENTER

1038 Superior Street NW   Nashville, TN 37189   Phone 615.555.5000

DIAGNOSTIC IMAGING SERVICES

Patient Name: Frances Southington   **Referring Physician**: A. Phipps, MD
Date of Procedure: March 16, ----   **Sex/Age**: F/52   **DOB**: June 1, ----

NAME OF PROCEDURE: CT of abdomen and pelvis with contrast.

HISTORY of gastric bypass surgery with RLQ pain. No known fever or leukocytosis.

TECHNIQUE: Helical imaging of the abdomen and pelvis with oral and uneventful angiodynamic administration of 105 mL Ultravist-370. Data was initially reconstructed at 5 mm slices; subsequently, the pelvic images were reconstructed at 2.5 mm slices.

FINDINGS: The visualized lung bases are clear.

ABDOMEN: Liver, spleen, gallbladder, pancreas, adrenal glands, and kidneys are normal. There has been previous gastric bypass surgery, and the gastrojejunostomy site appears normal. No evidence of adjacent free fluid or inflammatory change. The bowel is partially opacified. No bowel abnormalities are identified. The visualized portion of the appendix on images 62 and 63 appear normal. No evidence of inflammatory change or abnormal fluid elsewhere in the abdomen. No pathologic lymphadenopathy.

PELVIS: The urinary bladder is normal. Gynecologic organs are not optimally evaluated. However, there are 2 small uterine masses measuring up to 2.6 cm, suggestive of leiomyomata. The uterus appears somewhat bulky. The right ovary is slightly larger than the left, but no large ovarian cyst or mass is identified. No significant free fluid or inflammatory change evident in the pelvis. No osseous abnormality demonstrated.

IMPRESSION: No acute process identified. Visualized portion of the appendix appears normal. No evidence of inflammatory change or abnormal fluid.

The pelvic organs are not optimally evaluated. The uterus appears somewhat bulky and at least 2 small masses are evident, suggestive of leiomyomata. The right ovary appears slightly larger than the left without evidence of large cyst or mass. If further evaluation of the pelvis is needed, ultrasound would be helpful.

Status post gastric bypass surgery with no abnormality at the gastrojejunostomy site.

Electronically signed by Charles Tew, MD, Radiology, on 03/16/---- at 0830 hours.

CT:ds
D: 03/16/----
T: 03/16/----

C: Anderson Phipps, MD, Family Medicine/Geriatrics

Model Report No. 7: SOAP Note

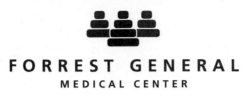

FORREST GENERAL
MEDICAL CENTER

1038 Superior Street NW   Nashville, TN 37189   Phone 615.555.5000

ARTHRITIS CLINIC—SOAP NOTE

Patient Name: Dana Sue Sandahl   **PCP**: Sandra Peebles, MD
Date of Visit: 10 August ----   **Sex/Age**: F/45   **DOB**: 9 July ----

SUBJECTIVE: Dana Sue, a 45-year-old white female who is being followed for inflammatory arthropathy, was seen 2 weeks ago after a lengthy hiatus. It was felt she had an exacerbation of her underlying systemic inflammatory arthropathy manifested by synovitis and dactylitis in her feet and her left knee. Evaluation undertaken previously was unremarkable in terms of laboratory studies. We completed her assessment by doing an anti-CCP antibody, which was negative. Arthrocentesis was performed on her left knee, which revealed only minimal inflammation with 610 white cells and no crystals. She was placed on 10 mg of prednisone and also had her left knee injected; she states that she is better but still has room for improvement. Her pain is now at a 4 to 5 level, and it had been at a 9. She is still having morning stiffness but clearly is much better. She has tolerated the prednisone without overt toxicity. She is having no nausea, vomiting, diarrhea, melena, or hematochezia.

OBJECTIVE: Vital signs are stable. General exam reveals her to be alert and in no acute distress. No skin rashes, lymphadenopathy, or focal neurologic deficits. No plural or pericardial rubs, no organomegaly. Rheumatologic assessment reveals synovitis of her second, third, and fourth MTPs on the left and dactylitis of digits 2 and 3 on the right. Trace synovitis, left knee. No peripheral clubbing, cyanosis, or edema. No ocular erythema or aphthous ulcerations.

ASSESSMENT: Inflammatory arthropathy, felt to be a recurrence of her prednisone-dependent reactive arthropathy.

PLAN: At this point, we will place Dana Sue back on methotrexate, which has controlled her problems in the past. She is to start with 10 mg per week along with 1 mg of folic acid daily. We went over side effects of methotrexate, including the possibility of bone marrow suppression, predisposing to bleeding, infection, and liver damage. She is to abstain from alcohol while on this drug regimen. The patient understands and agrees to the above plan. She is to return to Clinic in followup in 1 month.

_____

Faye Hampton, MD, Rheumatology

FH:ds
D: 8/10/----
T: 8/11/----

C: Sandra Peebles, MD, Internal Medicine

Model Report No. 8: HPIP Note

CARL E. LOFTIN
MEMORIAL CLINIC

9465 Enterprise Circle   Cookeville, TN 37269   Phone 931.555.4900

ORTHOPEDIC FOLLOWUP HPIP NOTE

Patient Name: Joseph L. Taylor   **Referring Physician**: Anderson Phipps, MD
Date of Visit: 20 April ----   **Sex/Age**: M/78   **DOB**: 28 July ----

HISTORY: Mr. Taylor, a 78 year old black male, came back in today for followup of the right hip. The patient dislocated the prosthesis last Thursday, 16 April ----. He had it reduced in a minor emergency center near his home. The patient reports he had the sensation of the hip wanting to sublux prior to dislocating. He dislocated the hip simply by rotating to his side while sitting.

PHYSICAL EXAMINATION: Lower Extremities: On exam today there is no erythema or warmth around the scar. The patient has a procession of instability as I externally rotate the hip. The limb lengths are equal. He is ambulating full weightbearing, and he has no pain with ambulation. He reports that since he had reduction of the hip last week, the pain has been less severe.

IMPRESSION: The patient had the CT arthrogram prior to this dislocation. This shows that he has dehisced the soft tissue repair with the anterior hip.

PLAN: I explained to Mr. Taylor that we have done extensive soft tissue reconstruction with sutures through drill holes in the trochanter, but apparently he tore that loose with the first dislocation. I explained that I do not think this hip is going to be stable without revision of that soft tissue reconstruction. If necessary, we can place a cerclage cable through the soft tissues to try to anchor these back to the trochanter. The patient is in favor of that, but he wants to wait on this a bit to make all his arrangements. We discussed the expected surgery, expected postoperative course, rehab, the pros and cons of the procedure, in addition to the risks of anesthesia. There were no barriers to communication, and the patient agreed to proceed as described. I will schedule him for surgery at Forrest General within the next 10 days.

_____

Olivia Glover, MD
Orthopedic Surgery

OG:ds
D: 4/20/----
T: 4/21/----

C: Anderson Phipps, MD
    Family Medicine/Geriatrics

Model Report No. 9: Office Procedure Note

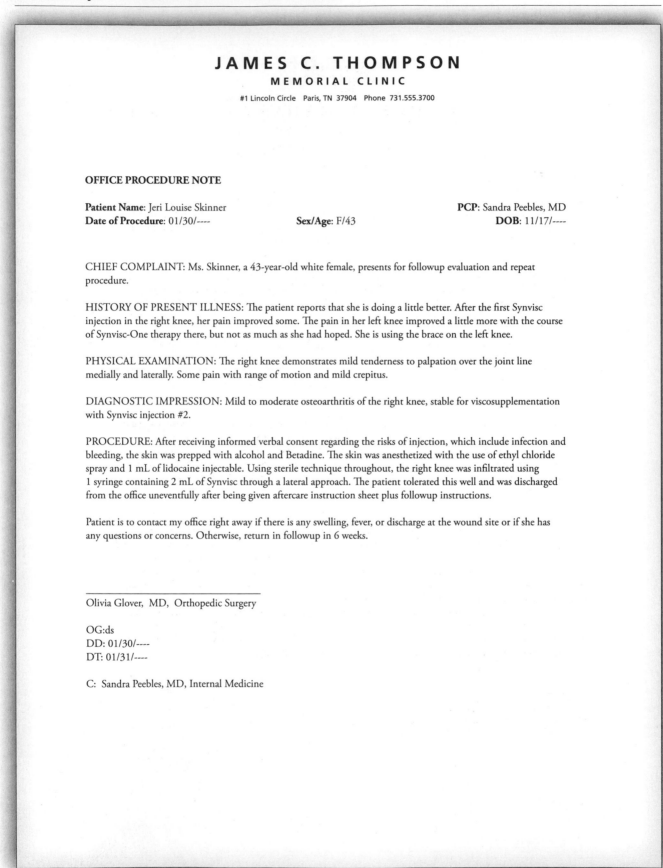

JAMES C. THOMPSON
MEMORIAL CLINIC
#1 Lincoln Circle   Paris, TN 37904   Phone 731.555.3700

OFFICE PROCEDURE NOTE

Patient Name: Jeri Louise Skinner   **PCP**: Sandra Peebles, MD
Date of Procedure: 01/30/----   **Sex/Age**: F/43   **DOB**: 11/17/----

CHIEF COMPLAINT: Ms. Skinner, a 43-year-old white female, presents for followup evaluation and repeat procedure.

HISTORY OF PRESENT ILLNESS: The patient reports that she is doing a little better. After the first Synvisc injection in the right knee, her pain improved some. The pain in her left knee improved a little more with the course of Synvisc-One therapy there, but not as much as she had hoped. She is using the brace on the left knee.

PHYSICAL EXAMINATION: The right knee demonstrates mild tenderness to palpation over the joint line medially and laterally. Some pain with range of motion and mild crepitus.

DIAGNOSTIC IMPRESSION: Mild to moderate osteoarthritis of the right knee, stable for viscosupplementation with Synvisc injection #2.

PROCEDURE: After receiving informed verbal consent regarding the risks of injection, which include infection and bleeding, the skin was prepped with alcohol and Betadine. The skin was anesthetized with the use of ethyl chloride spray and 1 mL of lidocaine injectable. Using sterile technique throughout, the right knee was infiltrated using 1 syringe containing 2 mL of Synvisc through a lateral approach. The patient tolerated this well and was discharged from the office uneventfully after being given aftercare instruction sheet plus followup instructions.

Patient is to contact my office right away if there is any swelling, fever, or discharge at the wound site or if she has any questions or concerns. Otherwise, return in followup in 6 weeks.

_____
Olivia Glover, MD, Orthopedic Surgery

OG:ds
DD: 01/30/----
DT: 01/31/----

C: Sandra Peebles, MD, Internal Medicine

Model Report No. 10: Autopsy Report

FORREST GENERAL
MEDICAL CENTER
1038 Superior Street NW   Nashville, TN 37189   Phone 615.555.5000

AUTOPSY REPORT

Patient Name: SANCHEZ, Delhi
Autopsy No.: A14-57   **Sex/Age**: F/78
Date of Admission: May 13, ----

Admitting Physician: Murray Travis, MD
DOB: July 29, ----
Date of Death: May 20, ---- at 2209 hours

GROSS DESCRIPTION
Autopsy was performed by Dr. Dominika Trigg on Saturday, May 21, ----, at Forrest General Medical Center
Morgue. Authority for examination of "the head only" was signed by the son of the deceased, Oscar M. Sanchez Jr.

EXTERNAL DESCRIPTION
The body is that of a well-developed, slightly obese, elderly Hispanic female identified by hospital wristband. The
head was normal in shape, covered with long black hair. The facial features are normal. The neck is symmetrical. The
chest is normal in shape with breasts slightly atrophic. The abdomen is slightly protuberant. The external genitalia are
normal adult female. The extremities are bilaterally symmetrical and grossly unremarkable.

CALVARIA
The scalp is reflected in the usual manner and the calvaria removed with a Stryker saw. There is a moderate amount
of blood-tinged fluid in the subdural space. The brain is removed, examined externally, and found to be grossly
symmetrical. There is a massive subarachnoid hemorrhage localized largely around the base of the brain and
extending over the cerebral hemisphere on both sides, more prominent on the right side. The vessels at the base
of the brain are largely encased and obscured by blood clot. The brain is placed in formalin; further dissection is
deferred pending adequate fixation.

GROSS BRAIN DISSECTION
On dissecting away clot from the base of the fixed brain, the vessels of the circle of Willis are found to be intact,
showing mild to moderate amounts of atherosclerosis with patent lumens. The clot is more severely impacted around
the right middle cerebral artery. On further dissection, the middle cerebral artery seems to disappear in a solid,
firm, dark red clot. Further dissection is carried out by multiple coronal sections through the temporal lobe and
the remainder of the brain. There is found to be a massive hemorrhage into the cerebral tissue, primarily involving
the anterior horn of the temporal lobe. The total area of the destructive hemorrhage is 4 cm in greatest diameter.
Surrounding cerebral tissue is soft and partially liquefied with a reddish gray appearance. Hemorrhage extends into
and fills the right lateral ventricle. The ventricle is slightly to moderately expanded in size; the lining has a reddish,
yellow-tinged discoloration. Examination of the terminating portion of the middle cerebral artery reveals no gross
dilatation or aneurysm formation. Gross diagnosis is pending microscopic description.

DT:pai
D: 5/21/----
T: 5/21/----

(Continued)

AUTOPSY REPORT
Patient Name: SANCHEZ, Delhi
Date of Death: May 20, ----

Page 2
Autopsy No.: A14-57

MICROSCOPIC DESCRIPTION

Sections through the involved area of the brain show massive hemorrhage replacing and disrupting cerebral tissue. Erythrocytes are largely laked, and there are layers of fibrin and platelets in some areas. Surrounding brain tissue shows blood staining and phagocytized pigmented material. Relatively few inflammatory cells are encountered. More remote areas of the brain show foci of verification and dilatation and engorgement of the blood vessels. Sections of the main vessels entering the area show a moderate amount of atherosclerosis with thickening of the wall, but the exact site of rupture cannot be identified; no histological evidence of aneurysm formation is seen.

COMMENT

The patient died as a result of a massive hemorrhage in the area of the right middle cerebral artery trifurcation. Aneurysm cannot be definitely demonstrated, though the hemorrhagic nature of the infarct indicated a spontaneous rupture of an arterial vessel. It is unknown whether or not the patient had hypertension; this may or may not have been a contributory factor. No evidence of a significant herniation of the brain is seen.

FINAL DIAGNOSES

1. Spontaneous intracerebral hemorrhagic infarction, predominantly right temporal lobe, area of the trifurcation of the right middle cerebral artery.
2. Cerebral atherosclerosis, mild to moderate.

_____

Dominika Trigg, MD, Pathology

DT:pai
D: 5/23/----
T: 5/23/----

C: Murray Travis, MD, OB/GYN

Model Report No. 11: Correspondence

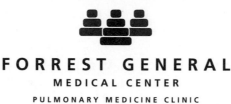

FORREST GENERAL

MEDICAL CENTER

PULMONARY MEDICINE CLINIC

1038 Superior Street NW   Nashville, TN 37189   Phone 615.555.5000

May 7, ----

Nashville Social Services Department
ATTN: Parker Mackey, MSW, Case Worker
100 Valley Parkway
Nashville, TN 37100

RE: Martha Bogart   DOB: 5/12/----

Dear Mr. Mackey:

I am writing this letter on behalf of my patient, Martha Bogart, who has a long history of excessive daytime sleepiness and loud snoring. She has suffered from these symptoms for many years, and her severe sleepiness has caused her to fall asleep while driving.

Ms. Bogart's sleep study done April 30, ----, was significant for a mild form of obstructive sleep apnea known as upper airway resistance syndrome (UARS), characterized by a significant number of respiratory effort-related arousals (RERAS), typically >10 per hour (16 per hour in her case), with normal oxygen saturation, making her apnea/hypopnea index (AHI) normal. The Respiratory Disturbance Index (RDI), when the respiratory effort-related arousals are included, is 16 per hour.

The upper airway resistance syndrome has been well described in the literature and is associated with severe sleepiness and significant morbidity (see references below). The implications of not treating this condition, particularly in someone having near misses while driving due to severe sleepiness, are profound. I am writing this letter requesting that you reconsider the decision made to deny coverage for CPAP therapy because of my patient's normal AHI.

Please give this matter your urgent attention, Mr. Mackey, and feel free to contact me if you have any questions.

Sincerely,

Robert Altman, MD
Pulmonary Surgery/Respiratory Medicine

RA:pai

References:

1. *Psychiatry Res. 2006 Apr; 40(3): 273-9.* Upper airway resistance syndrome: a long-term outcome study. Guilleminault C, Kirisoglu C, Poyares D, PalombiniL, Leger D, Farid-Moayer M, Ohayon MM.
2. *Sleep. 2000 Jun 15; 23 Supple 4:S197-200.* Upper airway resistance syndrome and its treatment. Guilleminault C, Kim YD, Palombini L, Li K, Powell N.

Model Report No. 12: Psychological Assessment

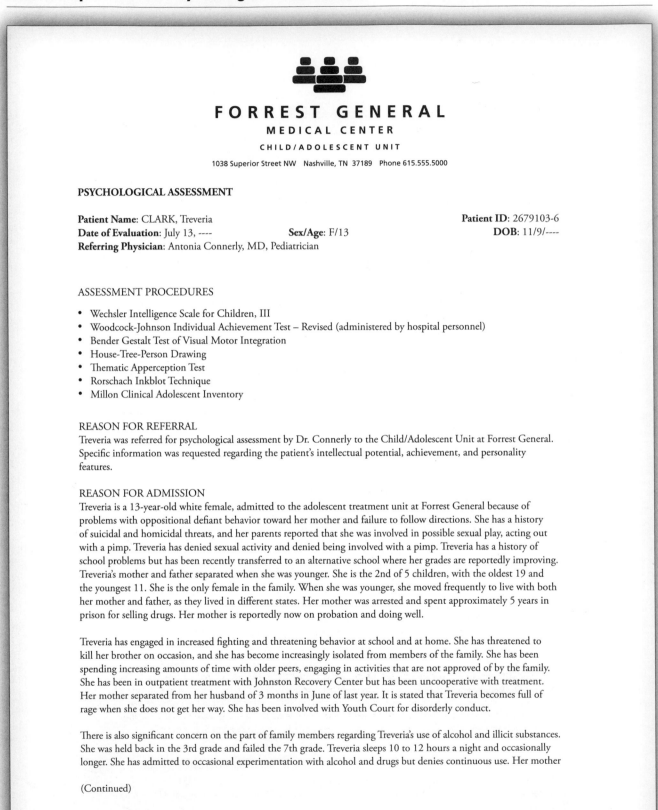

FORREST GENERAL
MEDICAL CENTER
CHILD/ADOLESCENT UNIT

1038 Superior Street NW   Nashville, TN 37189   Phone 615.555.5000

PSYCHOLOGICAL ASSESSMENT

Patient Name: CLARK, Treveria   **Patient ID**: 2679103-6
Date of Evaluation: July 13, ----   **Sex/Age**: F/13   **DOB**: 11/9/----
Referring Physician: Antonia Connerly, MD, Pediatrician

ASSESSMENT PROCEDURES

- Wechsler Intelligence Scale for Children, III
- Woodcock-Johnson Individual Achievement Test – Revised (administered by hospital personnel)
- Bender Gestalt Test of Visual Motor Integration
- House-Tree-Person Drawing
- Thematic Apperception Test
- Rorschach Inkblot Technique
- Millon Clinical Adolescent Inventory

REASON FOR REFERRAL

Treveria was referred for psychological assessment by Dr. Connerly to the Child/Adolescent Unit at Forrest General. Specific information was requested regarding the patient's intellectual potential, achievement, and personality features.

REASON FOR ADMISSION

Treveria is a 13-year-old white female, admitted to the adolescent treatment unit at Forrest General because of problems with oppositional defiant behavior toward her mother and failure to follow directions. She has a history of suicidal and homicidal threats, and her parents reported that she was involved in possible sexual play, acting out with a pimp. Treveria has denied sexual activity and denied being involved with a pimp. Treveria has a history of school problems but has been recently transferred to an alternative school where her grades are reportedly improving. Treveria's mother and father separated when she was younger. She is the 2nd of 5 children, with the oldest 19 and the youngest 11. She is the only female in the family. When she was younger, she moved frequently to live with both her mother and father, as they lived in different states. Her mother was arrested and spent approximately 5 years in prison for selling drugs. Her mother is reportedly now on probation and doing well.

Treveria has engaged in increased fighting and threatening behavior at school and at home. She has threatened to kill her brother on occasion, and she has become increasingly isolated from members of the family. She has been spending increasing amounts of time with older peers, engaging in activities that are not approved of by the family. She has been in outpatient treatment with Johnston Recovery Center but has been uncooperative with treatment. Her mother separated from her husband of 3 months in June of last year. It is stated that Treveria becomes full of rage when she does not get her way. She has been involved with Youth Court for disorderly conduct.

There is also significant concern on the part of family members regarding Treveria's use of alcohol and illicit substances. She was held back in the 3rd grade and failed the 7th grade. Treveria sleeps 10 to 12 hours a night and occasionally longer. She has admitted to occasional experimentation with alcohol and drugs but denies continuous use. Her mother

(Continued)

PSYCHOLOGICAL ASSESSMENT   Page 2
Patient Name: CLARK, Treveria   Patient ID: 2679103-6
Date of Evaluation: July 13, ----

reportedly used cocaine approximately 5 years ago during the time she was reportedly selling the substance. It was reported that Treveria's behavior has deteriorated dramatically since her mother's most recent divorce last August. Treveria's father reports that his relationship with Treveria is conflictual because of his strict rules.

Treveria's perinatal period was uneventful. She was born of a full-term gestation, vaginal delivery, without unusual features. Her developmental milestones occurred at appropriate ages; however, she spoke at 18 months of age. It was said that Treveria cursed, yelled, and threatened when she had temper tantrums, even as a young child.

OBSERVATION OF BEHAVIOR

Treveria presented as a 13-year-old white female of short and chunky build with long blond hair and green eyes. Treveria said she has not worn glasses in the past. She demonstrated no unusual gross or fine motor behaviors. She related verbally in a "slouchy" verbal style. She chewed on a plastic pen top throughout the assessment and spoke in garbled tones while chewing on this object. Her fingernails were noted to be bitten to the quick. She was also noted to have upside-down crosses on the outside end of each middle finger. This may raise questions regarding the possibility of her having been involved in satanic activities. Treveria frequently asked questions about the reasons for this assessment and made self-deprecatory comments about her abilities and skills. She occasionally asked whether or not she was doing well and on a couple of occasions she became frustrated and quit trying on difficult items. The test results obtained during this assessment appear to be valid estimates overall; however, the measure of intellectual potential may be an underestimate based on her lack of task persistence and depression.

TEST RESULTS

WECHSLER INTELLIGENCE SCALE FOR CHILDREN III

VERBAL TESTS		**PERFORMANCE TESTS**	
Information	7	Picture Completion	8
Similarities	7	Coding	9
Arithmetic	9	Picture Arrangement	10
Vocabulary	8	Block Design	2
Digit Span	5	Object Assembly	5
		Comprehension	8
VERBAL IQ	88	Factor Scores:	
PERFORMANCE IQ	80	Verbal Comprehension	80
FULL SCALE IQ	83	Perceptual Organization	79
		Freedom from Distractibility	84

Based on the scores obtained by Treveria on this instrument, she is apparently functioning overall with the low-average range of potential. A non-significant 8-point difference between verbal and performance scores was noted. Treveria scored highest on the subtest measuring her ability to put together pictures in the correct sequence so that they match common social interaction patterns. She scored lowest on the subtest measuring visual perceptual ability for abstract designs, short-term auditory memory, and visual perceptual ability for puzzles of familiar objects.

(Continued)

WOODCOCK-JOHNSON ACHIEVEMENT TEST - REVISED

	Raw Scale	Grade Equiv.	SS	%ile
Letter Word ID:	43	5.8	87	20
Passage Comp:	30	10.0	102	54
Math Calc	27	6.4	85	16
Applied Calc	39	8.0	95	38
Dictation:	41	7.4	93	32
Writing:	20	11.1	106	65

Based on the scores obtained by Treveria on this instrument, she is functioning within the average range in passage comprehension, applied problems, dictation, spelling, and writing. She is scoring within the low-average range in math calculation.

BENDER GESTALT TEST OF VISUAL MOTOR INTEGRATION
Treveria completed the Bender designs in much less time than is typical. Her manner of responding was impulsive and without due consideration for the task given her. Her errors were considered to be impulsive in nature rather than a reflection of her visual motor skills.

HOUSE-TREE-PERSON DRAWING
Treveria completed a drawing with the required picture elements. A large house dominated the page with prominent windows and curtains. The tree was also large with multiple curly lines used for foliage. The person was drawn in profile with excessive hair. Her drawing suggests that she is resistant to revealing herself and that she may be somewhat flamboyant in behavior. Sexuality may be an issue. The story told by Treveria to accompany her picture suggests that she is resistant and at least mildly oppositional.

THEMATIC APPERCEPTION TEST
Story themes generated by Treveria in response to the TAT materials suggest the following clinical hypotheses: Treveria appears to have feelings of discomfort regarding the aging of older relatives and their approaching death. She is quite capable of being verbally oppositional and impulsive. She seems to be angry regarding discipline and punishment which has been meted out toward her for no appropriate reason (in her perception). Her response to card number 16 clearly demonstrates her anger and opposition to the task at hand. She told a very brief story about a monkey who ate bananas, choked, and died.

RORSCHACH INKBLOT TECHNIQUE
The responses provided by Treveria to the Rorschach suggest the following clinical hypotheses: Treveria appears to miss essential details in her environment. She seems to look and either quickly decide what she is going to do or act impulsively without thinking. Her reality testing and perceptual accuracy appear to be adequate, and no evidence of a thought disorder was noted. She seems to have a tendency to be somewhat depressed and to exhibit poorly controlled emotions. She seems to have the capacity to understand the world in consensual ways.

(Continued)

PSYCHOLOGICAL ASSESSMENT   Page 4
Patient Name: CLARK, Treveria   Patient ID: 2679103-6
Date of Evaluation: July 13, ----

MILLON ADOLESCENT CLINICAL INVENTORY (MACI)

Responses provided by Treveria to the MACI resulted in a protocol that is questionable in terms of its validity. She did not respond in a particularly open manner to the items given her. The scores obtained from her responses suggest that she has a significant delinquent predisposition. Persons who score high on this scale demonstrate behavior that is likely to violate the rights of others. She appears likely to engage in a variety of behaviors which violate societal norms and rules. These behaviors may include threatening others, using weapons, being deceptive, lying persistently, stealing, and/or engaging in other anti-social behaviors. Her expressed concerns were all below clinical levels. Two scales, however, were notably higher than the others and near clinical levels. Those scales were social insensitivity and family discord. Persons who score high on these scales tend to be cool and indifferent to the welfare of others and have little empathy for others. In addition, persons who score high on these scales have considerable estrangement from their parents and feel that their families are tense and full of conflict. Personality patterns identified on the basis of her scores included submissive and unruly. These scales suggest that Treveria may be soft hearted, sentimental, and kindly. She may be reluctant to assert herself and she may avoid taking leadership roles. She may be inclined to be dependent and exhibit clinging behavior and fear separation. She may be likely to play down her own achievements and underestimate her abilities. In addition, she appears likely to act out in an anti-social manner and may resist the efforts of others who are trying to get her to follow socially acceptable standards of behavior. She may display a pervasively rebellious attitude that can bring her into conflict with parents and school or legal authorities.

SUGGESTED DIAGNOSES

AXIS I: Oppositional defiant disorder, dysthymia, rule out conduct disorder.
AXIS II: Developmental arithmetic calculation disorder and prominent dependent/anti-social
           personality features.

SUMMARY AND RECOMMENDATIONS

Treveria is a 13-year-old white female who was admitted to the adolescent treatment unit at Forrest General Medical Center because of escalating behavior problems, including difficulties at school, sexual acting out, threats to harm others, and increased isolation from her family. She has failed several grades and was recently placed in an alternative school where she is doing better. She has been in outpatient treatment but has been uncooperative. Her behavior has reportedly deteriorated since her mother divorced a husband after 3 months. She has been involved with Youth Court for disorderly conduct and has admitted experimentation with alcohol and illicit substances. She currently lives with her biological mother and 4 siblings. She is the only girl in a family of 5, and she is 2nd of 5 children. Treveria's mother reportedly was incarcerated for about 5 years for selling drugs when Treveria was younger. Her relationship with her father is said to be conflictual because of his strict rules.

Based on the information gathered during this assessment, Treveria appears to function intellectually overall within the low-average range of potential. Her measure of intellectual potential may be an underestimate of her actual abilities, however. Treveria's achievement was measured within the average range in all areas other than math calculation, which was within the low-average range. A specific learning disability in math calculation was suggested by her score pattern. No significant visual motor integration delays were noted. Personality features identified during the assessment include prominent oppositional and unruly personality traits coupled with a tendency to be dependent, clingy, and deny her independence of leadership. She appears quite resistant to revealing herself, and she may be flamboyant and involved in sexually provocative behaviors. Her reality testing and perceptual accuracy were found to be adequate; she appears to have a tendency to miss essential details when she tries to understand her environment. This pattern is prominent in children with ADHD.

(Continued)

PSYCHOLOGICAL ASSESSMENT   Page 5
Patient Name: CLARK, Treveria   Patient ID: 2679103-6
Date of Evaluation: July 13, ----

Based on the information gathered during this assessment, the following recommendations appear to be appropriate:

1. Treveria appears to need continued hospitalization in the adolescent treatment unit at Forrest General in order to take full advantage of the treatment milieu provided there.
2. Treveria appears to meet current SDE criteria for a specific learning disability in math calculation. The current test results may be submitted to the special education program developer in the school district where she currently attends classes so that eligibility determination can be pursued.
3. Treveria appears to be quite oppositional and noncompliant. She will likely engage in open complaints about tasks that she finds difficult or onerous. She appears to be capable intellectually in sight-oriented therapy; however, her approach to the surrounding environment will make such treatment approaches unfruitful. She appears more likely to benefit from activity-oriented, practical approaches, which emphasize behavior management and clear contingencies for inappropriate behaviors.
4. Further investigation of Treveria's possible participation in prostitution should be undertaken. Her scores on the MACI raise interesting questions regarding the personality traits necessary for such behavior. She scored in a manner suggestive of an unusual combination of anti-social and dependent personality patterns. It also appears reasonable to investigate whether or not she has been involved in satanic activities, as may be indicated by the upside-down crosses placed on the middle fingers of both hands.

Thank you, Dr. Connerly, for allowing me to participate in this most interesting child's evaluation. Please call me if I can offer any further evaluation or treatment possibilities.

_____
James Dustin Galbraith, MD, Psychology

JDG:pai
D: 6/16/----
T: 6/17/----

Model Report No.13: Routine Eye Examination

THE NASHVILLE
EYE CLINIC

Cataract & Lasik Surgery Center   7790 Iris Lane Suite 300   Nashville, TN 37758   Phone 615.801.8111

HISTORY AND PHYSICAL EXAMINATION

Patient Name: Lawrence V. Stewart   **Referring Physician**: Y. Rhodes, MD
Date of Exam: 1/28/----   **Sex/Age**: M/66   **DOB**: 9/10/----
Patient ID: 117651

CHIEF COMPLAINT/REASON FOR VISIT: New patient presents for complete eye exam. Vision is poor. Patient has blurred vision while reading, watching TV, and seeing road signs while driving at night.

HISTORY OF PRESENT ILLNESS
PROBLEM: Here for complete annual exam; having blurry vision.
ONSET: Gradual
LOCATION: Both eyes
QUALITY: No pain
SEVERITY: Mild to moderate, difficulty reading, difficulty seeing street signs at night, also watching TV
DURATION: Constantly
TIMING: Constant
AGGRAVATING: None
RELIEVING: None
ASSOCIATED SS: None
NOTES: Denies using eye drops

PAST MEDICAL HISTORY
OCULAR: Wears glasses.
PROCEDURES: No known ocular procedures.
INFECTIOUS: No known previous infections.
OCULAR SIGNIFICANT: Hypertension/high blood pressure, diabetes mellitus
ILLNESSES: High blood pressure, arthritis, diabetes mellitus.
SURGERIES: Appendectomy, hysterectomy, gallbladder, remote T&A.
HEAD/OCULAR TRAUMA: No known history of head or ocular trauma.

SOCIAL HISTORY
ALCOHOL: Denies drinking alcohol since college days.
SMOKING: Denies tobacco use.
OCCUPATION: Did not ask, retired.

FAMILY HISTORY
FAMILY: Cataract, diabetes mellitus on maternal side. Migraines, hypertension on
                          paternal side. Wife with osteoporosis and osteoarthritis; 2 children, L&W.

CURRENT MEDICATIONS
Actos   As directed.
Diovan   As directed.
Metformin   As directed.
Nexium   As directed.
Tricor   As directed.

(Continued)

HISTORY AND PHYSICAL EXAMINATION   Page 2
Patient Name: Lawrence V. Stewart   Referring Physician: Y. Rhodes, MD
Date of Exam: 1/28/----   Patient ID: 117651

ALLERGIES
Penicillin—it causes **hives**.

REVIEW OF SYSTEMS
GENERAL:	Good general health lately, recent weight gain.
RESPIRATORY:	Chronic or frequent cough, shortness of breath.
CARDIOVASCULAR:	Hypertension/high blood pressure.
GI:	Reflux.
GENITOURINARY:	Kidney stones.
MUSCULOSKELETAL:	Arthritis, joint pain, back pain.
ENDOCRINE:	Diabetes mellitus.

All other review of systems negative.

PHYSICAL EXAM
ORIENTATION, MOOD AND AFFECT: Alert and oriented x3.

	RIGHT EYE	**LEFT EYE**
UNCORRECTED VA	N/A	N/A
WEARING	+0.50 +0.50 x 007 add +2.50	+0.25 +0.75 x 172 add +2.50
MANIFEST REFRACTION	+1.50 +1.00 x 005 add +2.50	+1.00 SPHER add +2.50
AUTO REFRACTION	+1.25 +0.50 x 006	+0.75 +0.75 x 171
DR's FINAL REFRACTION	+1.50 +1.00 x 005 add +2.50	+1.00 SPHER add +2.50
CORRECTED VA	20/30 +2	20/20 SLOW
DOCTORS FINAL VA	20/20	20/20
DR's FINAL NEAR VA CHECK	J1+	J1+
PRESSURE METHOD:	Applantation	Applantation
PRESSURES:	14	14
DATE-TIME:	2:40 p.m.	2:40 p.m.
TECHNICIAN:	S. Fletcher	S. Fletcher
CONFRONTATION VF	Full to confrontation	Full to confrontation

EXTERNAL EYE EXAM
LID:	Normal for age	Normal for age
PUPIL:	Reactive with no APD	Reactive with no APD
ADNEXA:	Normal	Normal
MUSCLE BALANCE:	Orthophoric at distance and near	
OCULAR MOTILITY	Full	

(Continued)

HISTORY AND PHYSICAL EXAMINATION   Page 3
Patient Name: Lawrence V. Stewart   Referring Physician: Y. Rhodes, MD
Date of Exam: 1/28/----   Patient ID: 117651

SLIT-LAMP EXAM	**RIGHT EYE**	**LEFT EYE**
TEARFILM:	Good	Good
CONJUNCTIVA:	Pinguecula (N)	Pinguecula (N)
CORNEA:	Clear	Clear
ANTERIOR CHAMBER:	Deep and quiet	Deep and quiet
IRIS:	Normal pupil size and shape	Normal pupil size and shape
LENS:	Trace nuclear sclerosis	Trace nuclear sclerosis
ANTERIOR VITREOUS:	Normal	Normal

FUNDUS EXAM		
DILATION DROPS:	Paremyd both eyes on 1/28/---- at 2:40:17 p.m.	
CUP TO DISC:	.3	.3
OPTIC DISC:	No edema, no vascularization	No edema, no vascularization
	Good color (volk 90d)	Good color (volk 90d)
VITREOUS:	Clear	Clear
MACULA:	Normal contour and reflex for age	Normal contour and reflex for age
VESSELS:	2/3 ratio of arterioles/venules w/o tortuosity or abnormality	2/3 ratio of arterioles/venules w/o tortuosity or abnormality
PERIPHERY:	Flat, attached 360 degrees	Flat, attached 360 degrees

IMPRESSION

1. Senile Nuclear Cataract, both eyes.   366.16
2. Pinguicula, both eyes.   372.51
3. Hyperopia, both eyes.   367.0
4. Astigmatism, right eye.   367.20

DISCUSSION

• Explained today's visit in detail with the patient.
• Doctor states that patient is doing very well and both eyes look healthy.
• The nature of cataracts was discussed with patient and explained in detail. Explained that when daily activities are limited by vision, we may need to consider cataract surgery. The patient's questions were answered in full.

PLAN

• Patient to return in 1 year for complete exam.
• Surgery to be discussed at that time.

(Continued)

HISTORY AND PHYSICAL EXAMINATION   Page 4
Patient Name: Lawrence V. Stewart   Referring Physician: Y. Rhodes, MD
Date of Exam: 1/28/----   Patient ID: 117651

SPECTACLE PRESCRIPTIONS

	RIGHT EYE	**LEFT EYE**
MR REFRACTION:	+1.50 +1.00 x 005 add +2.50	+1.00 SPHER add +2.50

_____

Daniel Holcomb, MD, Ophthalmology

DH:xx
D: 1/29/----
T: 1/30/----

C: Yancy Rhodes, MD, Endocrinology

Model Report No. 14: Echocardiography Report

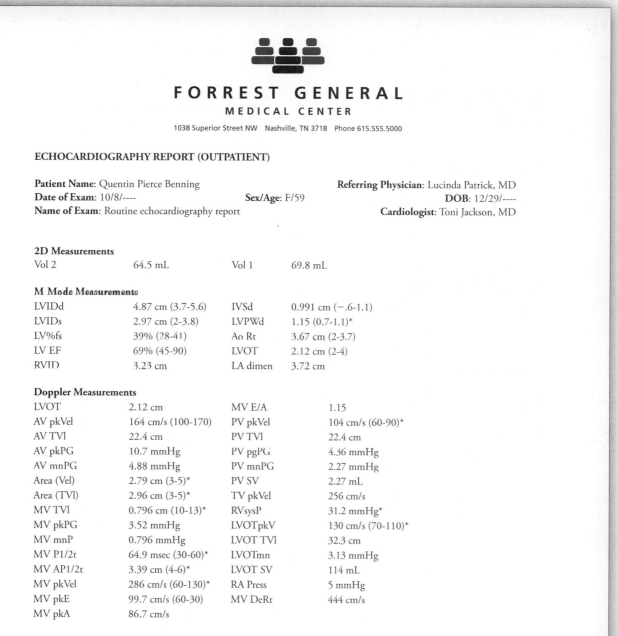

FORREST GENERAL
MEDICAL CENTER
1038 Superior Street NW   Nashville, TN 3718   Phone 615.555.5000

ECHOCARDIOGRAPHY REPORT (OUTPATIENT)

Patient Name: Quentin Pierce Benning   **Referring Physician**: Lucinda Patrick, MD
Date of Exam: 10/8/----   **Sex/Age**: F/59   **DOB**: 12/29/----
Name of Exam: Routine echocardiography report   **Cardiologist**: Toni Jackson, MD

2D Measurements

Vol 2	64.5 mL	Vol 1	69.8 mL

M Mode Measurements

LVIDd	4.87 cm (3.7-5.6)	IVSd	0.991 cm (−.6-1.1)
LVIDs	2.97 cm (2-3.8)	LVPWd	1.15 (0.7-1.1)*
LV%fs	39% (28-41)	Ao Rt	3.67 cm (2-3.7)
LV EF	69% (45-90)	LVOT	2.12 cm (2-4)
RVID	3.23 cm	LA dimen	3.72 cm

Doppler Measurements

LVOT	2.12 cm	MV E/A	1.15
AV pkVel	164 cm/s (100-170)	PV pkVel	104 cm/s (60-90)*
AV TVl	22.4 cm	PV TVl	22.4 cm
AV pkPG	10.7 mmHg	PV pgPG	4.36 mmHg
AV mnPG	4.88 mmHg	PV mnPG	2.27 mmHg
Area (Vel)	2.79 cm (3-5)*	PV SV	2.27 mL
Area (TVl)	2.96 cm (3-5)*	TV pkVel	256 cm/s
MV TVl	0.796 cm (10-13)*	RVsysP	31.2 mmHg*
MV pkPG	3.52 mmHg	LVOTpkV	130 cm/s (70-110)*
MV mnP	0.796 mmHg	LVOT TVl	32.3 cm
MV P1/2t	64.9 msec (30-60)*	LVOTmn	3.13 mmHg
MV AP1/2t	3.39 cm (4-6)*	LVOT SV	114 mL
MV pkVel	286 cm/s (60-130)*	RA Press	5 mmHg
MV pkE	99.7 cm/s (60-30)	MV DeRt	444 cm/s
MV pkA	86.7 cm/s		

Findings

LV: Left ventricular size is normal. Left ventricular function is normal. No abnormalities visualized in left ventricle. No left ventricular hypertrophy present. Wall motion is normal.

(Continued)

Name of Exam: Routine echocardiography report   Page 2
Patient Name: Quentin Pierce Benning   Referring Physician: Lucinda Patrick, MD
Date of Exam: 10/8/----

- RV: Right ventricular size is normal.
- LA: Left atrium size is normal.
- RA: Right atrium size is normal.
- IAS: Atrial septum is normal.
- AO: Aortic root is normal in size.
- AV: No structural atrioventricular abnormalities noted.
- MV: No structural mitral valve abnormalities noted. Trace mitral regurgitation.
- PV: No structural pulmonary valve abnormalities noted.
- TV: No structural tricuspid valve abnormalities. Trace tricuspid regurgitation.
- PERI: No pericardial effusion.

Summary

1. Normal left ventricular systolic function.
2. Left ventricular ejection fraction estimated at 67% to 70%.
3. Normal left ventricular relaxation.
4. Normal left ventricular filling pressures.
5. No evidence of hemodynamically significant valvular disease.

Electronically signed by Toni Jackson, MD, Cardiology, on 10 Oct ---- at 1532 hours.

TJ:xx
DD: 10/8/----
DT: 10/8/----

CC: Lucinda Patrick, MD, Internal Medicine

CHAPTER 2

CARDIOLOGY/ CARDIOVASCULAR SURGERY

Introduction

The *cardiovascular system* has numerous functions, two of which are carrying oxygen from the lungs to individual cells and transporting carbon dioxide from the cells back to the lungs. This system is composed of the *heart, blood vessels,* and *blood;* blood consists of *cells* and *plasma.*

The primary duty of the heart, which is the functional center of the system, is to act as a muscular pump propelling blood into and through the lungs (pulmonary circulation) and the rest of the body (systemic circulation). The heart beats in two phases. In *diastole,* or relaxation, the ventricle walls relax and blood flows into the heart from the venae cavae and pulmonary veins. When the walls of the right and left ventricles contract *(systole),* blood is pumped into the pulmonary artery and the aorta. This cycle of relaxation and contraction occurs approximately 100,000 times a day, pumping about 2000 gallons of blood through the body. After the heart performs the function of pumping the blood, the network of blood vessels *(vascular system)* carries the blood to all parts of the body.

The blood travels in a circular route beginning and ending at the same place. This course starts at the heart and is composed of the *arteries, arterioles, capillaries, vessels,* and *veins.* An artery is a blood vessel that carries blood away from the heart; a vein is a blood vessel that carries blood back to the heart. Capillaries are the tiny blood vessels connecting arterioles and venules.

The rhythm of the heart is controlled by the *sinoatrial node,* or pacemaker of the heart. Normal rhythm is called *sinus rhythm.* The force exerted on arterial walls by blood is called *blood pressure.* Medical personnel use a *sphygmomanometer* to measure blood pressure, which is reported in millimeters of mercury (mmHg) and recorded as a fraction with systolic pressure written over diastolic pressure. For example, a blood pressure reading of 120/80 mmHg is considered optimal for adults. A blood pressure reading of 140/90 mmHg or higher is considered elevated (hypertension).

Diagnostic procedures for treating heart problems consist of laboratory tests and clinical procedures. A *lipid profile* consists of a series of blood tests that measure the amounts of *cholesterol* and *triglycerides* in the serum. *Lipoprotein electrophoresis* is a laboratory test done on serum that separates lipoproteins (proteins that transport lipids). A *serum enzyme* or *cardiac enzyme* (i.e., CPK or LDH) test is used to measure enzymes released from the dying heart muscle into the bloodstream during a *myocardial infarction. Cardiac muscle protein troponins* are blood tests performed to determine heart muscle injury, which may or may not be detected by cardiac enzyme tests. Elevated levels can indicate a heart attack, even a mild one, for 10 to 14 days (Troponin I $\leq$ 9 days, Troponin T $\leq$ 14 days).

Critical Thinking Exercise

?

You work in the office of a local cardiologist. A friend calls you one night and says, "Jennifer told me she was going to see your cardiologist today. What did he find wrong with her?" How do you respond?

Clinical procedures employed to assess cardiovascular fitness or problems are x-rays, such as angiography and digital subtraction angiography. Other procedures include *echocardiogram, Doppler ultrasound, catheterization, cardiac scan, cardiac MRI, Holter monitoring, stress test,* and *angioplasty.* During angioplasty, physicians may insert either a balloon or a *stent* to open an occluded artery.

The specialty of cardiovascular surgery concerns itself with the diagnosis, repair, and reconstruction of the circulation: heart and blood vessel defects.

Cardiology/Cardiovascular Surgery Abbreviations

The abbreviations, acronyms, and terms in the following abbreviations and terminology sections are often dictated in this specialty. We offer abbreviated definitions here. Please see an unabridged medical dictionary and/or the suggested web sites in this chapter for more information on each term.

A2, A₂	aortic second sound
AAA	abdominal aortic aneurysm
ABG	arterial blood gas
ACLS	advanced cardiac life support
ACS	acute coronary syndrome
ACT	activated clotting time
AF, A fib	atrial fibrillation
A flt	atrial flutter
AI	aortic insufficiency
AICD/ICD	automatic implantable cardioverter defibrillator
AIVR	accelerated idioventricular rhythm
AMI	acute myocardial infarction
AR	aortic regurgitation/aortic insufficiency
AS	aortic stenosis
ASD	atrial septal defect
ASH	asymmetrical septal hypertrophy

ASHD	arteriosclerotic heart disease
ASPVD	atherosclerotic peripheral vascular disease
ATS	autotransfusion system
AV, A-V	atrioventricular (node)
AVB	atrioventricular block
AVG	aortic valve gradient
AVNRT	atrioventricular nodal re-entry tachycardia/atrioventricular node recovery time
AVR	aortic valve replacement
BBB	bundle branch block
BiVAD	biventricular assist device
BiVICD	biventricular implantable cardioverter defibrillator
BNP	brain natriuretic peptide
BVH	biventricular hypertrophy
CAB	coronary artery bypass/complete atrioventricular block
CABG	coronary artery bypass graft

CABRI	coronary artery bypass revascularization investigation
CAC	coronary artery calcium (score)
CAD	coronary artery disease
cardiac CTA	cardiac CT angiogram
cath	catheterization
CAVH	continuous arteriovenous hemofiltration
CC	cardiac catheterization/circular collapse
CCP	Certified Cardiovascular Perfusionist
CCU	coronary care unit
CHD	coronary heart disease
CHF	congestive heart failure
CI	cardiac index
CPB	cardiopulmonary bypass
CPK	creatine phosphokinase (released into bloodstream following injury to heart or skeletal muscles)
CPR	cardiopulmonary resuscitation
CRI	chronic renal insufficiency
CTR	cardiothoracic ratio
CTICU	cardiothoracic intensive care unit
CV	cardiovascular
CVA	cerebrovascular accident
CVP	central venous pressure
DCA	directional coronary atherectomy
DD	diastolic dysfunction
DHCA	deep hypothermic circulatory arrest
DILV	double-inlet left ventricle
DOE	dyspnea on exertion
DOLV	double-outlet left ventricle
DORV	double-outlet right ventricle
DSA	digital subtraction angiography
DVT	deep venous thrombosis/deep vein thrombosis
ECA	external carotid artery
ECC	extracorporeal circulation

ECD	endocardial cushion defect
ECG/EKG	electrocardiogram
ECHO	echocardiography
ECMO	extracorporeal membrane oxygenation
ECT	extracorporeal circulation technology
EECP	enhanced external counter pulsation
EF	ejection fraction
ERP	effective refractory period
ETT	exercise tolerance test
FHS	fetal heart sound
FLP	fasting lipid panel
FRP	functional refractory period
HCVD	hypertensive cardiovascular disease
HDL	high-density lipoproteins
H&L	heart and lungs
HOCM	hypotrophic obstructive cardiomyopathy
HPCD	hemostatic puncture closure device
HV	hallux valgus
HVD	hypertensive vascular disease
IAPB	intra-aortic balloon pump
IASD	interatrial septal defect
ICA	internal carotid artery
ICD	implantable cardioverter defibrillator
IMA	inferior mesenteric artery/internal mammary artery
IVC	inferior vena cava
IVCD	interventricular conduction defect
IVSD	interventricular septal defect
IVUS	intravascular ultrasound
LA	left atrium
LAD	left anterior descending coronary artery
LBBB	left bundle branch block
LDH	lactate dehydrogenase (enzyme released from dying heart muscle)
LDL	low-density lipoproteins
LIMA	left internal mammary artery

LM	left main
LV	left ventricle
LVAD	left ventricular assist device
LVEDP	left ventricular end diastolic pressure
LVEF	left ventricular ejection fraction
LVF	left ventricular failure
LVH	left ventricular hypertrophy
M2, M_2	mitral second sound
MI	mitral insufficiency/myocardial infarction
MIDCAB	minimally invasive direct coronary artery bypass
MR	mitral regurgitation
MS	mitral stenosis
MUGA	multigated angiogram (radioactive test of heart function)
MVP	mitral valve prolapse
NSR	normal sinus rhythm
NSTEMI	non-ST elevation myocardial infarction
OHS	open-heart surgery
OM	obtuse marginal
P2, P_2	pulmonic second sound
PA	pulmonary artery
PAC	premature atrial contraction
PAT	paroxysmal atrial tachycardia
PCI	percutaneous coronary intervention
PCWP	pulmonary capillary wedge pressure
PDA	patent ductus arteriosus
PICVA	percutaneous in situ coronary venous arterialization
PLB	posterior lateral branch
PMI	point of maximum impulse
PND	paroxysmal nocturnal dyspnea
PDA	patent ductus arteriosus/posterior descending artery
PT	prothrombin time/pro time
PTCA	percutaneous transluminal coronary angioplasty

PTT	partial thromboplastin time
PV	pulmonary valve
PVC	premature ventricular contraction
PVD	peripheral vascular disease
RA	right atrium
RAH	right atrial hypertrophy
RBBB	right bundle branch block
RCA	right coronary artery
RFA	radio frequency ablation
RHD	rheumatic heart disease
RI	ramus intermedius
RIMA	right internal mammary artery
RRP	relative refractory period
RSR	regular sinus rhythm
RV	right ventricle
RVH	right ventricular hypertrophy
SA, S-A	sinoatrial (node)
SACT	sinoatrial conduction times
SAM	systolic anterior motion
SCD	sudden cardiac death
SGOT	serum glutamic oxaloacetic transaminase
SGPT	serum glutamic pyruvic transaminase
STEMI	ST-elevation myocardial infarction
SV	stroke volume
SVC	superior vena cava
SVG	saphenous vein graft
SVPT	supraventricular premature contraction
TEE	transesophageal echocardiography
TGA	transposition of the great arteries
TI	tricuspid insufficiency/symbol for thallium
TIA	transient ischemic attack
TOF	tetralogy of Fallot
tPA	tissue-type plasminogen activator (drug used to prevent thromboses)
TR	tricuspid regurgitation

TS	triscupid stenosis	VLDL	very low-density lipoproteins
TV	triscupid valve	VPC	ventricular premature contraction
USA	unstable angina	VSD	ventricular septal defect
VAD	ventricular assist device	VT, V tach	ventricular tachycardia
VDH	valvular disease of heart	WPW	Wolfe-Parkinson-White syndrome
VEGF	vascular endothelial growth factor	XM, XMT	crossmatch/crossmatched
VHD	valvular heart disease		

Anatomic Illustrations

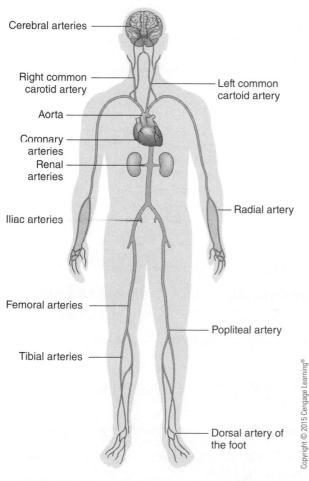

FIGURE 2-1   Arterial System of the Body

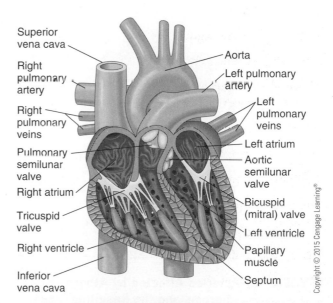

FIGURE 2-2   Pulmonary Arteries and Veins of the Heart

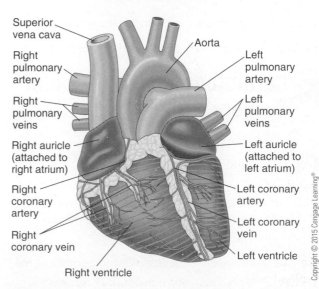

FIGURE 2-3   Heart and Great Vessels

Affected site   **Complication**

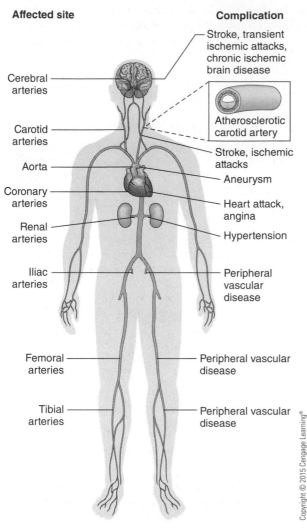

Stroke, transient ischemic attacks, chronic ischemic brain disease

Cerebral arteries

Carotid arteries

Atherosclerotic carotid artery

Aorta

Stroke, ischemic attacks

Coronary arteries

Aneurysm

Heart attack, angina

Renal arteries

Hypertension

Iliac arteries

Peripheral vascular disease

Femoral arteries

Peripheral vascular disease

Tibial arteries

Peripheral vascular disease

FIGURE 2-4   Arteries Affected by Athero-sclerosis and the Resulting Complications

Cardiology/Cardiovascular Surgery Terminology

ablation (uh-blā'-shun) – to remove or destroy tissue that is suspected of causing irregular heartbeats (arrhythmia)

anemia (ə-ne'me-ə) – a decrease in the number of red blood cells

aneurysm (an'-yoo-rizm) – ballooning out of a portion of a blood vessel (usually an artery) due to a congenital defect or a weakness in the wall of a blood vessel

aneurysmectomy (an"-yoo-riz-mek'-tuh-mē) – the surgical removal of an aneurysm by removing the sac

angina pectoris (an-jī'-nuh OR an'-jih-nah pek-tor'-is) – a paroxysmal thoracic pain with a feeling of suffocation and impending death due most often to anoxia of the myocardium and precipitated by effort or excitement

AngioJet Rheolytic™ thrombectomy system (an'-jē-ō-jet rē-ō-lih-tik throm-bec'-tuh-mē) – device that employs a minimally invasive catheter system to remove intravascular blood clots from leg and arm arteries and bypass grafts

angioplasty (an'-jē-ō-plas"-tē) – alteration of the structure of a vessel by surgical procedure or by dilating the vessel using a balloon inside the lumen

Angio-Seal™ (an'-jē-ō-sēl) – a hemostatic puncture closure device used after interventional or diagnostic vascular procedures to seal the arteriotomy

anticoagulant ([an"te-] an"ti-ko-ag'u-lənt) – a class of medication that prevents blood from clotting; a blood thinner

aorta (a-or'tə) – the body's largest artery, originating from the left ventricle of the heart

aortic atresia (ā-or'-tik uh-trē'-zē-uh) – small or undeveloped aortic valve

aortocoronary bypass (ā"-or-tō-kōr'-ō-nār-ē) – coronary bypass

aortotomy (ā"-or-tah'-tuh-mē) – surgical incision into the aorta

apex (a'peks) – the lower, rounded tip of the heart

arrhythmia (uh-rith'-mē-uh) – any variation from the normal heartbeat

arteriole (ahr-tēr'e-ōl) – a small arterial branch

arteriosclerosis (ar-tē"-rē-ō-skle-rō'-sis) – a group of diseases characterized by thickening and loss of elasticity of arterial walls

arteriotomy (ar"-tē-rē-ot'-uh-mē) – division or opening of an artery by surgery

asynchronous (ā-sing'-kruh-nus) – a fixed-rate type of pacemaker that discharges regular impulses despite the intrinsic rhythm or rate of the heart

atherectomy (ah-ther-ek'-tuh-mē) – procedure done to remove plaque from artery either by blade or rotation (rotablade); also known as directional coronary athrectomy (DCA)

atheromatous (ath"-er-ō'-muh-tus) – affected with a mass or plaque of degenerated, thickened arterial intima occurring in atherosclerosis

atrial fibrillation ('ā-trē-əl fib"rĭ-la'shən) – an irregular heartbeat; increases the risk of stroke and heart disease

atrial myxoma (mik-so'mə) – a tumor of the heart

atrial septal defect (sep'təl) – an abnormal hole located in the walls between the two upper chambers of the heart (atria)

atriotomy (ā"-trē-ot'-uh-mē) – surgical incision of an atrium of the heart

atrium (a'tre-əm) – one of the two smaller upper chambers or cavities of the heart

automatic implantable cardioverter defibrillator (AICD) (aw-tuh-mat'-ik im-plan'-tuh-bul car-dē-ō-ver'-tur dē-fih'-brih-lā-tur) – a device that is surgically implanted to monitor the heartbeat; if it senses rapid irregular heartbeats, it delivers an electric shock to the patient's heart

B

balloon angioplasty (an'je-o-plas"te) – a procedure performed to clean out clogged heart arteries; also known as percutaneous transluminal coronary angioplasty (PTCA)

beta-blocker (bā'-tuh-blä-kər) – a class of medication that slows heart rate, lowers blood pressure, controls angina, and protects patients with prior heart attacks

Beta-Cath System™ (bā'-tuh-kath) – device designed to prevent an artery from renarrowing following angioplasty or stent placement

bigeminy (bī-jem'-ih-nē) – any arrhythmia that occurs in pairs; sometimes refers to a normal beat followed by a premature beat

brachytherapy (brak"-ē-ther'-uh-pē) – a procedure that employs low-level radiation to reduce recurrence of blockage by scar tissue in previously stented arteries

bradycardia (brā"-dē-kar'-dē-uh) – abnormally slow heart rate (less than 60 beats per minute)

brain natriuretic peptide (BNP) (na"tre-u-ret'ik pep'tīd) – a test that measures the amount of the BNP hormone in the blood; this hormone is made by the heart, and a test for it is performed to check for heart failure

bundle branch – part of the electrical pathway of the heart that delivers electrical impulses to the ventricles of the heart to cause them to contract

bundle of His – this atrioventricular bundle, which forms a part of the conduction system of the heart, conducts electrical impulses from the AV node to the point of the apex of the fasicular branches

bypass surgery – a surgical procedure that redirects the blood supply around clogged arteries to improve oxygen and blood flow to the heart

calcium-channel blocker – a class of medication that reduces spasm of the blood vessels, lowers blood pressure, and controls angina

cardiac catheterization (kath"ə-tur"ĭ-za'shən) – a test to check blood flow in the coronary arteries, blood flow and pressure in the heart chambers, to determine how well the heart valves work, and to check for defects in the way the wall of the heart moves

cardiac perfusion scan (pər-fu'zhən) – a scan that measures the amount of blood in the heart muscle at rest and during exercise; done to determine the cause of chest pain

cardiac output (CO) – the amount of blood usually ejected by the left ventricle in one minute

cardiac reserve – the ability of the heart to increase its cardiac output during stress, normally 300% to 400% above resting values

cardiogenic shock (kar"-dē-ō-jen'-ik) – failure to maintain blood supply to tissues because of inadequate cardiac output

cardiomyopathy (kar"-dē-ō-mī-op'-uh-thē) – a general diagnostic term designating primary noninflammatory disease of the heart muscle; often of obscure or unknown etiology and not the result of ischemic, hypertensive, congenital, valvular, or pericardial disease

cardioplegia (kar"-dē-ō-plē'-jē-uh) – interruption of contraction of the myocardium as may be induced by the use of chemical compounds or of cold (cryocardioplegia) in the performance of surgery upon the heart

cardiopulmonary bypass (kar"-dē-ō-pul'-muh-nair-ē) – procedure employed during open-heart surgery whereby a heart-lung machine takes over the functions of the heart and lungs

CardioTek™ (kar'-dē"-ō-tek) – electrophysiologic tracer (a machine that prints out tracings during an EKG)

cardiotomy (kar"-dē-ot'-uh-mē) – surgical incision into the heart to repair cardiac defects

cardioversion (kar"-dē-ō-ver'-zhun) – the restoration of a normal rhythm of the heart by electric shock

cholesterol (kə-les'tər-ol") – an important type of fat (lipid) produced by the body that is necessary for it to function; however, excess amounts built up in blood vessels may lead to atherosclerosis, heart disease, and/or stroke. The two main forms are low-density lipoprotein (LDL) and high-density lipoprotein (HDL).

chorda (pl. chordae) ((kor'dā) (kor'dā-ē) – a tendinous or cord-like structure; there are many subcategories of chordae

chordae tendinae (of heart) (kor'dā-ē ten-'din-ē-ə) – thin cord-like structures that provide support to the tricuspid and mitral valves of the heart, helping them to open and shut properly

cineangiocardiography (sin"-ē-an"-jē-ō-kar"dē-og'-ruhfē) – study of the chambers of the heart and pulmonary circulation by the use of motion picture techniques (while the structures are in motion) following injection of radiopaque material

circulatory system – the system through which the blood is distributed through the body by way of the heart, arteries, capillaries, and veins

commissurotomy (kom"ĭ-shər-ot'ə-me) – a surgical procedure that aids in repairing the damage caused by defective heart valves

congestive heart failure (CHF) – inability of the heart to maintain normal circulation, resulting in shortness of breath and abnormal fluid retention

cordate (kor"-dāt) – heart shaped (*NB:* Do not confuse this word with chorda or chordae)

cor pulmonale (kōr pul'-mō-nal) – heart disease due to pulmonary hypertension secondary to diseases of the blood vessels of the lungs

coronary artery bypass graft surgery (CABG) – a procedure performed to bypass a diseased section of the coronary arteries with healthy artery or vein grafts in order to increase blood flow to the heart muscle

coupling interval (kup'-ling) – when utilizing a pacemaker to introduce a premature impulse, the time between the last normal beat and the premature beat

Crafoord™ clamps, scissors, forceps (krā'-foord) – surgical instruments used in heart and lung procedures

cyanosis (si"ə-no'sis) – a condition in which the body is not receiving enough oxygen-rich blood; causes a blue tint to the skin

defibrillation (dē-fib"-rih-lā'-shun) – the termination of ventricular fibrillation by electric shock

dextrocardia (deks"-trō-kar'-dē-uh) – location of the heart on the right side of the midline of the chest

diastolic blood pressure (di-ə-stol'ik) – the pressure of the blood in the arteries when the heart is filling

dyspneic (disp'-nē'-ik) – characterized by difficult or labored breathing

echocardiogram (ek"-ō-kar'-dē-ō-gram") – a diagnostic test used to measure the structure and function of the heart

effective refractory period (ERP) (rē-frak'-tuh-rē) – the same as absolute refractory period; that period of time just after depolarization when the cardiac cell cannot be stimulated

embolectomy (em"-bō-lek'-tuh-mē) – surgical removal of an embolus or clot from a blood vessel

embolus (em'bo-ləs) – a plug or clot originating in a vessel and carried by the blood to a smaller vessel, causing an obstruction

endarterectomy (end"-ar-ter-ek'-tuh-mē) – removal of the interior portion of an artery

endocardium (en"-dō-kar'-dē-um) – the innermost lining of the heart

endothelium (en"-dō-thē'-lē-um) – the monocellular lining of blood vessels, heart, and lymphatic system

epicardium (ep"ĭ-kahr'de-əm) – the external covering of the heart

External CounterPulsation™ therapy (ECP) (kown' ter puhl-sā'-shun) – a noninvasive procedure for chronic angina pectoris that stimulates the formation of small branches of blood vessels (collaterals), thereby increasing blood flow around blocked arteries

femoropopliteal bypass (fem"-ō-rō-pop-lit'-ē-ul) – vascular prosthesis that bypasses an obstruction in the femoral artery

fusion beat – the result of a normal and abnormal impulse stimulating the ventricles simultaneously

Glidewire™ (glīd'-wīr) – a coated, kink-resistant, guided wire used in endourology procedures; different types and other brand names are available

guidewire (gīd'-wīr) – a wire, thin and flexible and lubricated, that can be inserted into a confined space to act as a guide for subsequent placement of a larger, stiffer device or prosthesis, such as an intravascular angiographic catheter; different types of guidewires exist, including some brand names

(**NB**: Glidewire is a brand name and guidewire is generic; critical thinking skills must be employed before transcribing either term.)

heart-lung bypass machine – a machine that oxygenates the blood and circulates it throughout the body during surgery

heparinization (heh'-puh-rin-ih-zā'-shun) – treatment with an anticoagulant (heparin) to increase the clotting time of the blood

high-density lipoprotein (HDL) (lip"o- li"po-pro'tēn) – good cholesterol; deposits of cholesterol in the liver where it is excreted by the body

Holter™ monitor (hōl'tər) – a small recorder that is attached to electrodes on the chest; records the heart's rhythm continuously for 24 hours; the physician orders this test for as many hours as is deemed necessary—sometimes more than 24 hours

hyperlipidemia (hi"pər-lip"ĭ-de'me-ə) – high levels of lipids (fat) in the blood, such as cholesterol and triglycerides

hyperperfusion (hī"-per-per-fyoo'-zhun) – increased blood flow to an organ or tissue

hypertrophic cardiomyopathy (hī"-per-trō'-fik kar"-dē-ō-mī-op'-uh-thē) – disease of the myocardium produced by enlargement of the cells of the myocardium

hypoxia (hī-pok'-sē-uh) – oxygen deficiency

idioventricular rhythm (ih"-dē-ō-ven-trik'-yoo-lur) – relating to or affecting the cardiac ventricle alone

immunosuppressants (im"u-no-sə-pres'əntz) – class of drugs used to keep the body's immune system from rejecting a transplanted organ, such as the heart

implantable cardioverter defibrillator (ICD) (im-plant'ā-bəl kahr'de-o-vur"tər de-fib"rĭ-la'tər) – a surgically inserted electronic device that constantly monitors the heart rate and rhythm; if it detects a fast, abnormal heart rhythm, it sends electrical energy to the heart muscle to help it beat in a normal rhythm again.

infarct (in'fahrkt) – an area of necrosis due to lack of blood

interpolated (in"-ter-pō'-lā-ted) – refers to a premature beat that does not interrupt the regularity of the basic rhythm

intramyocardial (in"-truh-mī"-ō-kar'-dē-ul) – within the myocardium, the heart muscle

intravascular ultrasound (in"trə-vas'ku-lər) – an invasive procedure performed with catheterization, where a miniature sound probe on the tip of a catheter is threaded through the coronary arteries, and using high-frequency sound waves, produces detailed images of the interior walls of the arteries

ischemia (iss-kē'-mē-uh) – deficiency of blood to the heart muscle

joule (jool) – a unit of energy equivalent to 1 watt-second

12 leads – refers to the surface electrocardiogram (ECG) electrodes placed on the skin of the patient's extremities and chest. These are known as I, II, III, aVR, aVL, aVF, V1, V2, V3, V4, V5, and V6. The last six sequential leads are often referred to as the *V leads* or the *chest leads*. (**NB:** Roman numerals are used with these leads.)

LeGOO™ – brand name for a gel that surgeons use to temporarily stop blood flow during blood vessel surgery

lipoprotein (li"po-pro'tēn) – a combination of fat and protein that carries lipids in the blood

LOA cines (sin'-ēz) – abbreviation for left occipitoanterior position

low-density lipoprotein (LDL) – bad cholesterol; deposits of cholesterol into the lining of the artery

mitral insufficiency (in"sə-fish'ən-se) – the condition where blood in the left ventricle leaks back through the mitral valve into the left atrium and can back up into the lungs

mitral regurgitation (rē-gur"-jih-tā'-shun) – abnormal systolic backflow of blood from the left ventricle into the left atrium, resulting from imperfect closure of the mitral valve

mitral stenosis (stə-no'sis) – the condition where the mitral valve becomes narrowed or stenotic, thus preventing the easy flow of blood from the left atrium into the left ventricle

mitral valve – the valve between the left atrium and left ventricle

morphology (mor-fol'-uh-jē) – the structure and form, often meaning the form of an irregular heart rhythm (arrhythmia)

myocardial infarction (MI) (mi"o-kahr'de-əl in-fahrk'shən) – permanent damage to the heart muscle caused by a lack of blood supply to the heart for an extended time period

myocardium (mī"-ō-kar'-dē-um) – the middle and thickest layer of the heart; it lies between the endocardium (the inner lining) and the epicardium (the outer covering) of the heart; the heart muscle

myomectomy (mi"o-mek'tə-me) – a surgical procedure to remove abnormally thickened heart muscle

nodal (nō'-dul) – adj. referring to a node, such as the atrioventricular (AV) node, as in nodal enlargement or swelling

NOGA™ mapping system – diagnostic procedure that employs magnets to produce a three-dimensional, real-time image of the heart; appreciably reduces x-ray exposure of the patient

occlusion (ə-kloo'zhən) – blockage of a blood vessel

ostium secundum (os'-tē-um seh-kun'-dum) – an opening high in the septum primum of the embryonic heart, approximately where the foramen ovale will be later

pacemaker – a device implanted under the skin that sends electrical impulses to the heart muscle to stabilize heart rate and rhythm

palpitation (pal"pĭ-ta'shən) – a fluttering sensation in the chest that is often related to a missed heartbeat or rapid heartbeat; typically dictated in the plural, palpitations

Perclose ProGlide Suture-Medicated Closure System™ (pur'-klōz) – brand name for a specific closure system

perfusion (per-fyoo'-zhun) – the use of artificial blood pumps to propel blood through a patient's body tissue, replacing the function of the heart during open-heart surgery

perfusion scan (per-fyoo'-zhun) – a test to determine the status of blood flow to an organ

perfusion technologist (tek-nol'-uh-jist) – a health professional trained to operate the heart-lung machine and other life support devices

pericardial effusion (per"e-kahr'de-əl ə-fu'zhən) – an abnormal amount of fluid between the heart and the pericardium

pericardiocentesis (per"e-kahr"de-o-sen-te'sis) – a procedure performed to determine the cause of fluid buildup around the heart and to relieve pressure on the heart

pericarditis (pair"-ih-kar-dī'-tis) – inflammation of the pericardium

pericardium (per"ĭ-kahr'de-əm) – the membrane (sac) surrounding the heart

peroneal artery (per"-ō-nē'-ul) – artery located on the outer side of the leg; fibular artery

premature ventricular contraction (ven-trik'-yoo-lur) – an irregular heartbeat in which the lower chambers of the heart (ventricles) beat before they should

profunda femoris artery (prō-fun'-duh fem'-uh-ris) – deep femoral artery

pulmonary atresia (puhl'-muh-nair'-ē uh-trē'-zē-uh) – small or undeveloped pulmonary valve

Purkinje fibers or network (pur-kin'-j) – specialized cardiac muscle fibers that conduct the impulse from the right and left bundle branches to the ventricular muscle; this comprises the ventricular conduction system

quadrigeminy (kwod"-rih-jem'-ih-nē) – quadrigeminal or four-fold rhythm

rami communicans (rā'-mī kuh-myoo'-nih-kanz) – a communicating branch between two nerves; a branch connecting two arteries

ramus intermedius (ra'məs in"tər-me'de-əs) – intermediate branch of hepatic artery

reanastomosis (rē-uh-nas"-tuh-mō'-sis) – a reattachment between two vessels by collateral channels

regurgitation (re-gur"jĭ-ta'shən) – leaking or backward flow

restenosis (re"stə-no'sis) – the closing or narrowing of an artery that previously was opened by a cardiac procedure, such as angioplasty

revascularization (re-vas"ku-lər-ĭ-za'shən) – the restoration of an adequate blood supply to a part, such as with a bypass or angioplasty procedure

S

saphenous vein (suh-fē'-nus) – pertaining to or associated with a saphena, which is either of two larger superficial veins of the leg

septum – the muscular wall separating the right and left sides of the heart

sinoatrial (SA) (si"no-a'tre-əl) – a specialized cluster of cells in the heart that initiates the heartbeat; the heart's natural pacemaker

stenosis (stə-no'sis) – a narrowing or restriction of a blood vessel or valve that reduces blood flow

stent – a small mesh tube that is placed in an artery during a cardiac catheterization to assist in carrying blood away from the heart to other parts of the body

supraventricular (soo"-pruh-ven-trik'-yoo-lur) – a heartbeat originating "above" the ventricles

synchronous (sing'-krō-nus) – refers to an on-demand type of pacemaker

syncope (sing'-kuh-pē) – extreme dizziness or fainting due to lack of blood to the brain

systole (sis'-tuh-lē) – portion of the heart cycle in which the heart muscle fibers are contracting and forcing blood into the main blood vessels

tachycardia (tak"-ē-kar'-dē-uh) – a rapid heart rhythm of greater than 100 beats per minute

Takotsubo cardiomyopathy (tak ot su' bo kahr"de-o-mi-op'ə-the) – broken heart syndrome; during an episode of this disease of the heart muscle, it can be so severely affected that it cannot pump blood out to the body strongly enough. As a result, the patient may develop heart failure.

thallium exercise stress test (thal'e-əm) – a type of nuclear scanning technique (perfusion scan) that uses the radioactive substance thallium; it combines nuclear scanning with exercise on a treadmill or stationary bicycle to assess heart function and determine if there is adequate blood flow to the myocardium

thrombolytic medication (throm"bo-lit'ik) – a class of medication used to dissolve clots that may be obstructing blood flow in arteries and veins; clot-busting medication

thrombus (throm'bəs) – a plug or clot in a blood vessel or in one of the cavities of the heart, formed by coagulation of blood; remains at its point of formation

transesophageal echocardiogram (TEE) (trans"ə-sof"ə-je'əl ek"o-kahr'de-o-gram") – an invasive imaging procedure that produces a picture of the heart's movement, valves, and chambers using high-frequency sound waves that come from a small transducer passed through the throat and into the esophagus and stomach

transient ischemic attack (TIA) (tran'se-ənt is-kem'ik) – a stroke-like event that occurs when the brain is denied of oxygen-rich blood; however, the effects wear off completely after resumption of

blood flow; immediate intervention by healthcare professionals is required

transmyocardial revascularization (TMR) (tranz"-mī"-ō-kar'-dē-ul rē-vas"-kyoo-lar-ih-zā'-shun) – a state-of-the-art laser used during open-heart surgery to create new pathways in the heart muscle

tricuspid atresia (trī-kus'-pid uh-trē'-zē-uh) – small or undeveloped tricuspid valve

tricuspid valve (trī-kus'-pid) – the valve that lies between the right atrium and right ventricle

triglyceride (tri-glis'ər-īd) – a type of fat found in the blood that is a major source of energy; however, high levels may increase one's chance of developing coronary artery disease, atherosclerosis, and/or stroke

unifocal (yoo"-nih-fō'-kul) – an irregular heartbeat (arrhythmia) that has one point of origin

vagus nerve (vā'-gus) – this nerve slows the heart rate when stimulated; it is the tenth cranial nerve and part of the parasympathetic nervous system

Valsalva maneuver (val-sal'-vah muh"-noo'-ver) – bearing down, or a forced exhalation effort against a closed throat; this causes stimulation of the vagus nerve and usually slows the heart

valve – a fold or flap-like structure in the lining membrane of a canal or other hollow organ that prevents the backward flow of fluid

valve replacement – surgery to remove a badly damaged valve; the valve is replaced with either a plastic valve, a metal mechanical valve, or a bioprosthetic valve that may be made from pig tissue

valvuloplasty (val'-vyoo-lō-plas"-tē) – an operative procedure on a valve to improve function

valvulotomy (val"-vyoo-lot'-uh-mē) – an incision into a diseased and stenosed cardiac valve made to increase the valve area

vasodilator (vā"-zō-dī'-lā-tur) – any agent (usually a drug) that causes the blood vessels to dilate, thereby reducing the force against which the heart must pump the blood

vasopressor (vā"-zō-pres'-ur) – stimulating contraction of the muscular tissue of the capillaries and arteries; an agent that stimulates contractions of the muscular tissue of the capillaries and arteries

venotomy (vē-not'-uh-mē) – incision into a vein, as for the letting of blood (syn. phlebotomy)

ventricle (ven'trĭ-kəl) – one of the lower chambers on either side of the heart

ventricular fibrillation (ven-trik'-yoo-lur fih-bri-la'-shun) – rapid random quivering of the ventricles; essentially no blood is pumped during this arrhythmia, which leads to death unless reversed by electric shock (defibrillation)

ventricular tachycardia (tak"-ē-kar'-dē-uh) – an arrhythmia that originates in the ventricles at a rate of 150 to 250 beats per minute

Transcription Tips

When transcribing cardiology/cardiovascular surgery dictation, you will find the task easier if you are familiar with the structure of the heart and accompanying anatomic terms. For example, you should be able to recognize the chambers of the heart, the names of the valves, and the names and locations of arteries.

Heart chambers – right atrium, right ventricle, left atrium, and left ventricle

Valves – tricuspid, bicuspid or mitral, pulmonary semilunar, and aortic semilunar

Names and locations of main arteries –

- **radial** – radial (or thumb side) of the wrist
- **brachial** – in the bend of the elbow
- **carotid** – in the neck
- **temporal** – at the temple
- **femoral** – in the groin

Selected Diagnostic Tests

- coronary artery calcium (CAC) score
- catheterization
- cerebral angiogram
- coronary angiogram
- electrophysiology study

- MUGA scan
- stress test
- transtelephonic monitoring
- venogram

Selected Noninvasive or Minimally Invasive Tests/Services

ambulatory blood pressure monitoring as with the
Holter monitor
computed tomography (CT) scan or ultrafast CT scan
chest x-ray
echocardiogram
Types: one-dimensional (M-mode)
2-dimensional (cross-sectional)
Doppler ultrasound
stress, chemical stress
transesophageal

intravascular
elective cardioversions
electrocardiogram
exercise treadmill test
MRA (magnetic resonance angiography)
MRI (magnetic resonance imaging)
signal-averaged EKG
tilt-table test for syncope
ultrafast computed tomography

Selected Invasive Tests/Services

angiography
atherectomy
atrial fibrillation ablation procedure
cardiac mapping using NOGA
cardiac PET scan
cardiac output
diagnostic and therapeutic electrophysiology
procedures
hemodynamic studies
implantation of internal defibrillators
intra-aortic balloon pump insertion
intravascular ultrasound

MUGA scan myocardial biopsy
oxygen saturation studies
percutaneous transluminal angioplasty
pericardiocentesis
permanent and temporary transvenous pacing
right and/or left heart catheterization
SPECT test
stent placement
synchronized electrical cardioversion
thrombectomy (using AngioJet)
thrombolytic therapy
transesophageal echocardiogram (TEE)

Associated with Nuclear Imaging

exercise stress test
nuclear stress test
Adenosine stress test
Cardiolyte/thallium stress test

Debutamine stress test
Lexiscan stress test
radionuclide imaging

Selected Treatment Modalities

1. cardiac resynchronization therapy—stimulates both of the heart's lower chambers (and often one upper chamber) so they are "synchronized" and thereby are more efficient in pumping blood to the body
2. implantable cardioverter defibrillator—monitors heart rate and administers shock to heart in life-threatening situations
3. pacemaker therapy—an artificial cardiac pacemaker completely implanted into the subcutaneous tissue
4. radiofrequency ablation—for treatment of specific rhythm disturbances

Minimally Invasive Bypass Surgery

1. keyhole surgery (buttonhole surgery or laparoscopic bypass)
2. MIDCAB (minimally invasive direct coronary artery bypass)
3. OPCAB (off-pump bypass surgery)
4. port access bypass surgery

Supportive Web Sites

http://www.webmd.com/	Search for "Cardiology"; select the link "Glossary of Heart Disease Terms" for an extensive list of cardiology terms; open other links of interest.
http://www.centerwatch.com	Under "Drug Information" click on "New Medical Therapies." Select "Cardiology/Vascular Diseases" for results of all drug therapies in completed or ongoing clinical trials.
http://www.sjm.com/web-site-directory.aspx	Click on links of interest for more information on specific heart conditions.
http://www.heartcenteronline.com	Click on "heart quizzes," then "A to Z topic list" for links to deeper sites.
http://www.hgcardio.com	Click on the "procedures," "heart disease," "what's new," and "links" buttons for detailed information on heart-related topics.
http://www.nlm.nih.gov/	Click on links of interest on this page to take you to more specific information on heart-related conditions
http://www.novoste.com	Click on "patient" and "healthcare professional" links for access to other informative links.

Index of Cardiology/Cardiovascular Surgery Reports

Exercise#	Patient Name	Type of Report/Procedure
TE#1	Julia Paternoster	Consult (letter): Paroxysmal atrial fibrillation
TE#2	Mary Kramer	History and Physical Examination: Dyspnea
TE#3	Mary Kramer	Holter Monitor Report
TE#4	Mary Kramer	Discharge Summary: Acute diastolic heart failure
TE#5	Vivian Goff	Cardiac Consult: Myocardial infarction
TE#6	Vivian Goff	Coronary Artery Bypass
TE#7	Vivian Goff	Discharge Summary
TE#8	Vivian Goff	Cardiac Surgery SOAP Note
TE#9	Jonathan Olivier	Surgery: Right and left heart catheterization
TE#10	Margaret Miller	Surgery: Repair of thoracic aneurysm

CHAPTER 3
INFECTIOUS DISEASES

Introduction

Infectious diseases, also known as communicable diseases, contagious diseases, or transmissible diseases, are caused by microorganisms (germs) such as viruses, bacteria, fungi, or parasites. These diseases can be transmitted by various means, such as person to person via bites from insects or animals; by consuming contaminated food, water, or other infectious agents in the environment; via occupational risk (needle stick); and via blood/body fluid exposure. Infectious diseases of animals that can cause disease when transmitted to humans are known as zoonotic diseases.

Some of the more recognizable infectious diseases are AIDS, tuberculosis, Ebola hemorrhagic fever, West Nile Virus, and cholera. The hepatitis B virus (HBV) is one of the most common of all infectious diseases in the world. Infectious diseases are said to kill more people worldwide than any other single cause. Infectious diseases that are especially infective are sometimes called *contagious* and can be easily transmitted by contact with sick people or their secretions. An infection is not synonymous with an infectious disease, since some infections do not cause illness in a host. Infectious diseases may be contracted by different routes. These routes of transmission include contact (direct and indirect), droplet, and airborne.

Two types of infections are bacterial and viral. Bacterial infections are caused by bacteria, and viral infections are caused by viruses. Examples of bacterial infections are strep throat, staph infections, and tuberculosis. Diseases that result from viral infections include AIDS, chickenpox, and the common cold. For treatment of bacterial infections, antibiotic drugs are administered, since they usually kill the bacteria; however, they are not effective against viruses. Strains of bacterial disease have developed that are resistant to treatment with different types of antibiotic medications due to inappropriate and overuse of antibiotics—see MRSA, MRSE, and VRE below.

Because the HIV/AIDS virus lowers resistance to bacteria and parasites that are easily contained by normal defenses, *opportunistic infections* can occur. Examples of these infections are candidiasis, herpes simplex, Pneumocystis carinii pneumonia, and toxoplasmosis. *NB*: The cardinal signs of infection include calor (fever), dolor (pain), rubor (redness), and tumor (swelling). Patients must display at least one of these signs before infection can be diagnosed.

Some of the testing procedures for infectious diseases follow.

1. Cryptococcal infections. These fungal infections can be diagnosed in any of the following ways, depending upon where the infection lies in the body:

   - Fungal blood cultures, cerebrospinal fluid (CSF) fungal cultures, and sputum fungal cultures. Both the CSF fungal culture and the sputum fungal culture can include a fungal smear.
   - Cryptococcal antigen testing of either serum or CSF.
   - Cryptococcal India ink testing of CSF only.

2. Lyme disease, which is caused by the spirochete organism Borrelia burgdorferi, cannot be cultured. Tests available include complete blood count (CBC) with differential and a peripheral smear (blood). During a certain period of the infection, the spirochete can be seen on a peripheral smear. A total antibody test is available for screening, which can be done on serum and on CSF. If positive, then IgG and IgM antibody testing by Western blot is done. Also, Borrelia species DNA detection by PCR can be done.

3. MRSA and MRSE are diagnosed by microbiology culture. For routine screening or the detection of a possible carrier, the specimen can be a nasal culture. If there is a possible active infection, then a wound culture, an aerobic culture, or a blood culture would be done, depending on the type of infection and where it manifests itself.

A protocol to prevent the spread of infection is ever present in healthcare facilities, especially hospitals. Strict adherence to hand-hygiene practices, implementation of personal protective equipment (PPE), and utilizing best practice standards are examples of actions that healthcare workers perform with all patient care activities. Some examples of hospital-acquired conditions (HAC) include fractures, decubitus ulcers (greater than stage 2), central line bloodstream infections, and catheter-associated UTIs.

Selected infections/conditions are now reportable through the Centers for Disease Control (CDC) National Healthcare Safety Network (NHSN). These data are used by Centers for Medicare & Medicaid Services (CMS) to determine reimbursement amounts to facilities based on their rates of infections/conditions. CMS presently obtains reports of infections/conditions from NHSN as part of their Pay-for-Performance (P4P) Conditions of Participation regulations.

Healthcare documentation specialists (HDSs) are responsible for keeping their work stations clean, as many facilities employ shift workers who share this equipment; therefore, it is vital that HDSs have knowledge of proper infection-control procedures. Also, the HDS must employ critical thinking skills in order to edit a document accurately; the proofreading and editing process may include flagging and/or seeking clarification of questionable dictation. The HDS is the first member of the risk management team to have access to dictation errors.

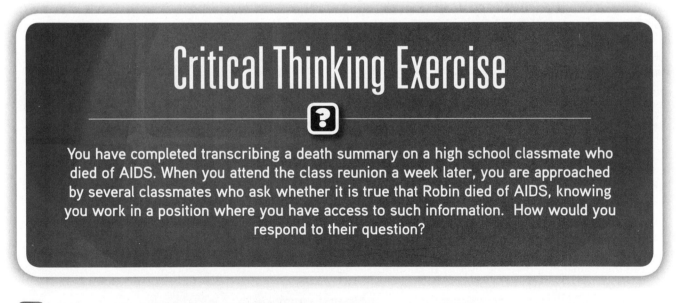

Critical Thinking Exercise

You have completed transcribing a death summary on a high school classmate who died of AIDS. When you attend the class reunion a week later, you are approached by several classmates who ask whether it is true that Robin died of AIDS, knowing you work in a position where you have access to such information. How would you respond to their question?

Infectious Diseases Abbreviations

The abbreviations, acronyms, and terms in the following abbreviations and terminology sections are often dictated in this specialty. We offer abbreviated definitions here. Please see an unabridged medical dictionary or the suggested web sites in this chapter for more information on each term.

Ad14	adenovirus 14		**CMV**	cytomegalovirus
AIDS	acquired immunodeficiency syndrome		**EBV**	Epstein-Barr virus
ARC	AIDS-related complex		**ELISA**	enzyme-linked immunosorbent assay (AIDS test)

ESBL	extended-spectrum beta lactamases
HAI	hospital-acquired infection/healthcare-associated infection
HIV	human immunodeficiency virus
MRSA	methicillin-resistant Staphylococcus aureus
MRSE	methicillin-resistant Staphylococcus epidermidis
NGU	nongonococcal urethritis
PCP	Pneumocystis carinii pneumonia
RMSF	Rocky Mountain spotted fever
RSV	respiratory syncytial virus
STD	sexually transmitted disease
TB	tuberculosis
TSS	toxic shock syndrome
UTI	urinary tract infection
VRE	vancomycin-resistant enterococci
VHFs	viral hemorrhagic fevers

Anatomic Illustrations

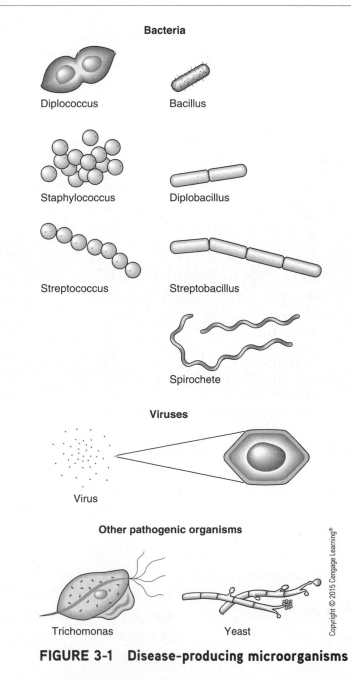

FIGURE 3-1 Disease-producing microorganisms

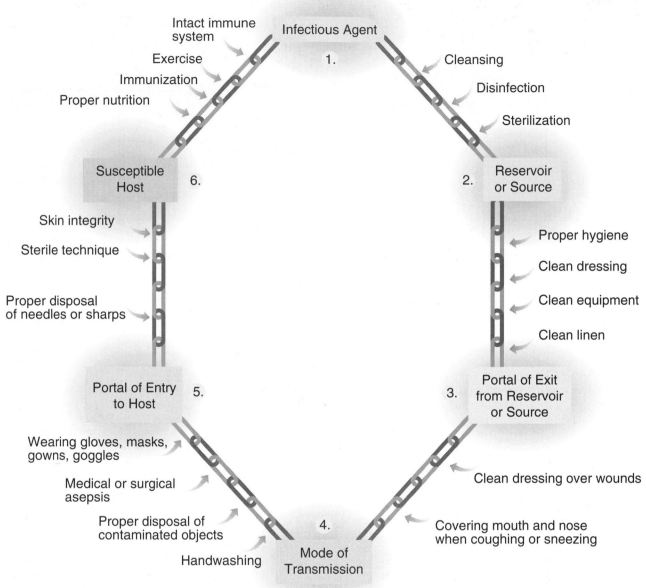

FIGURE 3-2 The chain of infection with preventive measures

Infectious Diseases Terminology

acquired immunodeficiency syndrome (AIDS) (ih"-myoo-no d -fish'-en-se) – condition resulting from suppression or deficiency of the immune response, caused by exposure to HIV (see below)

adenovirus 14 (ad'ə-no-vi"rəs) – called the "killer cold virus" due to the high incidence of hospitalizations and deaths attributed to this viral strain

anaphylaxis (an"-uh-fih-lak'-sis) – an exaggerated or unusual hypersensitivity to foreign protein or other substances

anthrax (an'thraks) – an infectious disease caused by infection with Bacillus anthracis

antigen (an'-tih-jen) – a molecule that can elicit antibody formation after a latent period (days or weeks)

B cells ('bē 'selz) – lymphocytes that change into plasma cells and secrete antibodies

botulism (boch'ə-liz-əm) – in humans, food poisoning with neurotoxicity resulting from eating food contaminated with Clostridium botulinum

carrier ('ker-ē-ər) – an apparently well person in whom pathogenic microorganisms live and multiply without apparent ill effect but who can disseminate disease to others

CD4+ lymphocytes (lim'fo-sītz) – helper T cells that carry the CD4+ protein antigen on their surface; HIV binds to CD4+ and infects and kills T cells bearing this protein

campylobacteriosis (kam"pə-lo-bak-tēr"e-o'sis) – bacterial infection with Campylobacter species; in humans, it is usually an intestinal condition acquired by eating inadequately cooked meat

Chagas disease (chah'gəs) – an infection caused by the protozoan parasite Trypanosoma cruzi that can cause acute inflammatory skin changes (chagomas) and may eventually cause infection and inflammation of many other tissues, especially those of the heart and intestinal tract

chickenpox (chĭk'ən-pŏks') – varicella; a highly contagious, infectious disease caused by human herpes virus 3, usually affecting children but also seen in those of any age who have not been vaccinated

cholera (kol'ər-ə) – an acute, infectious disease endemic in India and Southeast Asia that is spread by feces-contaminated water and food

coccidioidomycosis (kok-sid"e-oi"do-mi-ko'sis) – infection caused by inhaling spores of a fungus, Coccidioides immitis, found in desert regions

communicable disease (kə-mu'nĭ-kə-bəl) – an illness caused by a specific infectious agent or its toxic products that is transmitted directly or indirectly from an infected person or animal to a susceptible host

contagion (kən-ta'jən) – transmission of infection by direct contact, droplet spread, or contaminated fomites; e.g. objects, such as towels, utensils, or clothing that may harbor a disease agent

contamination (kən-,ta-mə-'nā-shən) – the presence of pathogenic microorganisms on a body or inanimate object

Cryptococcus (krip"to-kok'əs) – a type of fungus found in soil worldwide, usually in association with bird droppings

Cryptosporidiosis (krip"to-spo-rid"e-o'sis) – a waterborne disease caused by a parasite that spreads when a water source is contaminated, usually with the feces of infected animals or humans

cytomegalovirus (si"to-meg'ə-lo-vi"rəs) – one member of a group of large herpes-type viruses that can cause many diseases in persons with impaired immunity

cytotoxic cells (si"-to-tok'-sik) – killer cells (T cells) that promptly kill foreign cells; also called T8 cells

diphtheria (dif-thēr'e-ə) – an acute infectious disease caused by toxigenic strains of Corynebacterium diphtheriae; usually confined to the upper respiratory tract

E

Ebola virus hemorrhagic fever (eb'o-lə hem"- o -raj'- ik) – a severe, frequently fatal disease transmitted to humans by infected animals and animal materials

encephalitis (en-sef"ə-li'tis) – inflammation of the brain

endemic (en-dem'ik) – present in a community or among a group of people; said of a disease prevailing in a region

epidemic (ep-ih-DEM-ick) – a temporary and significant increase in the incidence of a disease above what is normally expected in a given time

enzyme-linked immunosorbent assay (ELISA) (en'zīm ih"-myoo-n -sor'-bunt as'a) – test used to screen blood for the antibody to the AIDS virus; because false-positive results can occur with this test, a backup test (Western blot) is used to confirm positive findings

filoviruses (fi'lo-vi"rəsez) – the Marburg and Ebola viruses, a genus of viruses of the family Filoviridae that cause hemorrhagic fevers

gangrene (gang'grēn) – death of tissue, usually in considerable mass and generally associated with loss of vascular supply

giardiasis (je"ahr-di'ə-sis) – a diarrheal illness caused by the organism Giardia intestinalis (also known as Giardia lamblia)

gonorrhea (gon"o-re'ə) – one of the most common infectious diseases caused by the bacterium Neisseria gonorrhoeae; transmitted most frequently through sexual intercourse (an STD)

helper cells – T cells that aid B cells in recognizing antigens and stimulating antibody production; also called T4 or CD$_4$+ cells (see above)

hepatitis (hep"ə-ti'tis) – inflammation of the liver usually due to viral infection but sometimes to toxic agents; there are many subcategories of hepatitis, but the three most common types are hepatitis A (HAV), hepatitis B (HBV), and hepatitis C (HCV)—hepatitis is a major public health problem in industrialized nations

herpes labialis (hur'pēz la"-b-al'-ihs) – infection caused by the herpes simplex virus; results in painful blisters (*cold sores* or *fever blisters*) on the skin of the lips, mouth, gums, external nares, or genitalia

human immunodeficiency virus (HIV) (im"u-no-də-fish'ən-se) – the virus (retrovirus) that causes AIDS

incubation period (in"ku-ba'shən) – the interval between invasion of the body by an infecting organism and the appearance of the first sign or symptom it causes; also, latent period

infection (in- fek' shun) – the entry and multiplication of an infectious agent in the body of humans or animals

infectious agent (in-fek'shəs) – a parasite capable of producing infection

infectious mononucleosis (mon"o-noo"kle-o'sis) – a common, acute, usually self-limited infectious disease caused by the Epstein-Barr virus

influenza (in"floo-en'zə) – a virus that attacks the human respiratory tract

interferons (in"-ter-f r'-ahnz) – antiviral proteins secreted by T cells; they also stimulate macrophages to consume bacteria

interleukins (in"-ter-loo'-kinz) – proteins that stimulate the growth of T-cell lymphocytes and activate immune responses

killer cells – T cells that envelop foreign cells, tumor cells, and bacteria; also called T8 cells

leishmaniasis (lēsh"mə-ni'ə-sis) – a disease spread by the bite of the sandfly and found mostly in tropical countries

leprosy (lep'r ə-se) – a slowly progressive, chronic infectious disease caused by Mycobacterium leprae and characterized by granulomatous or neurotrophic lesions in the skin

listeriosis (lis-te"re-o'sis) – serious infection caused by eating food contaminated with the bacterium Listeria monocytogenes

lymphogranuloma venereum (lim"fo-gran" u-lo'mə veh-ner'-ee-um) – an STD caused by the bacteria Chlamydia trachomatis

malaria (mə-lar'e-ə) – a mosquito-borne disease most common in tropical and subtropical areas

measles – a highly contagious viral disease caused by a paramyxovirus, common among children but also seen in those not vaccinated of any age

meningitis (men"-in-jʹ-tis) – an infection that causes inflammation of the membranes covering the brain and spinal cord

meningococcemia (mə-ning"go-kok-seʹme-ə) – an infection of the bloodstream caused by the bacterium Neisseria meningitidis

meningococcosis (mə-ning"go-kŏ-koʹsis) – any infection caused by meningococci, such as meningitis or pneumonia

mononucleosis (mon"o-noo"kle-oʹsis) – an acute infectious disease that results in enlarged lymph nodes and increased numbers of lymphocytes and monocytes in the bloodstream; caused by the Epstein-Barr virus (EBV)

necrotizing fasciitis (nekʹro-tīz"ing fas"e-iʹtis) – a fulminating subcutaneous soft tissue infection beginning with extensive cellulitis that rapidly spreads to involve the superficial and often the deep fascia

nosocomial infection (nos"o-koʹme-əl) – an infection or infectious disease that is contracted within a hospital or other institution

opportunistic infection (op"-ur-too-nisʹ-tik) – any of a number of infectious diseases associated with AIDS; examples include candidiasis, herpes simplex, Pneumocystis carinii pneumonia, toxoplasmosis

pathogens (pathʹo-jənz) – microorganisms capable of producing disease under favorable conditions

pneumonia (noo-mōnʹyə) – inflammation of the lung parenchyma caused by bacteria, viruses, fungi, or chemical irritants

Pneumocystis carinii pneumonia (pneumocystis) (noo"-m -sisʹ-tis kah-rinʹ ee-i noo-mōnʹyə) – pneumonia caused by Pneumocystis carinii fungi; the most common pneumonia in persons with advanced HIV disease and AIDs

rabies (raʹbēz) – an acute infectious disease of the central nervous system that can affect almost any mammal, caused by a virus of the genus Lyssavirus

respiratory syncytial virus (RSV) (sin-siʹ-sh(ē)-al) – any of a group of viruses belonging to the genus Pneumovirus; in humans, RSV causes respiratory disease that is particularly severe in infants

retrovirus (retʹro-vi"rəs) – an RNA virus that makes copies of itself by using the host cell's DNA; this is in reverse (retro) fashion because the regular method is for DNA to copy itself onto RNA; a retrovirus like HIV carries an enzyme called reverse transcriptase that enables it to reproduce within the host cell

Reye syndrome (riʹ) – a rare, sometimes fatal, disease of the brain accompanied by degeneration of the liver; occurs in children after acute viral infections, such as chickenpox or an influenza-type illness; also associated with taking medication containing aspirin during the illness

rheumatic fever (ru̇ -ʹma-tik) – an autoimmune disease that may occur following a group A streptococci throat infection; it causes inflammatory lesions of connective tissue, especially of the heart, blood vessels, and joints

Rocky Mountain spotted fever (ʹrä-kē ʹmau̇n-tən ʹspät'ted ʹfē-vər) – an acute, infectious, sometimes fatal disease caused by Rickettsia rickettsii, usually transmitted by the bite of an infected tick

Rotavirus (roʹtə-vi"rəs) – a genus of RNA viruses that includes the human gastroenteritis viruses, a major cause of infant diarrhea throughout the world

Salmonella (sal"mo-nelʹə) – a bacterium that causes one of the most common intestinal infections—salmonellosis; overall, it is the second most common bacterial food-borne illness reported

saprophytes (sap'ro-fitz) – microorganisms living on dead or decaying organic matter

scarlet fever (SCAR-let) – infection with group A β-hemolytic streptococci

sepsis (sep'sis) – the presence of various pus-forming and other pathogenic organisms, or their toxins, in the blood

sepsis syndrome (sep'sis SIN-drohm) – clinical evidence of acute infection, tachycardia, tachypnea, evidence of inadequate organ function; may have altered mental function, oliguria, or disseminated intravascular coagulation

septicemia (sep"tĭ-se'me-ə) – a common type of sepsis

shingles (shing'-gulz) – a painful illness caused by the varicella-zoster virus (the same virus that causes chickenpox)

sporadic (spə-rad'ik) – the occasional occurrence of a disease at a low level of incidence

Staphylococcus (staf"ə-lo-kok'əs) – a genus of non-motile, non-spore-forming, gram-positive cells that divide to form irregular clusters

strep throat – a common and contagious infection caused by group A streptococcus bacteria; it is especially common among children

suppressor cells (suh-pres'-er) – T-cell lymphocytes that inhibit the activity of B-cell lymphocytes

tetanus (tet'ə-nəs) – a bacterial infection caused by Clostridium tetani and which affects the nervous system; regular vaccinations against tetanus are required to maintain immunity

Toxic shock syndrome (TSS) – a rare, life-threatening illness caused by toxins (poisons) that circulate in the bloodstream

toxins (tok'sinz) – poisonous materials produced by bacteria

toxoplasmosis (tok"so-plaz-mo'sis) – an infection caused by a single-celled parasite called Toxoplasma gondii

TruGene™ test (troo'-jeen) – first FDA-approved test for analyzing genetic weaknesses in a patient's strain of HIV; assists physicians in choosing AIDS drugs that are likely to work best against the virus in that patient

tuberculosis (TB) (too-bur"ku-lo'sis) – an infectious disease caused the bacteria Mycobacterium tuberculosis

typhus (ti'fəs) – a bacterial disease spread by lice or fleas; caused by one of two types of bacteria: Rickettsia typhi or Rickettsia prowazekiis

vancomycin-resistant enterococci (VRE) (van"ko-mi'sin en"tər-o-kok'i) – bacteria called enterococci that have developed resistance to many antibiotics, especially vancomycin

viral hemorrhagic fevers (VHFs) (hem"- o - raj'-ik) – a group of illnesses that are caused by four distinct families of viruses: arenaviruses, filoviruses, bunyaviruses, and flaviviruses

Wegener granulomatosis (veg'-nerz gran"-yoo-lo"-muh-t '-sis) – an uncommon disease characterized by inflammation of the blood vessels (vasculitis)

Western blot – a test used to confirm the presence of antibodies to a specific organism in the serum; for example, HIV or Lyme disease

Transcription Tips

Transcribing dictation dealing with infectious diseases can be challenging. However, if you are familiar with infectious disease terminology, infection-causing microorganisms, parasites, fungi, viruses, and potential biological and chemical weapons, your task will be easier.

Microorganisms That Cause Infection (partial list)

Microorganism (genus)	Species
Acinetobacter	A calcoaceticus
Clostridium	C botulinum
	C perfringens
	C septicum
	C sporogenes
	C tetani
Enterobacter	E aerogenes
Escherichia	E cloacae
	E coli
Klebsiella	K pneumoniae
	K oxytoca
Mycobacterium	M avium-intracellulare
	M tuberculosis
Neisseria	N catarrhalis
	N gonorrhoeae
	N meningitides
Proteus	P mirabilis
	P vulgaris
Pseudomonas	P aeruginosa
Salmonella	S typhosa
Serratia	S marcescens
Spirochaeta	S plicatilis
Staphylococcus	S aureus
	S epidermidis
Streptococcus	S pneumonia

Parasites (singular, parasite) An organism that lives in or on another and draws its nourishment therefrom. A few examples include:

> autistic p.
> facultative p.
> heterogenic p.
> incidental p.
> obligate p.
> spurious p.
> temporary p.

Fungi (singular, fungus—from Latin for mushroom)
Fungi consist of yeasts and molds that are essential to the recycling of carbon and other elements. Fungi are important in the fermentation process in the development of substances of industrial and medical importance. Relatively few fungi are pathogenic for humans, whereas most plant diseases are caused by fungi. Some examples include:

> asexual f.
> f. cerebri

dematiaceous f.
imperfect f.
perfect f.
ray f.
yeast f.

Viruses (singular, virus) A term for a group of infectious agents that, with a few exceptions, are capable of passing through fine filters that retain most bacteria; viruses lack independent metabolism and are incapable of independent growth or reproduction apart from living cells. A few examples include:

Colorado tick fever v.
dengue v.
Desert Shield v.
monkeypox v.
tick-born encephalitis v.
varicella-zoster v.
West Nile v.

Potential Biological Weapons

anthrax – a bacterium that is contracted through the skin, by inhalation, or by eating infected meat; produces a toxin that can be fatal

botulism – a rare but serious paralytic illness caused by a nerve toxin produced by the bacterium Clostridium botulinum

Ebola – a filovirus that is usually fatal; causes fever, chills, headaches, muscle aches, loss of appetite, vomiting, bloody diarrhea, abdominal pain, sore throat; blood fails to clot and patients bleed from every orifice

plague – highly infectious disease caused by the bacterium Yersinia pestis; transmitted by flea bites or by eating contaminated animal tissue; types are bubonic, pneumonic, and septicemic (most deadly)

ricin – poison derived from castor bean plants; can be turned into an aerosol and released; can be inhaled or ingested from poisoned food or contaminated water supply

smallpox – acute, eruptive contagious viral disease that was a universal scourge, this disease has been extinct since the 1970s; vaccinations for military, healthcare, and other high-risk personnel have been resumed in case the smallpox virus should ever be used as a weapon of biologic warfare or bioterrorism

tularemia – acute, plague-like infectious disease; transmitted by insect bites, eating undercooked meat from an infected animal, or drinking contaminated water

viral hemorrhagic fevers (VHFs) – a severe, multisystem syndrome caused by four families of viruses (see above); affects multiple organ body systems; overall vascular system is damaged and body's regulatory ability is damaged

Potential Chemical Weapons

chlorine – greenish yellow, odorous gas that has a choking smell and is very poisonous; destroys cells that line the respiratory tract

hydrogen cyanide – colorless gas or pale blue liquid that blocks oxygen from reaching the blood; irritates and burns the skin and eyes; high exposure can cause sudden death

mustard gas – yellow to brown gas that smells like garlic; potentially deadly agent that attacks the skin and eyes; causes severe blisters and, if inhaled, can damage lungs and other organs; may cause death by respiratory failure

phosgene – colorless gas that causes the lungs to fill with water, resulting in choking and suffocation

sarin – highly toxic nerve gas that affects the signaling mechanism by which nerve cells communicate; causes death by suffocation

VX – a nerve agent that works like sarin but is more toxic; one milligram on the skin will kill a person

Supportive Web Sites

www.medscape.com/infectiousdiseases	Contains a link to "emerging infectious diseases"; also click on the "More" link for a list of terms/diseases.
http://www.apic.org	Search this site for links of interest.
http://medicalglossary.org/	Click on "organisms" and "diseases" for terms associated with these topics.
http://en.wikipedia.org/wiki/List_of_infectious_diseases	Gives extensive list of infectious diseases in humans.
http://www.aidsinfonet.org/	Click on "Fact Sheet Categories" or "Internet Bookmarks on AIDS" for helpful links.
http://www.cdc.gov/	Under "Diseases and Conditions," click on links of interest.
http://my.webmd.com/	Do a search for "Infectious disease"; click on links of interest.
http://www.nlm.nih.gov/	Search for "Infectious disease"; click on links of interest.

Index of Infectious Diseases Reports

Exercise#	Patient Name	Type of Report/Procedure
TE#1	Cara Reed	Consult: Pulmonary cryptococcosis
TE#2	Cara Reed	Operative Procedure: Flexible bronchoscopy
TE#3	Bipin Gupta	Correspondence: Lyme disease
TE#4	Donald Gardener	Consult: Wound infection
TE#5	Carmen G. Lombardi	Consult: Diabetic cellulitis
TE#6	Samuel Fairbrother	Discharge Summary: Endocarditis
TE#7	Samuel Fairbrother	Discharge Summary: Allergic reaction

CHAPTER 4

OTORHINOLARYNGOLOGY (ENT) & ORAL SURGERY

Introduction

The medical specialties of *otology, rhinology,* and *laryngology* refer to the structures, functions, and diseases of the ears, nose, and throat, respectively; these three specialties are usually practiced together. Physicians who are concerned with the medical and surgical diagnoses of diseases of the ears, nose, and throat are known as *otorhinolaryngologists.*

Separately, an *otologist* is a physician who is concerned with the medical and surgical diagnoses of the diseases of the ear. The ear is comprised of three basic parts—the *external* (or outer) ear, the *middle* ear, and the *internal* (or inner) ear. The outer ear is made up of the *pinna* and the *external auditory canal.* The middle ear consists of the *tympanic membrane,* the *malleus,* the *incus,* the *stapes,* and the *oval window.* The inner ear is made up of the *cochlea,* the auditory liquids and receptors in the organ of *corti,* the auditory nerve fibers, and the semicircular condyle for balance.

A *rhinologist* is a doctor who treats the nose and its diseases. The three basic parts of the nose are the *external nose,* the *internal nose,* and the *sinuses*—the openings that appear in the interior of the nose and occur in pairs, one for each side of the face. They are known as the *maxillary, frontal, ethmoid,* and *sphenoid* sinuses. *Sinusitis* is an inflammation of the sinuses.

A physician who studies the throat and the tracheobronchial tree is called a *laryngologist.* What the lay person calls the throat is referred to in medicine as the *pharynx,* which is composed of three natural divisions—the *nasopharynx,* the *oropharynx,* and the *laryngopharynx* (hypopharynx). Acute *pharyngitis* is an inflammation of the mucous membrane and underlying parts of the pharynx. Chronic pharyngitis can be classified as hypertrophic, atrophic, or chronic grandular.

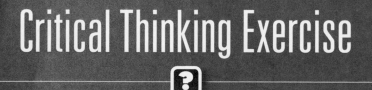

Critical Thinking Exercise

?

You are transcribing for an ENT specialist who states "Status post T&A on a 7-year-old male, the medication prescribed will be as follows: Augmentin 1000 mg p.o. b.i.d." You are aware that this dose is probably too high. How would you proceed?

▪ Otorhinolaryngology (ENT) & Oral Surgery Abbreviations

The abbreviations, acronyms, and terms in the following abbreviations and terminology sections are often dictated in this specialty. We offer abbreviated definitions here. Please see an unabridged medical dictionary or the suggested web sites in this chapter for more information on each term.

AC	air conduction
AD	right ear (AD is considered a dangerous abbreviation)
AS	left ear (AS is considered a dangerous abbreviation)
AU	both ears (AU is considered a dangerous abbreviation)
BC	bone conduction
AOM, BOM	acute otitis media, bilateral otitis media
dB	decibel
EES	erythromycin ethylsuccinate
ENG	electronystagmography
ENT	ears, nose, throat
ETF	eustachian tubal function
FESS	functional endoscopic sinus surgery
HD	hearing distance
HEENT	head, eyes, ears, nose, throat
Hz	hertz
IAC	internal auditory canal
IRT	infrared tympanic thermometry
LAM	laser-assisted myringotomy
MP	mouthpiece

NSR	nasal septal reconstruction
OM	otitis media
OME	otitis media with effusion
oto	otology
PE tube	polyethylene tube
PND	postnasal drip
PORP	partial ossicular replacement prosthesis
RD	respiratory disease
SAL	sensory acuity level
SD	septal defect
SISI	short increment sensitivity index
SMR	submucous resection
SOM	serous otitis media
staph	Staphylococcus
strep	Streptococcus
T&A	tonsils and adenoids; tonsillectomy and adenoidectomy
TM	tympanic membrane
TMJ	temporomandibular joint
TORP	total ossicular replacement prosthesis
URI	upper respiratory infection
ZMC	zygomaticomalar

Anatomic Illustrations

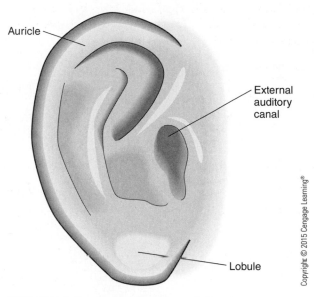

FIGURE 4-1   External view of the ear

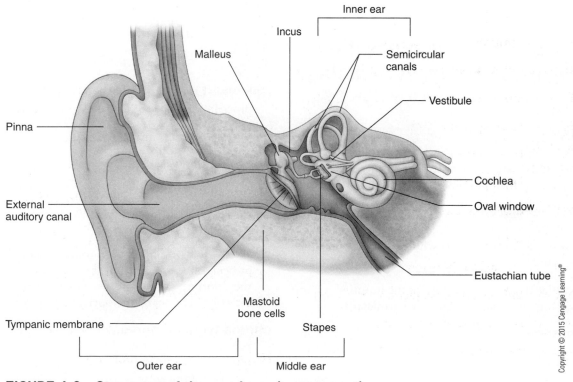

FIGURE 4-2   Structures of the ear shown in cross-section

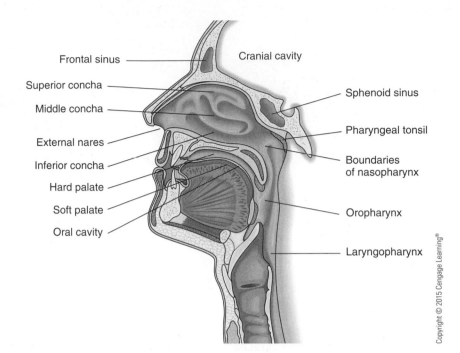

Cranial cavity

Frontal sinus

Superior concha

Middle concha

External nares

Inferior concha

Hard palate

Soft palate

Oral cavity

Sphenoid sinus

Pharyngeal tonsil

Boundaries
of nasopharynx

Oropharynx

Laryngopharynx

FIGURE 4-3   Sagittal section of the face and neck, showing the nose, nasal cavity, and pharynx

Otorhinolaryngology (ENT) & Oral Surgery Terminology

A

adenoidectomy (ad"-eh-noyd-ek'-tuh-mē) – surgical removal of adenoids

allergic rhinitis (ə-'lər-jik ri-ni'tis) – an allergic reaction caused by the pollens of ragweed, grasses, trees, and/or other plants whose pollen is spread by the wind

allergy (al'ər-je) – a sensitivity of the immune system to something that is ordinarily harmless

antrostomy (an-trahs'-tuh-mē) – surgical procedure whereby an opening into an antrum is created for purposes of drainage

attic (at'-ik) – a cavity situated on the tegmental wall of the tympanic cavity, just above the facial canal

auricle (aw"-ri-kl) – projecting shell-like structure on the side of the head (syn. pinna)

C

Caldwell-Luc operation (kald'-wel-look') – surgical procedure for the sinuses, done intraorally

cerumen (seh-roo'-men) – earwax

cheiloschisis (ki-los'kĭ-sis) – harelip

cheilosis (ki-lo'sis) – a condition marked by fissuring and dry scaling of the vermilion surface of the lips and angles of the mouth

cholesteatoma (ko"lə-ste"ə-to'mə) – a cystlike mass or benign tumor found in the middle ear behind the eardrum, generally caused by trauma or infection that heals improperly

chorda tympani nerve (kōr'-duh tim'-puh-nī) – a nerve originating from the facial nerve and distributed to the submandibular, sublingual, and lingual glands and the anterior two-thirds of the tongue

chorditis (kor-di'tis) – inflammation of a cord, usually a vocal cord

Chvostek sign (kvahs'-tek) – facial irritability or spasm resulting from a slight tap over the facial nerve just anterior to the external auditory meatus (ear canal)

cochlea (kok'le-ə) – the essential organ of hearing

concha (kong'kə) – a structure or part that resembles a shell in shape; as the pinna of the ear or a turbinate bone in the nose (pl. conchae)

corniculum laryngis (kōr-nik'-yoo-lum lār"-in'-jis) – a conical nodule of elastic cartilage surmounting the apex of each arytenoid cartilage

coryza (kō-rī'-zuh) – head cold

cricoid (krī'-koyd) – the cricoid cartilage; a ring-like cartilage forming the lower and back part of the larynx

cricoidectomy (krī"-koy-dek'-tuh-mē) – complete surgical removal of the cricoid cartilage

croup (krōop) – a condition resulting from acute partial obstruction of the upper airway, seen mainly in infants and children; characterized by a barking cough, hoarseness, and persistent high-pitched breath sounds

decibel (deh'-sih-bul) – a unit used to express the ratio of two powers; one decibel is equal to approximately the smallest difference in acoustic power that the human ear can detect

desensitization (dē-sen"-sih-tih-zā'-shun) – the reduction of allergic sensitivity or reaction to the specific antigen (allergen)

endolymphatic (en"-dō-lim-fat'-ik) – pertaining to the endolymph, the fluid contained in the membranous labyrinth of the ear

epiglottis (ep"-ih-glah'-tus) – the lid-like cartilaginous structure overhanging the entrance to the larynx; prevents food from entering the larynx and trachea while swallowing

epistaxis (ep"-ih-stak'-sis) – nosebleed

epitympanum (ep"-ē-tim'-puh-num) – the upper portion of the tympanic cavity above the tympanic

membrane; contains the head of the malleus and the body of the incus

ethmoidectomy (eth"-moy-dek'-tuh-mē) – removal of ethmoid cells that open into the nasal cavity

eustachian tube (auditory tube) (yoo-stā'-shun; aw'-dih-tōr"-ē) – a canal connecting the nasopharynx and the middle ear cavity

external auditory canal (aw'-dih-tōr-ē) – the canal that leads from the pinna to the tympanic membrane

extirpate (eks'-tur-pāt) – to completely remove an organ or a tissue

fauces (faw'sēz) – the space between the cavity of the mouth and the pharynx, bounded by the soft palate and the base of the tongue

faucial (faw' shul) – relating to the fauces, as in the faucial tonsils

fenestration (fen"-eh-strā'-shun) – the surgical creation of a new opening in the labyrinth of the ear for the restoration of hearing in cases of otosclerosis

follicular tonsillitis (fō-lik'-yoo-lur tahn"-sih-lī'-tis) – an acute inflammation of the tonsils and their crypts

fronto-occipital (frun"-tō-ok-sip'-ih-tul) – pertaining to the forehead and the occiput

frontoparietal (frun"-tō-pah-rī'-eh-tul) – pertaining to the frontal and parietal bones

frontotemporal (frun"-tō-tem'-pō-rul) – pertaining to the frontal and temporal bones

geniohyoid (je"ne-o-hi'oid) – pertaining to the chin and hyoid bone

genyantralgia (jen"-ē-an-tral'-jē-uh) – pain in the maxillary sinus

glossoepiglottic (glahs"-ō-ep-ih-glah'-tik) – pertaining to the tongue and epiglottis

glossopharyngeal (glah"-sō-făr-in'-jē-ul) – pertaining to the tongue and the pharynx

glossotomy (glah-sot'-uh-mē) – incision into the tongue

glue ear – a build up of fluid in the middle ear that becomes thick and glue-like

hemilaryngectomy (hem"-ē-lăr"-in-jek'-tuh-mē) – excision of one-half of the larynx

hyoid bone (hī'-oyd) – a horseshoe-shaped bone situated at the base of the tongue, just above the thyroid cartilage

hypopharynx (hī"-pō-făr'-inks) – the division of the pharynx that lies below the upper edge of the epiglottis and opens into the larynx and esophagus

in situ (in sī"-tyoo) – in position, in the natural or normal place

incudostapedial (ing"-kyoo-dō-stah-pē'-dē-ul) – pertaining to the incus and stapes

incus (ing'-kus) – the middle of the three bones of the ear; with the stapes and malleus, the incus conducts vibrations from the tympanic membrane to the inner ear; also called the *anvil*

Kiesselbach area (kē'-sul-bahk) – anterior nasal septal area, rich in capillaries; frequently the site of nose bleeds

L

labyrinth (lab'-ih-rinth) – a system of intercommunicating cavities or canals, especially that constituting the internal ear

labyrinthitis (lab"ə-rin-thi'tis) – inflammation of the internal ear; may be accompanied by hearing loss or vertigo

laryngitis (lăr"-in-jī'-tis) – an inflammation of the mucous membrane lining the larynx accompanied by edema of the vocal cords

laryngocentesis (lah-ring"-gō-sen-tē'-sis) – surgical puncture of the larynx

laryngopharyngectomy (lah-ring"-gō-făr"-in-jek'-tuh-mē) – surgical excision of the larynx and pharynx

laryngoscopy (lăr"-ing-gahs'-kuh-pē) – examination of the interior of the larynx, especially that performed with the laryngoscope

laser-assisted myringotomy (mir"ing-got'o-me) – procedure where a laser is used to create a small hole in the eardrum so that trapped fluid can drain; could reduce the need to place PE tubes in ears of those with chronic middle ear infections

lymphoepithelioma (lim"-fō-ep"-ih-thē"-lē-ō'-muh) – a poorly differentiated radiosensitive squamous cell carcinoma involving lymphoid tissue of the region of the tonsils and nasopharynx

malleus (mal'-ē-us) – the largest of the auditory bones and the one attached to the membrana tympani; also called the *hammer* because of its shape

membrana tympani (mem-brā'-nuh tim'-puh-nī) – eardrum

Ménière disease (mĕ-nyăr') – an affection characterized clinically by vertigo, nausea, vomiting, tinnitus, and hearing loss associated with endolymphatic hydrops

myasthenia gravis (mī"-as-thē'-nē-uh gra'-vis) – a syndrome of fatigue and exhaustion of the muscular system marked by progressive paralysis of muscles without sensory disturbance or atrophy; may affect any muscle of the body, but especially those of the face, lips, tongue, throat, and neck

myringotomy (mir"-in-got'-uh-mē) – surgical incision of the eardrum in an area that tends to heal readily; done to avoid spontaneous rupture at a site that rarely closes

nasolacrimal (nā"-zō-lak'-rih-mul) – pertaining to the nose and lacrimal apparatus

occipitomastoid (ok-sip"-ih-tō-mas'-toyd) – pertaining to the occipital bone and the mastoid process

olfactory center (ol-fak'-tuh-rē) – the center of smell

oropharynx (ō"-rō-fār'-inks) – division of the pharynx that lies between the soft palate and the upper edge of the epiglottis

ossicle (ahss'-ih-kul) – a small bone

otalgia (ō-tal'-jē-uh) – earache; pain in the ear

otitis media (ō-tī'-tis mē'-dē-uh) – inflammation of the middle ear

otorhinolaryngology (o"to-ri"no-lar"ing-gol'ə-je) – the branch of medicine dealing with diseases of the ear, nose, and throat; also called *otolaryngology*

otorrhagia (ō"-tō-rā'-jē-uh) – bleeding from the ear

otorrhea (ō"-tō-rē'-uh) – purulent drainage from the ear

otosclerosis (ō"-tō-skleh-rō'-sis) – a progressive condition in which the normal bone of the inner ear is replaced by abnormal osseous (bony) tissue

palatoglossal (pal"-uh-tō-glahs'-ul) – pertaining to the palate and tongue

palatopharyngeal (pal"-uh-tō-fah-rin'-jē-ul) – pertaining to the palate and pharynx

pansinusitis (pan"-sī-nuh-sī'-tis) – inflammation of all the sinuses

paracentesis tympani (pār"-uh-sen-tē'-sis tim'-puh-nī) – incision of the tympanic membrane for drainage or irrigation

parotid (puh-rot'-id) – situated or occurring near the ear, the gland beside the ear

parotitis (pār"-ō-tī'-tis) – inflammation of the parotid gland

perilymphatic (pār"-ē-lim-fat'-ik) – pertaining to the perilymph, or around a lymphatic vessel

peritonsillar abscess (pār"-ī-tahn'-sih-lur) – abscess near or around a tonsil; infection extends from the tonsil to form an abscess in surrounding tissue

pertussis (pər-tus'is) – an acute contagious infection of the respiratory tract that is usually seen in young children, but it can be seen in any unvaccinated population; also known as "whooping cough"

pharyngoplegia (fə-ring"go-ple'jə) – paralysis of the muscles of the pharynx

pinna (pin"-uh) – auricle (external ear)

piriform sinus (pēr'-ih-form) – pear-shaped sinus

preauricular (prē"-aw-rik'-yoo-lur) – situated in front of the auricle of the ear

presbycusis (prez"-bī-kyoo'-sis) – a progressive, bilateral hearing loss occurring with age

pseudocholesteatoma (soo"-dō-kō"-les-tē-uh-tō'-muh) – a mass of cornified epithelial cells resembling cholesteatoma in the tympanic cavity in chronic middle ear inflammation

Reinke edema (rīn'kə) – swelling of the vocal cords due to fluid collection; also known as polypoid degeneration

rhinitis (rī-nī'-tis) – an inflammatory condition of the mucous membranes of the nose and accessory sinuses

rhinorrhea (rī"-nō-rē'-uh) – a "runny" nose

Rosenmüller fossa (rō'-zen-mē"-ler fah'-suh) – a slit-like depression in the pharyngeal wall behind the opening of the eustachian tube

Scarpa membrane (skar'-puh) – secondary tympanic membrane

secretory otitis media (sē-krē'-tōr-ē) – thick, cloudy, viscous exudate in the middle ear containing cells and mucous strands

septoplasty (sep'-tō-plas"-tē) – plastic surgery on the nasal septum to correct defects or deformities

septorhinoplasty (sep"-tō-rī'-nō-plas"-tē) – a combined surgical procedure to repair defects or deformities of the nasal septum and of the external nasal pyramid

serous otitis media (sē'-rus) – thin, clear, amber fluid in the middle ear

Silastic™ tube (sī-las'-tik) – trademark for polymeric silicone substance having the properties of rubber; used in surgical prostheses

sinusitis (si"nəs-i'tis) – inflammation of a sinus, usually a paranasal sinus

sphenopalatine (sfē"-nō-pal'-uh-tīn) – pertaining to or in relation with the sphenoid and palatine bones

stapedectomy (stā"-pē-dek'-tuh-mē) – complete surgical removal of the stapes

stapes (stā'-pēz) – the innermost of the auditory ossicles, shaped somewhat like a stirrup; also called the *stirrup*

staphyledema (staf"-il-ē-dē'-muh) – an enlargement or swollen part of the uvula

Stensen duct, foramen (sten'-sen fō-rā'-men) – the duct that drains the parotid gland and empties into the oral cavity opposite the second superior molar

strep throat – a common and contagious infection caused by group A streptococcus bacteria; it is especially common among children

temporomandibular (tem"-pō-rō-man-dib'-yoo-lur) – pertaining to the temporal bone and the mandible

thyromegaly (thī"-rō-meg'-uh-lē) – enlargement of the thyroid gland; goiter

tinnitus (tih-nī'-tus) – the sensation of ringing, buzzing, roaring, and/or clicking sounds in one or both ears; can be a solid or an intermittent sound

tonsils – lymphoid tissue located in the depressions of the mucous membranes of the face and pharynx; the tonsils filter bacteria and aid in the formation of

white blood cells; referred to as faucial tonsils and palatine tonsils on dictation

tympanic membrane (tim-pan'-ik mem'-brān) – eardrum; the membrane separating the external from the middle ear

tympanitis (tim"-puh-nī'-tus) – inflammation of the eardrum

tympanocentesis (tim"pə-no-sen-te'sis) – the removal of fluid from behind the eardrum

tympanoeustachian (tim"-puh-nō-yoo-stā'-kē-un [OR -yoo-stā'-shun]) – pertaining to the tympanic cavity and auditory tube

tympanomandibular (tim"-puh-nō-man-dib'-yoo-lur) – pertaining to the middle ear and the mandible

tympanomastoiditis (tim'-puh-nō-mas"-toy-dī'-tus) – inflammation of the middle ear and the pneumatic cells of the mastoid process

tympanometry (tim"pə-nom'ə-tre) – a test to register the movement of the eardrum when an ear infection or other middle ear problem is suspected

tympanoplasty (tim'-puh-nō-plas"-tē) – surgical reconstruction of the hearing mechanism of the middle ear

tympanotomy tube (tim"-puh-naht'-uh-mē) – tube inserted into the membrane tympani

tympanum (tim'-puh-num) – middle ear

uvula (yoo'-vyoo-luh) – the soft, fleshy mass hanging from the soft palate

vallecula (vah-lek'-yoo-luh) – the depression between the epiglottis and the root of the tongue on either side

vestibular neuritis (ves-tib'u-lər no͞o-ri'tus) – inflammation of the vestibular nerve, which is in the inner ear; this nerve carries balance signals from the inner ear to the brain

vomer (vō'-mer) – the unpaired flat bone that forms the inferior and posterior part of the nasal septum

Wharton duct (hwor'tən) – the duct that drains submandibular fluid into the oral cavity under the tongue

W

Z

zygomaticomaxillary (zī"-gō-mat"-ih-kō-mak'-sih-lār"-ē) – pertaining to the zygoma and maxilla

Transcription Tips

When transcribing dictation in ENT and Oral Surgery, you should be familiar with the surgical equipment, tests, and procedures employed when evaluating the ears, nose, and throat areas, in either an office setting or an operative suite. An in-depth knowledge of ENT and Oral Surgery terminology and combining forms and root words will also be beneficial.

The nose is more than a passageway for movement of air into the lungs; it also preconditions the air by warming it, humidifying it, and cleaning it. The pharynx, commonly referred to as the throat, separates into the trachea and esophagus immediately above the larynx.

Some common surgeries performed by an oral surgeon include cleft lip and palate surgery, nasal reconstruction, ear reconstruction, congenital facial deformities, temporomandibular joint disease (TMJ) surgery, and congenital maxillofacial malformations. In performing some of these procedures, the oral surgeon might work with plastic and reconstructive surgeons.

Pertinent Equipment

audiophone – instrument that conducts sound to the auditory nerve through teeth or bone

esophagoscope – instrument used to examine the esophagus

laryngoscope – instrument used to examine the larynx

myringoscope – instrument used to examine the eardrum

nasal speculum – instrument used to examine the nose

otoscope – instrument used to examine the ear

rhinoscope – instriument used to examine the nasal passages

Thermoscan instant thermometer – device used to take the temperature in the ear

Tests and Procedures

acid-fast bacilli (AFB) – test performed on sputum to detect the presence of Mycobacterium tuberculosis; positive results indicate tuberculosis

auditory-evoked response – a hearing test for children too young for standard tests, for the autistic, hyperkinetic, and/or mentally challenged

audiogram – a record produced when hearing is measured

Bekesy, Bing, Doerfler-Stewart, Lombard, Rinne, Schwabach, and Weber – tests to check hearing, some of which utilize the tuning fork

culture of sputum, culture of throat – examination of sputum specimen or a throat swab in the microbiology lab to determine the presence of pathogenic microorganisms; abnormal results can indicate the presence of any of the infectious respiratory diseases (RD)

Supportive Web Sites

http://www.nlm.nih.gov/medlineplus/ earnoseandthroat.html	This site contains a visual of the head; click on the ear, nose, or throat to be directed to other links with detailed information on specific conditions.
http://www.mayoclinic.org/ent-rst/	Click on links of interest.
http://en.wikipedia.org/wiki/Otolaryngology	Click on "otology and neuro-otology," for example, to view other links with detailed information on conditions.
http://www.webmd.com/a-to-a-guides/ commontopics/default.htm	Search for "ENT"; then click on links of interest.

Index of Otorhinolaryngology (ENT) & Oral Surgery Reports

Exercise#	Patient Name	Type of Report/Procedure
TE#1	Stephanie Brown	History and Physical Examination
TE#2	Stephanie Brown	CT scan of sinuses
TE#3	Stephanie Brown	Discharge Summary
TE#4	Ruby Moreno	Office Visit—Immediate care
TE#5	Alfonse Petrozello	Microlaryngoscopy, vocal cord polyps
TE#6	Nancy Eklund	Pierre Robin and cleft palate procedure
TE#7	Roger E. Siskall	LeFort I surgical procedure
TE#8	Parker H. Donaldson	LeFort II surgical procedure
TE#9	Cheryl Crane	Partial parotidectomy
TE#10	Jeffrey Finegold	Tonsillectomy and adenoidectomy

CHAPTER 5
ENDOCRINOLOGY

Introduction

The endocrine system is a system of glands, each of which produces a type of hormone that goes directly into the bloodstream and is transported to tissues and organs throughout the body. These hormones regulate the body's growth, metabolism, sexual development, and purpose. This system works with the nervous system, kidneys, reproductive system, stomach, liver, pancreas, and fat to help control and maintain various bodily functions.

Glands comprising the endocrine system consist of the following: adrenal, pineal, pituitary, hypothalamus, ovaries, testes, pancreas, thyroid, and parathyroid. Each of these glands performs a specific, vital function in the body. If any gland develops a minor glitch in function, the delicate balance of hormones in the body can be disturbed and lead to an endocrine disorder or endocrine disease. For example, hormones may be released in amounts that are too great or too small for the body to work normally.

Endocrine disorders are generally grouped into two categories: (1) endocrine disease resulting from a gland producing too much or too little of a hormone, called a hormone imbalance; and (2) endocrine disease resulting from the development of lesions, such as tumors or nodules in the endocrine system. Examples of endocrine diseases or disorders include adrenal insufficiency, hyperthyroidism, hypothyroidism, and polycystic ovary syndrome. Endocrine cancers can include papillary thyroid carcinoma, follicular thyroid carcinoma, and adrenal cancer. Some endocrine nodules can be noncancerous and may not spread to other parts of the body; however, they may interfere with the gland's hormone production.

The physician who studies and treats endocrine disorders is called an *endocrinologist*. A disorder in the function of an endocrine gland is referred to as an *endocrinopathy*. One of the most prevalent disorders treated by the endocrinologist is diabetes mellitus. Adult-onset or type 2 diabetes mellitus, gestational diabetes, and insulin-dependent diabetes mellitus are three ways in which diabetes presents. In order to identify a specific problem, the physician will normally have blood and urine tests done to check hormone levels and to help locate or pinpoint a nodule or tumor.

Treatment of an endocrinopathy can be complicated, as a change in one hormone level can throw off another. In chronic diseases, like Hashimoto thyroiditis or diabetes mellitus, life-long medication is required. Routine blood work is normally ordered by the physician to determine if the medication or treatment that has been prescribed needs to be adjusted.

Critical Thinking Exercise

[?]

You are transcribing a note for a 47-year-old female patient with Graves disease. "CT scan revealed a mass on the left adrenal. Fine-needle biopsy aspiration on the right adrenal also showed questionable malignant cytology. I recommend further evaluation. The patient is scheduled for laparoscopic evaluation and possible removal of the left kidney." What is wrong with the above dictation, and how do you proceed?

Endocrinology Abbreviations

The abbreviations, acronyms, and terms in the following abbreviations and terminology sections are often dictated in this specialty. We offer abbreviated definitions here. Please see an unabridged medical dictionary or the suggested web sites in this chapter for more information on each term.

ACTH	adrenocorticotropic hormone	LHRH	luteinizing hormone-releasing hormone
ADH	antidiuretic hormone; vasopressin	MTC	medullary thyroid carcinoma
CRH	corticotropic-releasing hormone	PCOS	polycystic ovary syndrome
DI	diabetes insipidus	PRL	prolactin
DKA	diabetic ketoacidosis	PTC	papillary thyroid carcinoma
DM	diabetes mellitus	RIA	radioimmunoassay
FSH	follicle-stimulating hormone	TRH	thyrotropin-releasing hormone
FTC	follicular thyroid carcinoma	TSH	thyroid-stimulating hormone
GC	glucocorticoid	TBG	thyroxine-binding globulin
GH	growth hormone	T_4	thyroxine
GnRH	gonadotropin-releasing hormone	T_3	triiodothyronine
ICSH	interstitial cell-stimulating hormone	VP	vasopressin
LH	luteinizing hormone		

Anatomic Illustrations

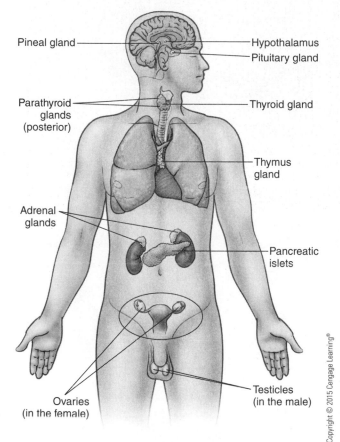

FIGURE 5-1 **Structures of the endocrine system**

Pineal gland
Hypothalamus
Pituitary gland
Parathyroid glands (posterior)
Thyroid gland
Thymus gland
Adrenal glands
Pancreatic islets
Ovaries (in the female)
Testicles (in the male)

Copyright © 2015 Cengage Learning®

Endocrinology Terminology

acromegaly (ak"ro-meg'ə-le) – a chronic disease of adults caused by hypersecretion of growth hormone; characterized by marked enlargement and elongation of the bones of the face, jaw, and extremities

Addison disease (ad'ĭ-sən) – an autoimmune disease that causes the adrenal glands to produce too little of the hormone *cortisol*; also referred to as primary adrenal insufficiency

adenoma (ad"ə-no'mə) – a benign tumor of a gland, such as a parathyroid adenoma

adrenaline (ə-dren'ə-lin) – the hormone produced by the central part (medulla) of the adrenal gland

anaplastic thyroid carcinoma (an"ə-plas'tik thi'roid) – a rare, highly malignant thyroid tumor composed of spindle cells or giant cells; it is an undifferentiated carcinoma of the thyroid

antithyroid drugs (an"te-thi'roid) – medications that slow down the thyroid gland's ability to generate thyroid hormone

beta blocking drugs – medications that helps block the symptoms caused by excess thyroid hormone, such as heart palpitations and tremors

calcitonin (kal"sĭ-to'nin) – a hormone; in the normal state, calcitonin is produced only by the thyroid; it increases the deposition of calcium and phosphate in bone and lowers the level of calcium in blood

cancer (kan"-ser) – general term frequently used to indicate any of various types of neoplasms, most of which invade surrounding tissues; may spread to other sites, are likely to recur after attempted removal, and are likely to kill the patient unless treated adequately

carcinoma (kar' sin o" muh) – any of various types of malignant neoplasm derived from epithelial cells, chiefly glandular or squamous cells; the most commonly occurring type of cancer

cortex (kor'teks) – the outer layer of an organ or other body structure

cortisol (kor'tĭ-sol) – the primary stress hormone; produced by the adrenal cortex, it provides an anti-inflammatory effect and helps the body cope during times of stress.

Cushing syndrome/disease (koosh'ing) – a disorder that occurs when the adrenal gland produces too much cortisol. It can be caused by dysfunction of the pituitary gland producing too much ACTH.

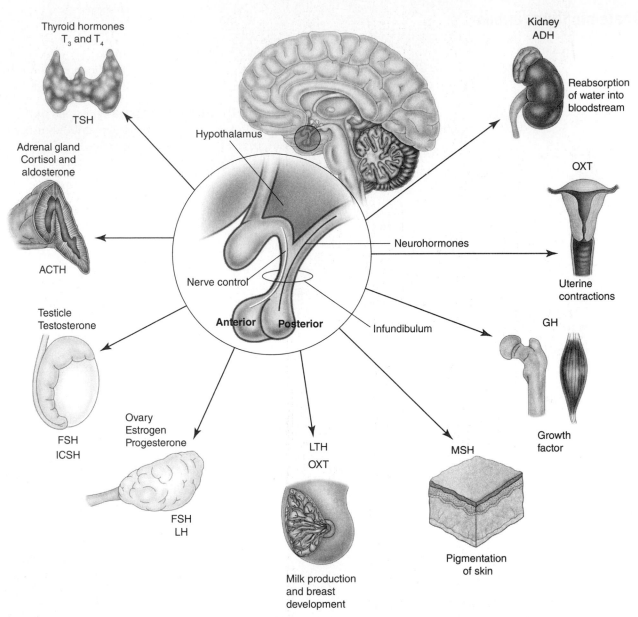

FIGURE 5-2 **The pituitary gland secretes hormones that control the activity of other endocrine glands. Hormones are often referred to by their abbreviations.**

de Quervain thyroiditis (də kār-vă' thi"roid-i'tis) – inflammation of the thyroid gland causing enlargement and pain (syn. subacute granulomatous thyroiditis)

diabetes mellitus, type 1 (di"ə-be'tēz me-lə-təs) (formerly called juvenile diabetes) – an autoimmune disease that occurs when the body's own immune system destroys the insulin-producing cells of the pancreas, called beta cells

diabetes mellitus, type 2 (non-insulin-dependent diabetes) – the most common form of diabetes; patients with this type of diabetes produce insulin, but either the pancreas does not produce enough or the body cannot use the insulin adequately (insulin resistance)

diabetic retinopathy (di"ĭ-bet'ik ret"-nop'ə-the) – retinal changes sometimes associated with diabetes mellitus of long duration

endocrine (en'do-krin) – refers to glands that secrete hormones into the bloodstream through which they travel to and affect distant organs

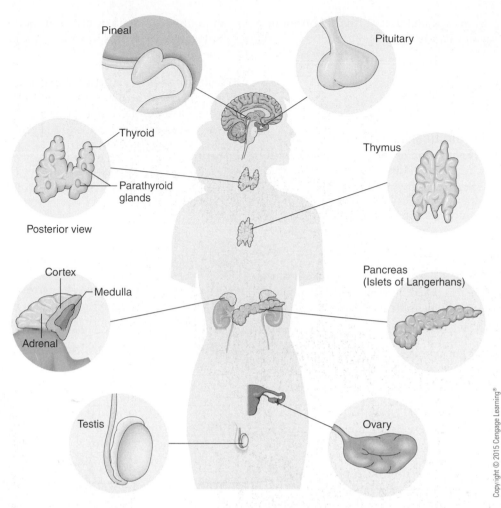

FIGURE 5-3 The endocrine glands and their locations in the body

enzymes (en'zīmz) – proteins that act as catalysts in mediating and speeding a specific chemical reaction

estrogen (es'trə-jen) – a female hormone produced by the ovaries and that is responsible for the development of the secondary female sex characteristics

exocrine (ek'so-krin) – pertaining to the secretion of a substance outwardly through a duct, as opposed to *endocrine*

exophthalmos (ek"sof-thal'mos) – abnormal condition characterized by marked protrusion of one or both eyeballs; bilateral exophthalmos is usually seen in thyroid disease

follicular carcinoma (fə-lik'u-lər kahr"sĭ-no'mə) – carcinoma of the thyroid that can be difficult to distinguish from adenoma; the criteria include

blood vessel invasion and the finding of metastatic follicular thyroid tissue in other structures, such as cervical lymph nodes and bone

gestational diabetes (je-'stā-shən-el) – a condition characterized by carbohydrate intolerance during pregnancy that resolves after delivery

glucose (gloo'kōs) – the simple sugar that serves as the chief source of energy in the body; it is the principal sugar the body makes from proteins, fats, and carbohydrates

goiter (goi'tər) – a chronic, benign enlargement of the thyroid gland, causing a swelling in the front of the neck

Graves disease – a type of autoimmune disease that causes the thyroid to produce too much thyroid hormone; this overproduction of thyroid hormone is called *hyperthyroidism*

Hashimoto thyroiditis (hah"she-mo'to thi"roid-i'tis) – diffuse infiltration of the thyroid gland with lymphocytes, resulting in diffuse goiter, progressive destruction of the parenchyma, and *hypothyroidism*

hormone – chemical substance produced by the endocrine glands that controls and regulates the activity of certain cells or organs

Hürthle cell tumor (hērt'lə) – a rare neoplasm of the thyroid gland, also called Hürthle cell carcinoma; the cell pattern may be follicular, papillary, or undifferentiated

hyperglycemia (hi"pər-gli-se'me-ə) – abnormally increased glucose levels in the blood, such as in diabetes mellitus

hyperparathyroidism (hi"pər-par"ə-thi'roid-iz-əm) – a condition caused by excessive amounts of parathyroid hormone, causing elevated serum calcium

hyperthyroidism (hi"pər-thi'roid-iz-əm) – a condition caused by excessive secretion of thyroid hormones; a condition that can affect many body systems

hypoglycemia (hi"po-gli-se'me-ə) – low blood sugar levels

hypopituitarism (hi"po-pǐ-too'ǐ-tə-riz"əm) – a condition due to diminished activity of the pituitary gland with inadequate secretion of one or more anterior pituitary hormones

hypothyroid (hi"po-thi'roid) – marked by reduced thyroid function (see hypothyroidism)

hypothyroidism (hi"po-thi'roid-iz-əm) – diminished production of thyroid hormone, leading to decreased basal metabolic rate, slow mentation, fatigue, dryness, loss of hair, and/or lethargy

immune system (ǐ-mūn') – a complex system that is responsible for distinguishing the human body from everything foreign; for protecting the human body against infections and foreign substances; it works to seek and kill invaders of the human body

insulin (in'sə-lin) – a natural hormone made by the pancreas that regulates the metabolism of glucose, carbohydrates, fats, and proteins in the cells; used in the management of diabetes mellitus

isthmus (is'məs) – a narrow passage connecting two larger cavities; the narrow portion of the thyroid connecting the larger right and left lobes

medulla (mə-dul'ə) – any soft, narrow-like structure, especially in the center of a part; in endocrinology, it refers to the innermost part of the adrenal gland.

medullary thyroid carcinoma (MTC) (med'ə-lar"e) – this malignant thyroid neoplasm arises from the parafollicular calcitonin-secreting cells of the thyroid gland

melatonin (mel"ə-to'nin) – a hormone produced by the pineal gland that is involved in circadian rhythms, i.e., the sleeping and waking cycles

metabolism (mə-tab'ə-liz"əm) – refers to the breakdown of food and its transformation into energy

myxedema (miks"ə-de'mə) – the most severe form of hypothyroidism, it is characterized by marked edema of the face, stiff hair, and a somnolent look to the face; it literally means condition of mucus swelling—without treatment, coma and death can occur

neoplasm (ne'o-plaz"əm) – abnormal tissue in which growth is uncontrolled and progressive; it usually forms a distinct mass of tissue that may be either benign (benign tumor) or malignant (cancerous tumor)

osteoporosis (os"te-o-pə-ro'sis) – a condition characterized by atrophy of skeletal tissue; it occurs in postmenopausal women and elderly men and results in bone that is scanty, thin, and porous

oxytocin (ok"se-to'sin) – a hormone made in the hypothalamus that stimulates uterine contraction during childbirth and stimulates the release of milk during suckling

panhypopituitarism (PHP) (pan-hi"po-pǐ-too'ǐ-tə-riz-əm) – a condition in which the secretion of all anterior pituitary hormones is either inadequate or absent

papillary thyroid carcinoma (pap'ǐ-lar"e) – papillary tumors of the thyroid are the most common form of thyroid carcinoma to result from exposure to radiation; papillary carcinoma appears as an irregular solid or cystic mass in normal thyroid parenchyma

parathyroid glands (par"ə-thi'roid) – endocrine glands, located beside the thyroid gland, which regulate calcium

pheochromocytoma (fe"o-kro"mo-si-to'mə) – a usually benign, well-encapsulated, lobular, vascular tumor of chromaffin tissue of the adrenal medulla

progesterone (pro-jes'tə-rōn) – a female hormone that prepares the lining of the uterus to receive and sustain the fertilized egg; released during the second half of the menstrual cycle

prolactin (pro-lak'tin) – a hormone secreted by the pituitary gland that stimulates lactation and plays an important role in the maintenance of the immune system

somatostatin (so"mə-to-stat'in) – growth-inhibiting hormone produced by islet cells of the pancreas; regulates endocrine and nervous system function by inhibiting the secretion of several other hormones

testosterone (tes-tos'tə-rōn) – the major androgenic hormone produced by the interstitial cells (Leydig cells) of the testes; male hormone responsible for secondary sex characteristics and masculinization

thyroiditis (thi"roid-i'tis) – inflammation of the thyroid gland

thyroxine (T_4) – primary hormone produced by the thyroid gland; maintains and regulates the basal metabolic rate (BMR)

tri-iodothyronine (T_3) – hormone produced by the thyroid gland; influences the basal metabolic rate

(***NB***: Both T_4 and T_3 can be transcribed on the line or as subscripts.)

vasopressin (VP) (va"zo-o-pres'in) – hormone produced by the hypothalamus and stored in the posterior lobe of the pituitary gland; also called antidiuretic hormone (ADH)—helps conserve and regulate the balance of water within the body

Transcription Tips

Transcription of endocrinology reports will be easier if you are familiar with the abbreviations and terminology presented in this chapter as well as the endocrine glands and their functions, together with laboratory and diagnostic testing procedures relating to this specialty.

Endocrinologists can deal with conditions/disorders such as adrenal cancer, varied types of thyroid cancers, goiters, growth disorders, and pituitary disorders. In addition, they also treat benign diseases, like thyroid disease, diabetes, amyloidosis, and disorders of calcium, sodium, and potassium imbalance.

Information gained from perusing the web sites listed at the end of this chapter can provide valuable information on common endocrine disorders and a visual of the endocrine system.

Endocrine Glands and Their Functions

1. **Pituitary** – sometimes called the "master gland" be-cause of its influence on the other body organs. Two parts—anterior and posterior—comprise this gland.

   The *anterior* pituitary produces the following hor-mones:

   - Prolactin (PRL) stimulates milk production follow-ing childbirth and can affect sex hormone levels in both men and women.

   - Growth hormone (GH) stimulates growth in child-hood and assists in maintaining muscle and bone mass in adults.

   - Adrenocorticotropin (ACTH) stimulates production of cortisol (stress hormone) by the adrenal glands and helps to control both blood pressure and blood glucose levels.

   - Thyroid-stimulating hormone (TSH) stimulates the thyroid gland to make hormones that regulate body metabolism, energy, growth and development, and the activity of the nervous system.

   - Luteinizing hormone (LH) regulates production of estrogen in women and testosterone in men.

   - Follicle-stimulating hormone (FSH) promotes sperm production in men and stimulates the ovaries to release eggs in women.

   The *posterior* pituitary produces the following hormones:

   - Oxytocin causes milk letdown in nursing mothers and contractions during childbirth.

   - Antidiuretic hormone (ADH) regulates water bal-ance in the body, therefore affecting the kidneys.

2. **Adrenal** – comprised of two parts: The outer por-tion (*adrenal cortex*) that sits on top of each kidney and the inner portion (*adrenal medulla*). Hormones produced by the adrenal cortex are essential for life, whereas hormones secreted by the adrenal medulla are not essential.

   - The adrenal cortex generates glucocorticoids (such as cortisol) that help the body control blood sugar, boost the burning of fats and proteins, and react to stressors like major illness, injury, and fever. It also produces mineralocorticoids (such as aldosterone) that assist in controlling blood volume and regulat-ing blood pressure.

   - The adrenal medulla produces epinephrine (adrenaline), which is emitted by nerve endings and boosts the heart rate, improves blood flow to muscles, and opens airways to improve oxygen intake—usually when one is excited, under stress, and/or scared.

3. **Thyroid** – a small, butterfly-shaped gland inside the neck that is located in front of the trachea. Hormones produced by the thyroid control metabolism, which is the body's ability to break down food and store it as energy. In addition, it stimulates body heat production and bone growth. The thyroid produces both tri-iodothyronine (T_3) and thyroxine (T_4).

   Disorders of the thyroid can result from either underactive or overactive thyroid production, which means either too little or too much thyroid hormone is being produced. When the thyroid produces too much hormone, the resulting condition is *hyperthyroidism*. This can result from the development of Graves disease. Symptoms may include weight loss, anxiety, rapid heart rate, or diarrhea. When too little hormone is produced, the condition is known as *hypothyroidism*. This can cause lack of energy, slow heart rate, dry skin, constipation, and feeling cold all the time. In adults, hypothyroidism can cause weight gain and the possible development of a goiter.

4. **Parathyroid** – comprised of four tiny glands located in the neck that produce a hormone called parathor-mone (or parathyrin); most commonly just called parathyroid hormone. This hormone regulates calcium and phosphorus metabolism.

5. **Pineal** – located near the center of the brain, the pineal gland is believed to secrete melatonin, which may affect the body's sleep-regulating apparatus.

6. **Hypothalamus** – part of the brain that is located just above the pituitary gland. The function of this gland is to tell the pituitary gland when to discharge the hormones that control body temperature, hunger, and thirst.

7. **Pancreas** – a large gland situated behind the stom-ach, between the spleen and the duodenum. Some cells in the pancreas secrete the hormone insulin that controls the use of glucose by the body. Additionally, it secretes glucagon and somatostatin into the bloodstream.

8. **Ovaries** – a pair of oval or almond-shaped glands lying on either side of the uterus, they produce eggs or "ova" as well as the female sex hormones estrogen and progesterone.

9. **Testes** – the male reproductive glands that produce sperm and sex hormones, such as testosterone.

Laboratory and Diagnostic Testing

Some routine tests ordered by an endocrinologist consist of the following:

catecholamines – Test performed on urine determines the amount of epinephrine and norepinephrine present. These adrenal hormones are increased by stress.

fasting blood sugar (FBS) – Test performed on blood to determine the level of sugar in the blood stream.

glucose tolerance test (GTT) – Test performed on blood done at specified intervals after a glucose challenge to diagnose diabetes mellitus.

Hb A$_{1C}$ test – Hemoglobin A$_{1C}$ test is done on blood and is used to diagnose diabetes mellitus.

radioactive iodine uptake – Test measures the ability of the thyroid gland to concentrate ingested iodine.

radioimmunoassay (RIA) – Used in the clinical laboratory to measure hormone levels, for therapeutic drug monitoring, and in substance abuse screening.

thyroid scan – Test to detect tumors and functional status of nodules of the thyroid gland. The patient is given radioactive iodine, which localizes in the thyroid gland. It is then visualized with a scanner device.

total calcium – Test performed on blood serum to determine the amount of calcium present.

ultrasonography (US) – Use of high-frequency sound waves as either a screening test or a diagnostic test.

Supportive Web Sites

http://www.umm.edu/endocrin/	Contains good information about the glands in the endocrine system.
http://www.hormone.org/Public/ endocrinologist.cfm	Presents a definition of the endocrine system and a description of the role of endocrinologists.
http://www.endocrineweb.com/	Provides a list of common endocrine disorders; click on links to the disorders for more information.
http://www.emedicinehealth.com/anatomy_ of_the_endocrine_system/article_em.htm	Contains informative data on the endocrine system and includes a visual of the system.
http://www.endocrineweb.com/conditions	Contains a composite list of endocrine disorders.

Index of Endocrinology Reports

Exercise#	Patient Name	Type of Report/Procedure
TE#1	Cortez Tatum	Thyroid ultrasound
TE#2	Jody Gamble	FNA of left thyroid nodule
TE#3	Zachary Beckman	Consult (Letter): Intrauterine growth retardation
TE#4	Kathleen Modanski	HPIP Note: Euthyroid
TE#5	Andrew Julian Frost	SOAP Note: Low serum testosterone
TE#6	George M. Huda	SOAP Note: Hypogonadism
TE#7	Ruby Denmark	Radioactive iodine therapy
TE#8	Mrs. Tanya Mishenko	Correspondence regarding diabetes

CHAPTER 6
GASTROENTEROLOGY/ GASTRIC SURGERY

Introduction

Gastroenterology, a subspecialty of internal medicine, is the branch of medical science concerned with the study of the physiology and pathology of the *stomach, intestines,* and related structures such as the *esophagus, liver, gallbladder,* and *pancreas.* The liver, gallbladder, and pancreas contribute hormones, enzymes, and bile—all vital to digestion. These components make up the digestive system.

The main functions of the digestive system are the *digestion, absorption,* and *elimination* of food. These processes occur in the gastrointestinal tract, or alimentary canal, which is a tube approximately 30 feet long in adults; it begins at the mouth and ends at the anus.

When food is taken into the mouth, it travels through the pharynx into the esophagus. Next it goes into the stomach, where the digestive process begins. Gastric juices and hydrochloric acid break the food down into a semiliquid state (called *chyme*), and in this state the food passes into the small intestine in stages. The small intestine is composed of the *duodenum,* the *jejunum,* and the *ileum.* While in the small intestine, the food is mixed with bile from the liver and gallbladder and juice from the pancreas.

After nutrients have been absorbed by tiny capillaries and lymph vessels, the food passes into the large intestine where the digestive and absorption process continues.

Components of the large intestine are the *cecum;* ascending, transverse, descending, and sigmoid colon; the *rectum;* and the *anal canal.* The waste products of digestion are expelled from the body through the rectum and anus.

Physicians who treat diseases of the gastrointestinal tract are known as *gastroenterologists.* Among the procedures performed by gastroenterologists are *esophagogastroduodenoscopy* (EGD), *endoscopic biopsy, small-bowel biopsy, esophageal dilatations, esophageal* and *rectal manometry, laparoscopy, endoscopic retrograde cholangiopancreatography* (ERCP), and *endoscopic removal of foreign bodies.*

The following are some of the surgical procedures performed by *gastric surgeons:*

Abdominal wall reconstruction	Appendectomy
Endocrine surgery	Endoscopy
Gallbladder removal	Gastrointestinal surgery
Laparoscopic hernia repair	Islet cell transplantation
Laparoscopic liver resection	Laparoscopic pancreas resection
Therapeutic neck dissections	Thyroidectomy
Roux-en-Y Gastric bypass (RGB)	Laparoscopic sleeve gastrectomy
Whipple procedure	Gastric balloon

Critical Thinking Exercise

?

You are teaching a healthcare documentation specialty class and are asked if there are any prerequisites or conditions necessary before a patient undergoes gastric bypass surgery. How would you respond?

Gastroenterology/Gastric Surgery Abbreviations

The abbreviations, acronyms, and terms in the following abbreviations and terminology sections are often dictated in this specialty. We offer abbreviated definitions here. Please see an unabridged medical dictionary or the suggested web sites in this chapter for more information on each term.

a.c.	before meals		**BS**	bowel sounds, barium swallow, breath sounds
ACBE	air contrast barium enema		**Bx**	biopsy
A/G	albumin/globulin (ratio)		**CCK**	cholecystokinin
ALP/alk phos	alkaline phosphatase		**CEA**	carcinoembryonic antigen
ALT/ SGPT	alanine transaminase/serum glutamic pyruvic transaminase (enzyme tests of liver function)		**CHO**	carbohydrate
			chol	cholesterol
AMA	antimitochondrial antibody		**CPK**	creatine phosphokinase
ANA	antinuclear antibodies		**CRC**	colorectal cancer
AST/ SGOT	aspartic acid transaminase/serum glutamic oxaloacetic transaminase (enzyme tests of liver function)		**C&S**	culture and sensitivity
			CUC	chronic ulcerative colitis
Ba	barium		**E coli**	Escherichia coli
BE	barium enema		**EE**	erosive esophagitis, esophageal endoscopy
BMR	basic metabolic rate		**EGD**	esophagogastroduodenoscopy
BRBPR	bright red blood per (through) rectum		**ERCP**	endoscopic retrograde cholangiopancreatography

ESR	erythrocytic sedimentation rate
FBS	fasting blood sugar
FOBT	fecal occult blood test
GB	gallbladder
GERD	gastroesophageal reflux disease
GFR	glomerular filtration rate
GGT	gamma-glutamyl transpeptidase
GI	gastrointestinal
GTT	glucose tolerance test
HAV	hepatitis A virus, hepatitis A vaccine
HbA	hemoglobin adult
HbF	hemoglobin fetal
HbS	hemoglobin sickle cell
HBsAg	hepatitis B surface antigen
HBsAb	hepatitis B surface antibody
HBeAg	hepatitis Be antigen
HBeAb	hepatitis Be antibody
HBcAb	hepatitis B core antibody
HBIG	hepatitis B immune globulin
HBV	hepatitis B virus, hepatitis B vaccine
HCL	hydrochloric acid
HCV	hepatitis C virus, hepatitis C vaccine
H&H	hemoglobin and hematocrit
HH	hiatal hernia, hiatus hernia
IBD	inflammatory bowel disease
IBS	irritable bowel syndrome
KCl	potassium chloride
KVO	keep vein open
LDH	lactic dehydrogenase
LES	lower esophageal sphincter
LFTs	liver function tests—alk phos, bilirubin, AST (SGOT), ALT (SGPT)
MCV	mean clinical value or mean corpuscular volume
N&V	nausea and vomiting
NG	nasogastric (tube)
NH4	ammonia
n.p.o.	nothing by mouth (nil per os)
O&P	ova and parasites
OCG	oral cholecystography
OCP	ova, cysts, parasites
p.c.	after meals
PBC	primary biliary cirrhosis
PEG	percutaneous endoscopic gastrostomy
PKU	phenylketonuria
PND	paroxysmal nocturnal dyspnea
p.o.	by mouth (per os)
PP	postprandial (after meals)
PSC	primary sclerosing cholangitis
PT	prothrombin time or pro time
PTC	percutaneous transhepatic cholangiography
PTT	partial thromboplastin time
PUD	peptic ulcer disease
RDA	recommended dietary (daily) allowance
TPN	total parenteral nutrition
UGI	upper gastrointestinal
ZES	Zollinger-Ellison syndrome

Anatomic Illustrations

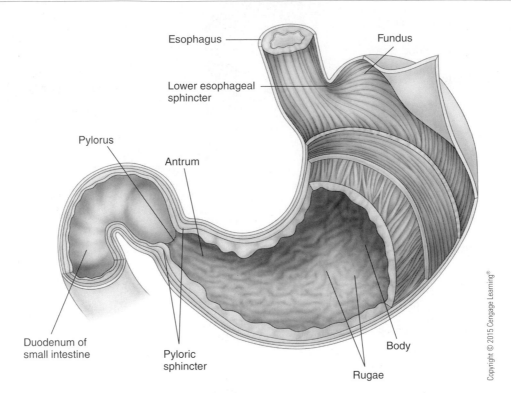

FIGURE 6-1   Structures of the stomach

Gastroenterology/Gastric Surgery Terminology

A

achalasia (ā"-kuh-lā'-zē-uh) – a failure to relax of the smooth muscle fibers of the gastrointestinal tract at any point of their junction of one part with another

achlorhydria (ā"-klōr-hī'-drē-uh) – absence of hydrochloric acid in the gastric juices

achylia (ā-kī'-lē-uh) – absence of gastric juices

adenomatous polyp (ad"-ē-nō'-muh-tus pahl'-ip) – a grape-shaped growth on the lining of the colon and rectum; can become cancerous

aerophagia (ā"-er-ō-fā'-jē-uh) – spasmodic swallowing of air followed by eructations

alimentary canal (āl"-ih-men'-tuh-rē) – the digestive tract

amebiasis (am"-ē-bī'-uh-sis) – the state of being infected with amebae

amylase (am'-ih-lāss) – one of the three digestive enzymes produced by the pancreas

amylasuria (am"-ih-lāss-yoo'-rē-uh) – an excess of amylase in the urine; a sign of pancreatitis

anal fissure (fish'ǝr) – a painful linear ulcer or tear at the margin of the anus

ancylostomiasis (an"-sih-lō-stō-mī'-uh-sis) – hookworm disease

anhidrosis (an"-hī-drō'-sis) – an abnormal deficiency of sweat

apepsinia (ā"-pep-sin'-ē-uh) – total absence or lack of secretion of pepsinogen by the stomach

aperistalsis (ā"-per-ih-stal'-sis) – absence of peristaltic action

appendix (uh-pen'-diks) – the worm-like appendage attached to the cecum (vermiform appendix)

ascites (uh-sī'-tēz) – an accumulation of fluid in the abdominal cavity

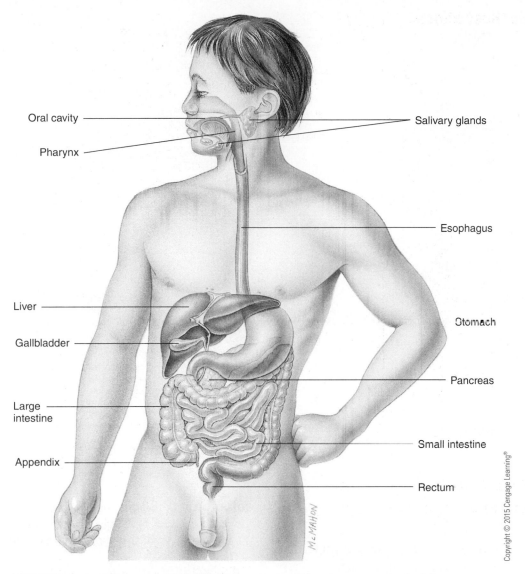

FIGURE 6-2   The gastrointestinal tract, or alimentary canal, and its accessory organs

B

bacteremia (bak-ter"-ē'-mē-uh) – the presence of bacteria in the blood

buccal (buk'əl) – pertaining to, adjacent to, or in the direction of the cheek

C

carcinoid (kar'-sih-noyd) – a yellow circumscribed tumor occurring in the small intestine, appendix, stomach, or colon

cardia (kar'-dē-uh) – the opening of the esophagus into the stomach

catecholamines (kat"-eh-kō'-luh-mēnz) – chemical substances secreted by the adrenal gland; major elements in responses to stress

celiac disease (se'le-ak) – a malabsorption syndrome including the inability to digest gluten-containing foods with diarrhea, weight loss, and electrolyte depletion

cholangiolitis (kō-lan"-jē-ō-lī'-tis) – inflammation of the cholangioles, the fine terminal elements of the bile duct system

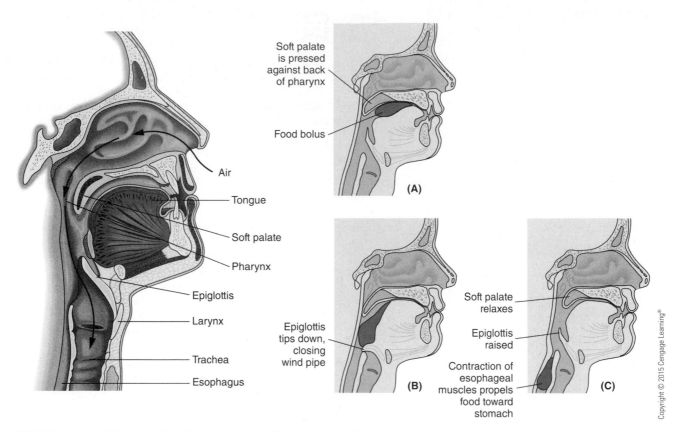

Soft palate
is pressed
against back
of pharynx

Food bolus

(A)

Air

Tongue

Soft palate

Pharynx

Epiglottis

Larynx

Trachea

Esophagus

Epiglottis
tips down,
closing
wind pipe

(B)

Soft palate
relaxes

Epiglottis
raised

Contraction of
esophageal
muscles propels
food toward
stomach

(C)

FIGURE 6-3   The swallowing sequence into the esophagus

cholangitis (ko"lan-ji'tis) – inflammation of the walls of the bile ducts

cholecystogastric (kō"-leh-sis"-tō-gas'-trik) – referring to the gallbladder and stomach

choledocholithotomy (kō-led"-ō-kō-lih-thot'-uh-mē) – incision of the common bile duct for the removal of a stone or stones

choledochoplasty (kō-led"-ō-kō-plass'-tē) – rearrangement of tissues of the common bile duct

cholemia (kō-lē'-mē-uh) – the occurrence of bile or bile pigment in the blood

cholestasis (kō"-leh-stā'-sis) – stoppage or suppression of the flow of bile

cholesterosis (kō-les"-ter-ō'-sis) – a condition in which cholesterol is deposited in tissues in abnormal quantities

chyme (kīm) – the mixture of gastric juices with food

colon – segment of the large intestine that extends from the cecum to the rectum

colostomy (kuh-lahss'-tuh-mē) – surgical procedure that creates an opening from the colon through the abdominal wall; this allows waste products to move out of the body

Crohn disease (krōn) – regional enteritis; inflammation of the small intestine

Cruveilhier-Baumgarten syndrome (kroo-vāl-yā'-bom'-gar-ten) – cirrhosis of the liver with portal hypertension, associated with congenital patency of the umbilical or paraumbilical veins

cystadenocarcinoma (sis-tad"-eh-nō-kar"-sih-nō'-muh) – adenocarcinoma characterized by tumor-lined cystic cavities occurring usually in the ovaries

defecation (def"-eh-kā'-shun) – the passage of stool

deglutition (dē"-gloo-tih'-shun) – swallowing

dehydrogenase (dē-hī"-drah'-jen-āz) – an enzyme

diverticulitis (di"vər-tik"u-li'tis) – inflammation of diverticula, which are tiny pockets or pouches in the lining of the bowel

diverticulosis (di"vər-tik"u-lo'sis) – presence of a number of diverticula in the intestine, common in middle age

diverticulum (dī"-ver-tik'-yoo-lum) – singular noun, a pouch opening from a tubular organ, such as the esophagus or intestine; plural diverticula

duodenoileostomy (doo"-ō-dē'-nō-il"-ē-ahs'-tuh-mē) – surgical formation of a new communication between the duodenum and ileum

duodenojejunostomy (doo"-ō-dēh'-nō-jeh"-joo-nahs'-tuh-mē) – surgical formation of a new communication between the duodenum and jejunum

duodenum (doo"-ō-dē'-num OR doo-ahd'-eh-num) – the first part of the small intestine

dysentery (dis'-en-ter"-ē) – an intestinal disease characterized by inflammation of the mucous membrane

dyspepsia (dis-pep'-sē-uh) – indigestion

emesis (em'-eh-sis) – vomiting

enzyme (en'-zīm) – a macromolecule that acts as a catalyst to induce chemical changes in other substances, while itself remaining unchanged

eructation (ē-ruk-tā'-shun) – the act of belching

esophagoscope (ē-sof'-uh-gō-skōp) – an endoscope for internal examination of the esophagus

fecal impaction (fē'-kul ī-pak'-shun) – feces firmly lodged in the colon or rectum

fecalith (fe'-kah-lth) – a fecal concretion

fundoplication (fun"-dō-plih-kā'-shun) – surgically wrapping the fundus of the stomach around the lower end of the esophagus to relieve reflux esophagitis; also called fundic wrapping

galactosemia (guh-lak"-tō-sē'-mē-uh) – a hereditary disorder of galactose metabolism

gastrectomy (gas-trek'-tuh-mē) – surgical excision of all or part of the stomach

gastrojejunostomy (gas"-trō-jē-joo-nahs'-tuh-mē) – surgical creation of an anastomosis between the stomach and jejunum

gastroparesis (gas"tro-pə-re'sis) – paralysis of the stomach, usually from damage to its nerve supply

gastrorrhea (gas"-trō-rē'-uh) – excessive secretion of mucus or gastric juices in the stomach

gastrosuccorrhea (gas"-trō-suk"-ō-rē'-uh) – excessive and continuous secretion of gastric juices

Given™ diagnostic imaging system – diagnostic technique that uses an imaging capsule to examine the small bowel; the capsule is swallowed by the patient

hemochromatosis (hē"-mō-krō"-muh-tō'-sis) – an excess of iron absorption and the presence of iron-containing deposits in the liver, pancreas, kidneys, adrenals, and heart

hemorrhoid (hem'-uh-royd) – a large varicose vein within the rectum or anus

hepatitis (hep"ə-ti'tis) – inflammation of the liver; there are many types including, but not limited to, hepatitis A, B, C, D, and E

hepatomalacia (hep"-uh-tō-muh-lā'-shē-uh) – softening of the liver

hepatomegaly (hep"-uh-tō-meg'-uh-lē) – enlargement of the liver

hepatorrhea (hep"-uh-tō-rē'-uh) – a morbidly excessive secretion of bile; any morbid flow from the liver

hiatal hernia (hī-ā'-tul her'-nē-uh) – produced when the esophageal hiatus weakens and stretches so that part of the stomach and/or esophagus intrudes into the chest cavity; hiatus hernia is sometimes dictated, which is equally acceptable

hiatus (hi-a'təs) – a gap, cleft, or opening

Hirschsprung disease (hersh'-sprung) – excessive enlargement of the colon associated with an absence of ganglion cells in the narrowed bowel wall distally

hyperalimentation (hī"-per-al"-ih-men-tā'-shun) – often dictated "hyper al," this refers to the ingestion of excessive quantities, as in bulimia and binge eating

hyperinsulinism (hī"-per-in'-suh-lin-izm") – excessive secretion of insulin by the pancreas, resulting in hypoglycemia; insulin shock

hypochlorhydria (hī"-pō-klōr-hī'-drē-uh) – deficiency of hydrochloric acid in the gastric juice

icterus (ik'-ter-us) – jaundice

ileitis (il"-ē-ī'-tis) – inflammation of the ileum

ileocolitis (il"-ē-ō-kō-lī'-tis) – inflammation of the ileum and colon

jaundice (jawn'dis) – a yellow appearance of the skin, mucous membranes, and sclerae; also called icterus

jejunum (jē-joo'-num) – the second part of the small intestine

kalemia (kah-lē'-mē-uh) – the presence of potassium in the blood

Laennec cirrhosis (lā"-en-nek sih-rō'-sis) – cirrhosis of the liver closely associated with chronic, excessive alcohol ingestion

leukocytosis (loo"-kō-sī-tō'-sis) – an increase in the number of leukocytes in the blood, resulting from various causes

leukopenia (loo"-kō-pē'-nē-uh) – reduction in the number of leukocytes in the blood

lingua (ling'-gwuh) – the tongue

lipase (lip'-āz OR lī'-pāz) – one of the three digestive enzymes produced by the pancreas

lipomatosis (lip"-ō-muh-tō'-sis) – a condition characterized by abnormal localized or tumor-like accumulations of fat in the tissues

lymphangioma (lim-fan"-jē-ō'-muh) – a tumor composed of newly formed lymph spaces and channels

M2A Swallowable Imaging Capsule™ (swal'-ō-uh-bul) – a capsule containing a camera; after the patient swallows it (like a regular pill), the camera transmits images of the GI tract to an external device worn on a belt

maduromycosis (mad-yoor"-ō-mī-kō'-sis) – a chronic infection caused by a variety of fungi affecting the skin, subcutaneous tissue, and bone (syn. mycetoma)

mastication (mas"-tih-kā'-shun) – the act of chewing

megacolon (meg"-uh-kō'-lun) – abnormally large or dilated colon

mononucleosis (mon"-ō-noo"-klē-ō'-sis) – the presence of an abnormally large number of mononuclear leukocytes in the circulating blood

oxyuriasis (ok"-sē-yoo-rī'-uh-sis) – pinworm

pancreatitis (pan"kre-ə-ti'tis) – inflammation of the pancreas, which may be acute or chronic

paralytic ileus (pār"-uh-lit'-ik il'-ē-us) – paralysis of the intestines that causes distention and symptoms of acute obstruction and prostration

parenteral (puh-ren'-ter-ul) – outside the alimentary tract

pellagra (peh-lag'-ruh) – skin lesions, mental and nervous disorders that may be caused by a poor diet or alcoholism or some other disease-impairing nutrition

peptic ulcer (pep'tik) – an ulcer of the mucous membrane of the alimentary tract caused by action of acidic gastric juice

peristalsis (pār"-ih-stahl'-sis) – the rhythmic-like contractions of the tubes of the alimentary tract and other tubular structures

peritonitis (pār"-ih-tō-nī'-tis) – inflammation of the peritoneum

polyposis (pol"-ē-pō'-sis) – presence of several polyps

postprandial (post-pran'-dē-ul) – occurring after dinner or after a meal

primary biliary cirrhosis (bil'e-ar-e sĭ-ro'sis) – a disease of the bile ducts inside the liver whereby chronic inflammation causes scaring that eventually blocks and destroys the bile ducts

primary sclerosing cholangitis (sklə-rōs'ing ko"lan-ji'tis) – a disease primarily of the bile ducts, both inside and outside the liver where inflammation causes scarring and hardening that narrows the bile ducts

psychogenic (sī"-kō-jen'-ik) – having an emotional or psychologic origin

ptyalocele (tī-al'-ō-sēl) – cystic tumor of a salivary gland

pylorectomy (pī"-lōr-ek'-tuh-mē) – excision of the pylorus

pyloric sphincter (pī-lōr'-ik sfingk'-ter) – the ring of muscle at the distal region of the stomach

pyloroplasty (pī-lōr'-ō-plas"-te) – a surgical procedure to relieve pyloric obstruction or to accelerate gastric emptying

pyrosis (pī-rō'-sis) – heartburn

rugae (roo'-jē) – folds, ridges, creases, or wrinkles (singular ruga, pronounced with a hard "g")

salivary gland (sal'-ih-vār-ē) – a gland that secretes saliva

sialaden (sī-al'-ah-den) – a salivary gland

sialoadenectomy (sī"-ul-ō-ad"-ē-nek'-tuh-mē) – surgical excision of a salivary gland

sialozemia (sī"-ul-ō-zē'-mē-uh) – involuntary flow of saliva

sideropenia (sid"-er-ō-pē'-nē-uh) – iron deficiency

sigmoid colon (sig'-moyd) – the S-shaped segment of the colon between the descending colon and the rectum

singultus (sing-gul'-tus) – hiccup(s); this spelling is correct in both singular and plural usage

Stretta procedure (streh'-tuh) – outpatient, non-surgical procedure for treatment of gastroesophageal reflux disease; uses electrosurgical coagulation

toxicosis (tok"-sih-kō'-sis) – any disease condition due to poisoning

trypsin (trip'-sin) – one of the three digestive enzymes produced by the pancreas

ulcerative colitis (ul'-ser-ā"-tiv kō -lī'-tis) – an inflammatory process of the inner lining of the large intestine

uvula (yoo'-vyoo-luh) – the small fleshy mass hanging from the soft palate

volvulus (vol'-vyoo-lus) – intestinal obstruction due to a knotting and twisting of the bowel

Transcription Tips

You will find transcription in gastroenterology/gastric surgery easier if you are familiar with the names of the organs of the digestive system, can locate them on a chart, and can describe their functions. Knowledge of the digestive hormones and enzymes, confusing terms, roots and combining forms, and diagnostic and laboratory tests also make the transcription process easier.

Organs of the Digestive System

The digestive system is composed of the mouth, pharynx, esophagus, stomach, and intestines. The accessory organs include the teeth, salivary glands, liver, gallbladder, and pancreas.

  The gastrointestinal tract, or alimentary canal, has three functions: (1) the digestion of food, (2) the absorption of food, and (3) the excretion of the waste products of digestion from the large intestine.

Digestive Hormones

cholecystokinin

gastric inhibitory peptide

gastrin

insulin

pancreozymin

secretin

vasoactive intestinal polypeptide

villikinin

Digestive Enzymes

bile

gastric juice

intestinal juice

pancreatic juice

saliva

Diagnostic and Laboratory Testing

toxicology – test performed on blood serum or plasma to calculate levels of alcohol or drugs

ammonia – test conducted on plasma to determine the level of ammonia

barium enema – test performed by administering barium through the rectum and viewing via x-ray to ascertain the condition of the colon

bilirubin blood test – test performed on blood serum to determine the level of bilirubin in the blood

carcinoembryonic antigen (CEA) – test done on whole blood or plasma to discover the presence

of antigens originally segregated from colon tumors

cholangiography – x-ray examination of the common bile duct, cystic duct, and hepatic ducts to assess presence of obstruction, stones, and/or tumors

cholecystography – x-ray examination of the gallbladder

colonoscopy – test performed using a colonoscope to view the colon; a fiberoptic colonoscopy

endoscopic retrograde cholangiopancreatography (ERCP) – x-ray exam of the biliary and pancreatic ducts to assess presence of such things as cysts, stones, fibrosis, or pancreatitis; uses a flexible endoscope to inject contrast into the biliary and/or pancreatic ducts in order to take x-rays

esophagogastroduodenoscopy (EGD) – an endoscopic exam of the esophagus, stomach, and small intestine

fecal occult blood test (FOBT) – test for detection of blood in the stool

gamma-glutamyl tranferase (GGT) – test conducted on blood serum to determine the level of GGT, an enzyme found in the liver, kidney, prostate, heart, and spleen

gastric analysis – test performed to assess quality of secretion, amount of free and combined HCl, and absence or presence of blood, bacteria, bile, and fatty acids

gastrointestinal (GI) series – fluoroscopic examination (following ingestion of barium) of the esophagus, stomach, and small intestine

Hemoccult test – a qualitative assay test that detects heme (the iron-containing portion of hemoglobin) in the stool

liver biopsy – surgical procedure performed to obtain a sample of liver tissue for pathologic examination and diagnosis

occult blood – test done on feces to determine GI bleeding that is invisible to the human eye

ova and parasites (O&P) – test conducted on stool to identify ova and parasites

stool culture – test done on stool in microbiology (a culture) to determine the presence of bacterial organisms

ultrasonography, gallbladder – a test performed to image the gallbladder by using high-frequency sound waves

ultrasonography, liver – test done to image the liver by using high-frequency sound waves

Supportive Web Sites

http://gicare.com/Diseases/diseaseinner.aspx	This site lists diseases of the gastrointestinal tract.
http://www.acg.gi.org/	Under "Patient Information," click on "Common GI Problems."
http://www.gastro.com	In the introductory paragraph, click on the "gastroenterology," "liver disease," and " endoscopes" links for helpful information.
http://www.gastromd.com	Click on "Medications and Prescriptions," "Liver Function Tests," "Radiographic Studies."
http://www.mayoclinic.com	Click on the "Diseases and Conditions" link and then on related gastroenterology links; search on the home page for "gastroenterology."
http://www.medmark.org	Click on "Gastroenterology" and items of interest under the "For Consumers" link.
http://www.mtdesk.com	Click on "WORD LISTS (by specialty)," then on "Digestive/Gastroenterology terms."
http://www.my.webmd.com	Click on the "Diseases and Conditions" link and then select links of interest; search for gastroenterology or specific conditions.

Index of Gastroenterology/Gastric Surgery Reports

Exercise#	Patient Name	Type of Report/Procedure
TE#1	Barbara C. Anello	Esophagogastroduodenoscopy (EGD) Report
TE#2	Doris Dean Richards	Colonoscopy Procedure Report
TE#3	Patrick O'Donnell	Followup Letter—Dysphagia
TE#4	Frances Southington	CT abdomen/pelvis with contrast
TE#5	Henry Chin	Abdominal surgical report: Aneurysm
TE#6	Julianne Pontillo	Letter—Ulcerative colitis, on steroids
TE#7	Connie Roseberry	Laparoscopic Nissen fundoplication
TE#8	Beverly T. O'Neal	Bravo Catheter-free pH study
TE#9	Keith A. Yuen	Colonoscopy with anoscopy and polypectomy
TE#10	Ryan Fletcher	Esophageal stricture, EGD
TE#11	Angela Dale Bullock	EGD with TTS balloon dilatation
TE#12	Anderson Lowery	Lap cholecystectomy w/cholangiogram

CHAPTER 7
HEMATOLOGY/ONCOLOGY

Introduction

Hematology means the study of the blood or hematopoietic system in humans, which consists of several interconnected components: the peripheral blood, the bone marrow, and the lymph nodes. The circulating blood, consisting of some five liters in a man (almost 10 percent less in a woman) comprises a fluid component (the *plasma*) and makes up some 55 percent of total blood volume. The plasma contains the three basic cell types: *erythrocytes* (red cells), *leukocytes* (white cells), and *thrombocytes* (platelets).

The *erythrocytes* are largely concerned with oxygen transport; the *leukocytes* play various parts in defense against infection and tissue injury; and the *thrombocytes* are involved in maintaining the integrity of blood vessels and the prevention of blood loss by helping the blood to clot.

An abnormal condition of blood is called blood *dyscrasia* or disease. Diseases of red and white blood cells, bone marrow, and disorders of blood clotting are examples of blood dyscrasias. *Anemia, hemochromatosis,* and *polycythemia vera* are diseases of red blood cells. Diseases of white blood cells include *leukemia* and *granulocytosis.* Two disorders of blood clotting are *hemophilia* and *purpura.*

Lymph, the other main fluid in the body, does not circulate as does the blood. Lymph travels in one direction through lymph vessels, which drain into large veins of the circulatory system situated in the neck region. Although lymph does not contain erythrocytes or platelets, it does contain *lymphocytes* and *monocytes.*

Lymph capillaries, lymphatic vessels, lymphatic ducts, and lymph nodes form the lymphatic system. This system serves as a drainage medium to transport needed proteins and fluid that have leaked out of the blood capillaries back to the bloodstream via the veins. In addition, the lymphatic vessels absorb *lipids* (fats) from the small intestine and carry them to the bloodstream. The lymphatic system also assists the immune system in protecting the body by producing antibodies or by engulfing and destroying foreign matter.

Though they are not specific parts of the lymphatic system, the *spleen, faucial tonsils,* and *thymus* are closely related to it by virtue of the functions they perform in the body. Of particular importance is the thymus, which manufactures infection-fighting *T cells.* These cells play a very important role in the body's immune response. T-cell lymphocytes also form in stem cells in the bone marrow.

A practicing hematologist spends a great deal of time treating patients suffering from blood malignancies. One of the most common forms of blood tumor is lymph-node cancer (*Hodgkin disease* and *non-Hodgkin lymphoma*).

Oncology is a word derived from the Greek *onchos,* meaning a lump or tumor. *Oncology* is the study of cancer. An *oncologist* is a physician who specializes in the diagnosis and treatment of cancer.

Cancer is a proliferation of cells that grow in an uncontrolled manner, invading local tissues and spreading widely through the blood or lymphatics to produce secondary deposits, or *metastases,* in distant parts of the body. The cells composing the tumor reproduce faster than normal cells. More than 200 different types of cancer have been identified; however, these different types can be divided into three main groups based on the tissue from which the tumor cells originate—carcinomas, sarcomas, and mixed-tissue tumors.

Carcinomas comprise the largest group and are malignant tumors that arise from the epithelial tissues that line internal and external body surfaces. For example, lung carcinoma arises from the epithelium lining the main airways, or bronchi; breast carcinoma develops from the ductal tissue in the breast; stomach and colon carcinomas originate from their epithelial linings.

Sarcomas develop from supportive and connective tissue such as cartilage, bone, muscle, fat, and bone marrow, as well as from cells of the lymph system. Another word for bone sarcomas is osteosarcomas; fat sarcomas are called liposarcomas. Sarcomas are commonly seen in children and spread via the bloodstream, whereas carcinomas are more commonly seen in adults and usually spread via the lymphatics.

Mixed-tissue tumors originate in tissue that can separate into both epithelial and connective tissue. When cancer occurs simultaneously in adjacent tissue types, it is known as a mixed-tissue tumor.

The method of classifying tumors involves establishing the tumor's *grade* (degree of maturity) and its *stage* (extent of metastasis) within the body. The aggressiveness of tumor malignancy is classified using the Broders index on a scale of 1 to 4. A *grade 1* tumor indicates the most differentiation and best prognosis, whereas a *grade 4* indicates the least differentiation and poorest prognosis. Other classification systems are used to describe malignancies in different parts of the body; for example, Dukes A, B, and C are used to classify the extent of operable adenocarcinoma of the colon or rectum, and FIGO stages describe gynecologic malignancies, particularly carcinomas of the ovary. FIGO stages are expressed using roman numerals.

Although the evolution of a normal cell into a cancerous one is not understood fully, the genetic material deoxyribonucleic acid (DNA) of the cell holds the key. DNA contains genes (codes) that direct the production of new cells. During cell division, DNA replicates itself to pass the same genetic material to two new cells. This process is called *mitosis.* Sometimes during mitosis the process is disrupted because the DNA stops making the codes that allow cells to function normally. Instead, the cells begin to make new signals that cause them to move and invade adjacent tissue and *metastasize* or spread. These are malignant cells. As these malignant cells reproduce, the *mutations* (cell changes) are passed on to the new cells, and the process is replicated over and over, leading to malignant growths.

Chemicals, drugs, radiation, and some viruses can cause DNA changes that lead to cancer. Heredity can also predispose a person to certain types of cancer. Although cancer occurs frequently in the elderly, it can occur at any age and can affect any body tissue.

Each type of cancer requires a specific type of therapy. The four basic methods used to treat cancer are chemotherapy, surgery, radiation therapy, and biological therapy. At times a combination of these methods is used for the most effective treatment plan.

Chemotherapy employs drugs to treat cancer. Chemotherapeutic agents fall into five classifications: alkylating agents, antibiotics, antimetabolites, plant derivatives, and steroids. *Surgery* removes the cancerous tissue from the body through excision. *Radiation therapy* involves the use of radiation to the tumor tissue; high doses damage DNA. *Biological therapy* uses the body's own immune system to fight tumor cells.

As cancer research continues to be aggressively pursued, new treatment methods continue to emerge. Research and development being done all over the world plays the most important role in finding new drugs and treatment methods to not only help treat cancer but also to ultimately find a cure for it.

Critical Thinking Exercise

?

Dictation reads "A 57-year-old male presents with worsening cough, no fever. CT scan, fine-needle biopsy, and PET scan reveal SCC, T3N2M0." Can these abbreviations be transcribed if dictated? What do they mean?

Hematology/Oncology Abbreviations

The abbreviations, acronyms, and terms in the following abbreviations and terminology sections are often dictated in this specialty. We offer abbreviated definitions here.

Please see an unabridged medical dictionary or the suggested web sites in this chapter for more information on each term.

adeno-CA	adenocarcinoma
AHF	antihemophilic factor
ALL	acute lymphocytic leukemia
AML	acute myelogenous leukemia
AVM	arteriovenous malformation
BAC	blood-alcohol concentration
baso	basophils
BL	Burkitt lymphoma
BMT	bone-marrow transplant
CA	cancer or carcinoma
CEA	carcinoembryonic antigen
CFS	chronic fatigue syndrome
chemo	chemotherapy
CLL	chronic lymphocytic leukemia
CMF	cytoxan, methotrexate, 5-fluorouracil (combination chemotherapy)
CML	chronic myelogenous (myelocytic) leukemia
CMV	cytomegalovirus
CR	complete response
DES	diethylstilbestrol
Diff	differential (count)
DNA	deoxyribonucleic acid
eos	eosinophil(s)
ER	estrogen receptors
ESR	erythrocyte sedimentation rate
Ga	Gallium
Hct	hematocrit
HD	Hodgkin disease
Hgb, Hg	hemoglobin

Hp	haptoglobin
HTLV	human T-cell leukemia-lymphoma virus
IgA, IgD	immunoglobulin A, immunoglobulin D
IgE, IgG	immunoglobulin E, immunoglobulin G
IgM	immunoglobulin M
IL-2	interleukin-2
LAK	lymphokine-activated killer (cells)
LGV	lymphogranuloma venereum
lymphs	lymphocytes
MCH	mean corpuscular hemoglobin—average amount of hemoglobin per cell
MCHC	mean corpuscular hemoglobin concentration—average concentration of hemoglobin in a single red cell
MCL	mantle cell lymphoma
MCV	mean corpuscular volume—average volume or size of a single red blood cell
mets	metastasis/metastases
NED	no evidence of disease
NHL	non-Hodgkin lymphoma
NSCLC	non-small-cell lung cancer
PCV	packed cell volume
PMN, PMNL	polymorphonuclear neutrophil
poly	polymorphonuclear leukocyte
PR	partial remission
prot.	protocol
PSA	prostate-specific antigen
PT, pro time	prothrombin time
PTT	partial thromboplastin time

R&D	research and development
Rh	Rhesus (factor)
RIA	radioimmunoassay
RNA	ribonucleic acid
sed rate	erythrocyte sedimentation rate
segs	segmented, mature white blood cells
TNF	tumor necrosis factor
TNM	tumor, node, metastasis
VIP	vasoactive intestinal peptides
WBRT	whole-brain radiation therapy
XRT	radiation therapy
YSC	yolk sac carcinoma

Anatomic Illustrations

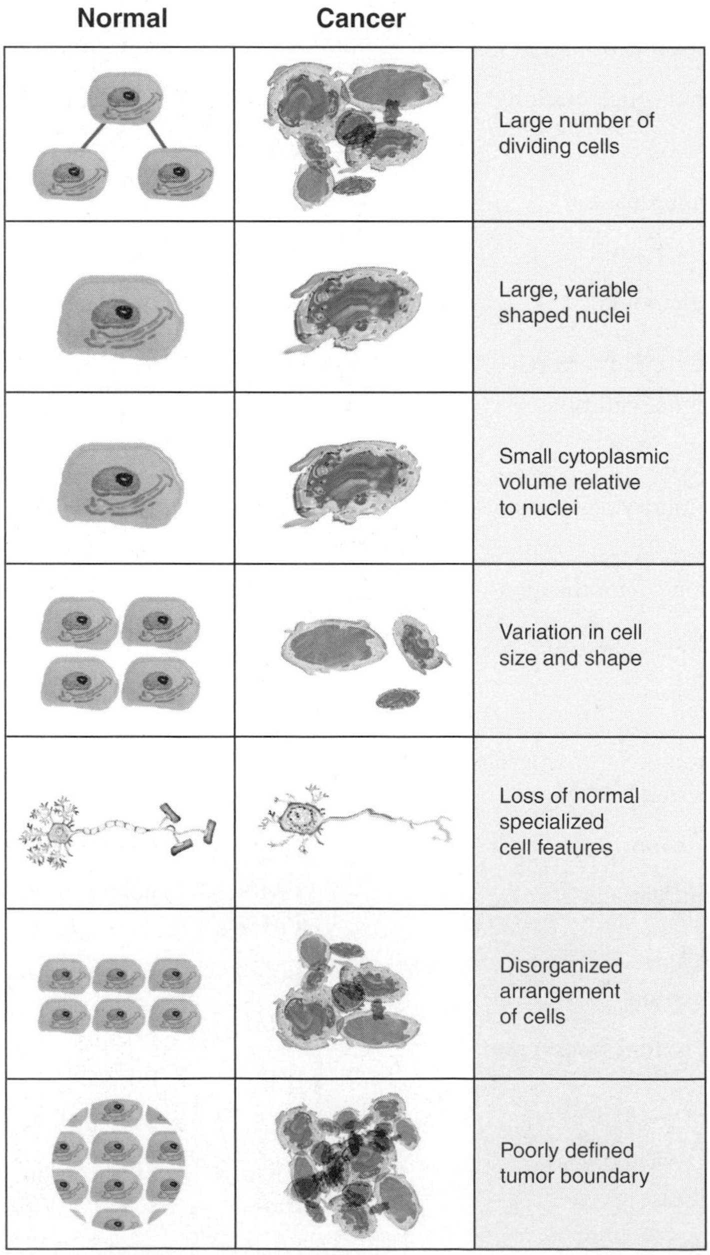

Courtesy of National Cancer Society

Figure 7-1 Comparison of normal cells to cancerous cells

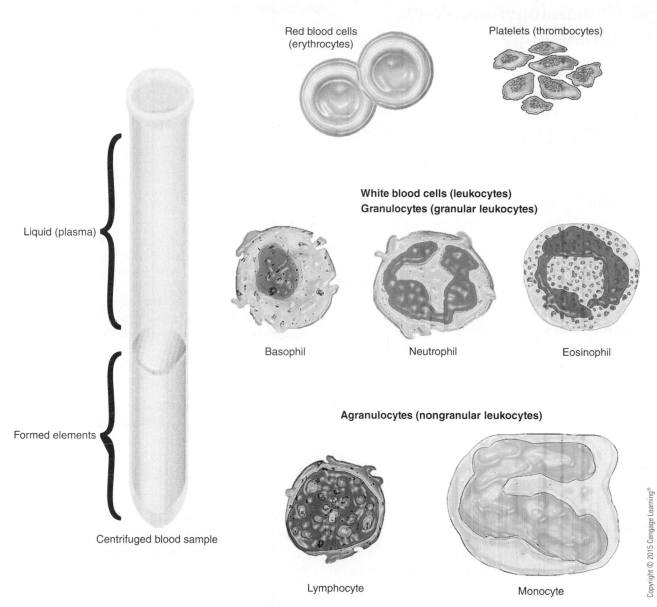

Red blood cells
(erythrocytes)

Platelets (thrombocytes)

Liquid (plasma)

White blood cells (leukocytes)
Granulocytes (granular leukocytes)

Basophil

Neutrophil

Eosinophil

Formed elements

Agranulocytes (nongranular leukocytes)

Lymphocyte

Monocyte

Centrifuged blood sample

Figure 7-2 Cellular elements of the blood

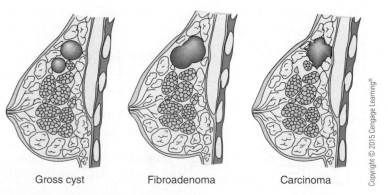

Gross cyst

Fibroadenoma

Carcinoma

Figure 7-3 Characteristics of common breast masses

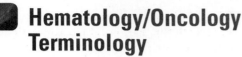

Hematology/Oncology Terminology

adenoacanthoma (ah-de"-nō-ak"-an-thō'-muh) – an adenocarcinoma in which some of the cells exhibit squamous differentiation

adenocarcinoma (ah-dē"-nō-kar"-sih-nō'-muh) – a malignant new growth derived from glandular tissue or in which the tumor cells form recognizable glandular structures

adenomyosarcoma (ah-dē"-nō-mī"-ō-sar-kō'-muh) – a mixed mesodermal tumor in which striated muscle cells are one component

adjuvant therapy (ad'-joo-vent) – the use of drugs (chemotherapy) along with surgery or radiation to attack cancer cells

agglutination (uh-gloo"-tih-nā'-shun) – the clumping of blood when incompatible blood types are mixed; this is fatal to the recipient because it stops the flow of blood

albumin (serum albumin) (al-byoo'-min) – a protein found in blood that maintains the proper amount of water in the blood

alkylating agent (al'-kih-lāt"-ing) – a synthetic compound that disrupts the process of DNA synthesis

anemia (uh-nē'-mē-uh) – a deficiency in erythrocytes or hemoglobin; there are many types of anemia, including familial, hemolytic, microcytic, pernicious, sickle cell, and target cell anemia

amelanotic melanoma (ā"-mel-uh-not'-ik mel"-uh-nō'-muh) – an unpigmented malignant melanoma

ameloblastoma (uh-mel"-ō-blas-tō'-muh) – a tumor of the jaw arising from enamel-forming cells

antihemorrhagic (an"-tī-hēm"-ō-raj'-ik) – preventing or stopping hemorrhage

antimetabolites (an"-tī-meh-tab'-uh-lītz) – drugs used in cancer chemotherapy that block the formation of substances necessary to make DNA

apheresis (af"-er-ē'-sis) – a procedure in which blood is separated into its parts

aplastic anemia (ā-plass'-tik uh-nē'-mē-uh) – characterized by a lack of formation of bone marrow cells

apoptosis (ap"-op-tō'-sis) – disintegration of cells into membrane-bound particles that are then ingested by other cells; process may be important in limiting growth of tumors

astrocytoma (ass"-trō-sī-tō'-muh) – a tumor composed of astrocytes

basophil (ba'-zō-fil) – a type of white blood cell containing coarse granules that stain readily with basic dyes

basosquamous carcinoma (bā'-zōo skwā'-mus kar"-sih-nō'-muh) – carcinoma that histologically exhibits both basal and squamous elements

Brenner tumor (bren'-er) – a benign fibroepithelioma of the ovary

bronchogenic carcinoma (brong-kō-jen'-ik) – carcinoma originating in the bronchus

cancer (kan(t)-sər) – a group of neoplastic diseases in which there is a transformation of normal cells into malignant cells where they proliferate in an abnormal way resulting in a malignant, cellular tumor

carcinoid (kar'-sih-noyd) – a yellow circumscribed tumor occurring in the small intestine, appendix, stomach, or colon

carcinoma in situ (kar-sih-nōh'-mah in-'sī-tü) – a condition in which the tumor cells of a neoplastic entity still lie within the epithelium of origin, without invasion of the basement membrane

carcinosarcoma (kar"-sih-nō-sar-kō'-muh) – a malignant tumor composed of both carcinomatous and sarcomatous tissues

cellular oncogenes (ong'-kō-jēnz) – broken or dislocated pieces of human DNA

chondroblastoma (kahn"-drō-blas-tō'-muh) – a benign neoplasm in which the cells resemble cartilage cells, and the tumor appears to be cartilage

chondrosarcoma (kahn"-drō-sar-kō'-muh) – a malignant tumor derived from cartilage cells or their precursors

chordoma (kor-dō'-muh) – a rare tumor that occurs any place along the vertebral column

choriocarcinoma (ko"-rē-ō-kar"-sih-nō'-muh) – an extremely rare, malignant neoplasm, usually of the uterus but sometimes at the site of an ectopic pregnancy

chronic myelogenous leukemia (mī"-eh-lah'-jeh-nus loo-kē-'mē-uh) – a malignant cancer of the bone marrow

creatinemia (krē"-ah-tih-nē'-mē-uh) – an excess of creatine in circulating blood

cryosurgery (krī"-ō-sur'-jer-ē) – procedure that uses cold to freeze and destroy cancerous tissue, often used to treat brain and bladder tumors

cystosarcoma (sis"-tō-sahr"-kō'-muh) – a sarcoma in which cysts have formed

cystosarcoma phyllodes (sis"to-sahr-ko'mə fəl-o'dēz) – infiltrating fibroadenomatous tumor that may be either benign or malignant, partly cystic, of the breast, prostate, or other organs

dermatofibrosarcoma protuberans (der"-muh-tō-fī"-brō-sahr-kō'-muh prō-too'-ber-enz) – a fibrosarcoma of the skin

dysgerminoma (dis"-jer-mih-nō'-muh) – a malignant neoplasm of the ovary

electrophoresis (ē-lek"-trō-fō-rē'-sis) – the method of separating substances by electrical charge

en bloc resection (awn blahk' rē-sek'-shun) – process whereby a malignant tumor is removed in a lump or whole, sometimes along with a large area of surrounding tissue and/or lymph nodes

eosinophil (ē"-ō-sin'-ō-fil) – a granular leukocyte that stains readily with the acid stain eosin

ependymoma (eh-pen"-dī-mō'-muh) – a tumor arising from fetal inclusion of ependymal elements

epidermoid carcinoma (ep"-ih-der'-moyd) – carcinoma in which the cells tend to differentiate in the same way that the cells of the epidermis do

epithelioma (ep"-ih-thē"-lē-ō'-muh) – a malignant tumor, consisting mainly of epithelial cells, that originates in the epidermis of the skin or in a mucous membrane

erythroblast (ē-rith'-rō-blast) – an immature red blood cell

erythrocytosis (ē-rith"-rō-sī-tō'-sis) – an abnormal condition in which there is an increase in red blood cells

erythropathy (er"-ih-throp'-uh-thē) – disease of the red blood cells

erythropenia (ē-rith"-rō-pē'-nē-uh) – deficiency in the number of red blood cells

erythropoiesis (ē-rith"-rō-poy-ē'-sis) – the formation of red blood cells

erythropoietin (ē-rith"-rō-poy'-eh-tin) – hormone secreted by the kidney that stimulates production of erythrocytes

Ewing sarcoma (yoo'-ing sar-kō'-muh) – a malignant tumor of the bone that arises in medullary tissue, occurring more often in cylindrical bones; pain, fever, and leukocytosis are prominent symptoms

exenteration (eks-en"-ter-ā'-shun) – process of surgically removing a tumor together with the organ from which it originated plus all surrounding tissue in the body space

fibrin (fī'-brin) – threads of protein that form the basis of a blood clot

fibromatosis (fī"-brō-muh-tō'-sis) – the formation of a fibrous, tumor-like nodule arising from the deep fascia, with a tendency to local recurrence

Gamma Knife™ – minimally invasive radiosurgical system used in the treatment of benign and malignant intracranial neoplasms and arteriovenous malformations (AVMs)

glioblastoma multiforme (glī"-ō-blas-tō'-muh mul"-tih-for'-muh) – a neoplasm of the central nervous systems, especially the cerebrum, consisting of a variety of cellular types

glucagonoma (gloo'-kuh-guh-nō"-muh) – pancreatic tumor that is usually malignant

granulocytic leukemia (gran'-yoo-lō-sit"-ik) – myelocytic leukemia; leukemia arising from myeloid tissue in which the granular, polymorpho-nuclear leukocytes and their precursors predominate

granulocytosis (gran"-yoo-lō-sī-tō'-sis) – occurs when there is an abnormal increase in granulocytes in the blood, which may result from infection or inflammation of any type

H

hemangioblastoma (hē-man"-jē-ō-blas-tō'-muh) – a capillary hemangioma of the brain consisting of proliferated blood vessel cells or angioblasts

hemangiosarcoma (hē-man"-jē-ō-sar-kō'-muh) – a malignant tumor formed by proliferation of endo-thelial and fibroblastic tissue

hematogenous (hē"-uh-tahj'-eh-nus) – produced by or derived from the blood; disseminated by circula-tion or through the bloodstream

hemocytoblasts (stem cells) (hē"-mō-sī'-tō-blasts) – immature cells

hemoglobin test (hē"-mō-glō'-bin) – lab test that measures the total amount of hemoglobin in a sample of peripheral blood

hemolysis (hē-mol'-ih-sis) – the destruction of red blood cells

hemolytic anemia (hē"-mō-lit'-ik uh-nē'-mē-uh) – occurs when red cells are reduced due to excessive destruction

hemophilia (hē"-mō-fil'-ē-uh) – an inherited disorder of blood coagulation characterized by a permanent tendency to hemorrhage, spontaneously or trau-matically, due to a deficit in the blood coagulating mechanism; there is hemophilia A, hemophilia B, and hemophilia C, each of which lacks a specific blood clotting factor

hepatoblastoma (hep"-uh-tō-blas-tō'-muh) – a malignant intrahepatic tumor occurring in infants and young children and consisting chiefly of embry-onic hepatic tissue

hepatocellular carcinoma (hep"-uh-tō-sel'-yoo-lur) – a malignant tumor of the liver

hepatoma (hep"-uh-tō'-muh) – a tumor of the liver

Hodgkin disease (hahj'-kin) – a malignant neo-plasm of lymphoid cells of uncertain etiology producing chronic enlargement of the lymph nodes, spleen, and often the liver

human T-cell leukemia-lymphoma virus (HTLV) – the first virus known to cause cancer in humans

humoral immunity (hyoo'-mur-ul ih-myoo'-nih-tē) – an immune response in which B cells change into plasma cells and secrete antibodies

Hürthle cell tumor (hert'-el) – a tumor of the thyroid and composed of Hürthle cells (large eosinophil-staining cells occasionally present in the thyroid gland)

hypercapnia (hī"-per-kap'-nē-uh) – an increased amount of carbon dioxide in the blood

hyperlipemia (hī"-per-lih-pē'-mē-uh) – an excessive quantity of fat in the blood

hypersplenism (hī"-per-splen'-izm) – a syndrome characterized by enlargement of the spleen

I

iatrogenic (ī"-at-rō-jen'-ik) – any adverse mental or physical condition induced in a patient by the effects of treatment by a physician or surgeon

immunoglobulins (ih"-myoo-nō-glob'-yoo-linz) – specific types of gamma globulin that are capable of acting as antibodies; examples are IgG (found in high concentration in the plasma) and IgA (found in breast milk, saliva, tears, and respiratory mucus); other immunoglobulins include IgM, IgD, and IgE

immunotherapy (ih-myoo"-nō-thār'-uh-pē) – includes nonspecific systemic stimulation, adjuvant, active specific immunotherapy, and adoptive im-munotherapy; new forms include the use of mono-clonal antibodies

interferon (in"-ter-fĕr'-on) – substance produced by lymphocytes that either directly blocks tumor growth or stimulates the immune system and other body defenses

interleukin (in"-ter-loo'-kin) – substance that stimulates the immune system to destroy tumors

islet cell carcinoma (ī'-let) – a tumor of the islands of Langerhans; such tumors may result in hyperinsulinism

IsoMed Infusion Pump™ (ī'-sō-med) – The IsoMed constant flow infusion system, manufactured by MedTronic, uses a catheter to deliver small doses of medication directly into the cerebrospinal fluid for the management of chronic pain

Kaposi sarcoma (kap'-uh-sē) – a multifocal, metastasizing, malignant reticulosis with features resembling those of angiosarcoma, mainly involving the skin, manifest as reddish blue or brownish soft nodules and tumors; the signature lesion of patients with full-blown AIDS

Krukenberg tumor (kroo'-ken-berg) – a special type of carcinoma of the ovary, usually metastatic from cancer of the gastrointestinal tract, especially of the stomach

leiomyosarcoma (lī"-ō-mī"-o-sar-kō'-muh) – a sarcoma containing large spindle cells of smooth muscle, most commonly of the uterus or retroperitoneal region

leukemia – progressive proliferation of abnormal white blood cells found in the blood and other organs; there are many types of leukemia, including adult T cell, hairy cell, mast cell, mixed cell, plasma cell, Rieder cell, splenic, stem cell

leukopenia (loo"-kō-pē'-nē-uh) – an abnormal decrease in leukocytes

leukocytopenia (loo"-kō-sī"-tō-pē'-nē-uh) – leukopenia; a reduction of the number of leukocytes in the blood to a count of 5000 or fewer

Leydig cell tumor (lī'-dig) – the most common non-germinal tumor of the testis, derived from the Leydig cells of the testis; such tumors are rarely malignant

liposarcoma (lip"-ō-sar-kō'-muh) – a malignant tumor derived from primitive or embryonal lipoblastic cells that exhibit varying degrees of lipoblastic and/or lipomatous differentiation

lymphadenitis (lim-fad"-eh-nī'-tis) – inflammation of one or more lymph nodes

lymphadenopathy (lim-fad"-eh-nop'-uh-thē) – disease of the lymph nodes

lymphadenotomy (lim-fad"-eh-not'-uh-mē) – surgical incision into a lymph node

lymphangiogram (lim-fan"-jē-ō-gram) – test in which contrast medium is injected into lymph vessels in the foot, and x-rays are taken to show the path of lymph flow as it moves into the chest region; often used in the staging and diagnosis of lymphoma

lymphangiography (lim-fan"-jē-ahg'-ruh-fē) – x-ray of the lymphatic vessels following the injection of a contrast medium

lymphangiosarcoma (lim-fan"-jē-ō-sar-kō'-muh) – a malignant tumor of lymphatic vessels, usually arising in a limb that is the site of chronic lymphedema

lymphosarcoma (lim"-fō-sar-kō'-muh) – a general term applied to malignant neoplastic disorders of lymphoid tissue, not to include Hodgkin disease

lymphangiology (lim-fan"-jē-ol'-uh-jē) – the study of the lymphatic system

lymphocytopenia (lim"-fō-sī"-tō-pē'-nē-uh) – condition of fewer than normal lymphocytes in the blood

lymphoid organs (lim'-foyd) – lymph nodes, spleen, and thymus gland

lymphopoiesis (lim"-fō-poy-ē'-sis) – the formation of lymphocytes or of lymphoid tissue

macrophages (mak'-rō-fā-jez) – cells in the spleen, liver, and bone marrow that destroy worn-out erythrocytes (red blood cells)

malignant fibrous histiocytoma (his"-tē-ō-sī-tō'-muh) – a malignant fibrous tumorlike nodule of the dermis

malignant schwannoma (muh-lig'-nent shwon-nō'-muh) – a malignant neoplasm of the white substance of Schwann (i.e., of a nerve sheath)

mediastinal nodes (mē"-dē-uh-stī'-nul) – lymph nodes in the area between the lungs in the thoracic cavity

medulloblastoma (meh-dul"-ō-blas-tō'-muh) – a cerebellar tumor composed of undifferentiated neuroepithelial cells

megakaryocytes (meg"-uh-kār'-ē-ō-sītz) – giant cells from which platelets (syn. thrombocytes) are formed in the bone marrow

melanoma (mel"-uh-nō'-muh) – a tumor made up of melanin-pigmented cells; the term can refer to malignant melanoma

meningioma (meh-nin"-jē-ō'-muh) – a hard, slow-growing, usually vascular tumor that originates in the arachnoidal tissue

mesenchymal tumor (mez-eng'-kī-mul) – a tumor composed of tissue that resembles mesenchymal cells

mesenchymoma (mez"-eng-kī-mō'-muh) – a neoplasm containing a mixture of mesenchymal and fibrous tissue

mesonephroma (mez"-ō-neh-frō'-muh) – a relatively rare malignant tumor of the female genital tract, most often the ovary

mesothelioma (mez"-ō-thē"-lē-ō'-muh) – a tumor developed from mesothelial tissue

metastasis (pl. metastases) (meh-tass'-tuh-sis OR meh-tass'-tuh-sees) – the process by which cancer spreads from a primary site to a secondary one

modality (mō-dal'-ih-tē) – method of treatment

morbidity (mōr-bid'-ih-tē) – the condition of being diseased or morbid

mucinous tumor (myoo'-sih-nus) – a cyst (open space filled with fluid) containing thick, sticky fluid

multiple myeloma (mī"-eh-lō'-muh) – a malignant tumor of bone marrow

mycosis fungoides (mi-kō'-sis fung-goy'-dēz) – a rare, chronic, malignant, lymphoreticular neoplasm of the skin and, in the late stages, the lymph nodes and viscera

myeloma (mī"-eh-lō'-muh) – a tumor originating in cells of the hematopoietic portion of bone marrow

myosarcoma (mī"-ō-sar-kō'-muh) – cancerous tumor of muscle tissue

nephroblastoma (neh"-frō-blas-tō'-muh) – a rapidly developing malignant mixed tumor of the kidneys, made up of embryonal elements (Wilms tumor); usually affects children before age 5

neuroblastoma (nyoo"-rō-blas-tō'-muh) – sarcoma of nervous system origin, composed mainly of neuroblasts and affecting mostly infants and children up to 10 years of age

neuroepithelioma (nyoo"-rō-ep"-ih-thē"-lē-ō'-muh) – a relatively rare tumor of neuroepithelium in a nerve of special sense

neurofibromatosis (nyoo"-rō-fi"-brō-muh-tō'-sis) – a condition in which there are tumors of various sizes on peripheral nerves

oligodendroglioma (ol"-ih-gō-den"-drō-glī-ō'-muh) – a malignant tumor occurring mainly in the cerebrum, consisting mostly of neuroglial cells

oncogene (ong'-kō-jēn) – a piece of DNA that has the ability to cause a cell to become malignant

oncogenic (ong"-kō-jen'-ik) – relating to the ability to give rise to tumors, especially malignant tumors

osteoblastoma (ah"-stē-ō-blas-tō'-muh) – a benign, rather vascular tumor of bone characterized by the formation of osteoid tissue and primitive bone

osteogenic sarcoma (ah"-stē-ō-jen'-ik) – a malignant primary tumor of bone composed of a malignant connective tissue stroma with evidence of malignant osteoid, bone, and/or cartilage formation

osteosarcoma (ahss"-tē-ō-sar-kō'-muh) – osteogenic sarcoma

Paget disease (paj'-et) – an inflammatory cancerous affection of the areola and nipple, usually associated with carcinoma of the lactiferous ducts and deeper structures of the breast; occurs mainly in middle-aged women

palliative (pal'-ē-uh-tiv) – refers to a form of treatment that relieves symptoms without curing

pancytopenia (pan"-sī-tō-pē'-nē-uh) – deficiency of all cell elements of the blood; aplastic anemia

peritoneoscopy (pār"-ih-tō"-nē-ahs'-kuh-pē) – examination of the peritoneal cavity by an instrument inserted through the abdominal wall

pernicious anemia (per-nish'-us uh-nē'-mē-uh) – develops when there is an insufficient number of mature erythrocytes; caused by an inability to absorb vitamin B12 into the body

phagocytosis (fag"-ō-sī-tō'-sis) – the process that occurs when phagocytes ingest and digest bacteria and particles

pheochromocytoma (fē-ō-krō"-mō-sī-tō'-muh) – a well-encapsulated, lobular, vascular tumor of chromaffin tissue of the adrenal medulla or sympathetic paraganglia

pinealoma (pin"-ē-ul-ō'-muh) – a tumor of the pineal body (glandlike structure in the brain), usually encapsulated

pituitary adenoma (pih-tyoo'-ih-tār"-ē ad"-eh-nō'-muh) – an adenoma of the pituitary gland

plasmapheresis (plaz"-muh-fer-ē'-sis) – the process of removing blood from the body and separating the cellular elements from the plasma by centrifuge

pleomorphic (plē"-ō-mōr'-fik) – occurring in various distinct forms

polycythemia vera (pahl"-ē-sih-thē'-mē-uh vē'-ruh) – chronic condition referring to an increased number of red blood cells; sometimes called polycythemia rubra vera

radiocurable tumor (rā"-dē-ō-kyoor'-uh-bul) – a tumor that can be completely eliminated by radiation therapy; usually a tumor that has not metastasized

radioresistant tumor (rā"-dē-ō-rē-zis'-tent) – a tumor that requires large doses of radiation to kill the malignant cells; the high doses of radiation may kill surrounding healthy cells

radiosensitive tumor (rā"-dē-ō-sen'-sih-tiv) – a tumor in which radiation can kill cells without doing serious damage to surrounding healthy tissue

radiosensitizers (rā"-dē-ō-sen"-sih-tī'-zerz) – drugs that boost the sensitivity of tumors to x-rays

reticulocyte (reh-tik'-yoo-lō-sīt) – a developing red blood cell

reticulosarcoma (reh-tik"-yoo-lō-sar-kō'-muh) – a cancerous tumor of the lymphatic system

retinoblastoma (ret"-ih-nō-blas-tō'-muh) – a cancerous tumor of the retina

Rh factor – antigen normally located on the surface of red blood cells of Rh-positive individuals

rhabdomyoma (rab"-dō-mī-ō'-muh) – a striated muscular tissue tumor

rhabdomyosarcoma (rab"-dō-mī"-ō-sar-kō'-muh) – an extremely malignant neoplasm originating in skeletal muscle

sarcoma (sar-kō'-muh) – cancer arising from connective tissue such as muscle or bone; may affect the bones, bladder, kidneys, liver, lungs, parotid glands, and spleen

scirrhous carcinoma (skēr'-us) – a form of cylindrical carcinoma with a firm, hard structure

seminoma (seh"-mih-nō'-muh) – a cancerous tumor of the testis

serodiagnosis (sē"-rō-dī"-ug-nō'-sis) – diagnosis made by observing the reactions of blood serum

sickle cell anemia – a hereditary condition characterized by crescent or sickle-shaped erythrocytes caused by an abnormal type of hemoglobin in the red cell; occurs most commonly in people of African descent

sideropenia (sid"-er-ō-pē'-nē-uh) – a lack of iron in the blood

splenemia (splē-nē'-mē-uh) – condition in which the spleen is clogged with blood

teratocarcinoma (teh"-rat-tō-kar"-sih-nō'-muh) – a carcinoma thought to originate from primordial germ cells or misplaced blastomeres; contains tissues from all embryonic layers, such as bone, muscle, cartilage, nerve, tooth buds, and various glands

teratoma (tār"-uh-tō'-muh) – congenital tumor containing one or more of the three primary embryonic germ layers

thalassemia (thal"-ah-sē'-mē-uh) – an inherited defect in the ability to produce hemoglobin; occurs most frequently in persons of Mediterranean background

thrombocyte (throm'-bō-sīt) – clotting cell (syn. platelet)

thrombogenic (throm"-bō-jen'-ik) – formation of a blood clot

thrombolysis (throm-bahl'-ih-sis) – destruction of a blood clot

thrombophlebitis (throm"bo-flə-bi'tis) – condition where there is both inflammation and a blood clot in a vein; can occur in either superficial or deep veins

thromboplastin (throm"-bō-plas'-tin) – a protein released at the site of an injury when platelets clump; helps promote the formation of a fibrin clot

thymectomy (thī-mek'-tuh-mē) – surgical removal of the thymus gland

villous adenoma (vil'-us ad"-eh-nō'-muh) – a large soft papillary polyp on the mucosa of the large intestine

VIPoma (vī-pō-muh) – vasoactive intestinal peptide-producing tumor; pancreatic endocrine tumor

xerostomia (zē"-rō-stō'-mē-uh) – condition of mouth dryness caused by chemotherapy or radiation therapy

Transcription Tips

Transcribing dictation dealing with hematology/oncology can be challenging. However, if you are familiar with blood diseases, lab and diagnostic tests, surgical procedures used in the treatment of cancer, and the main categories of chemotherapy drugs used to fight cancer, your task will be easier.

diseases of red blood cells – anemia and its types—aplastic, pancytopenia, hemolytic, pernicious, and sickle-cell

diseases of white blood cells – leukemia (acute myelogenous, acute lymphocytic, chronic myelogenous, and chronic lymphocytic) and granulocytosis

Diagnostic and Laboratory Testing

antiglobulin test (Coombs test) – test performed to demonstrate whether the patient's erythrocytes are coated with antibody; used to determine the presence of antibodies in infants of women with Rh-negative blood

antinuclear antibodies (ANA) – blood test to identify antigen-antibody reactions

bleeding time – test that is performed to determine the time required for blood to stop flowing—a prick of the earlobe or a finger stick provides sufficient blood for the test

blood typing – test to determine an individual's blood type and Rh factor

bone marrow aspiration – test for aplastic anemia, leukemia, certain cancers, and polycythemia; performed by aspirating (removing) bone marrow via a lumbar puncture

coagulation time – test conducted to determine the time required for venous blood to clot in a test tube; normally less than 15 minutes

complete blood count (CBC) – blood test that yields a hematocrit, hemoglobin, red and white blood cell count, and differential

erythrocyte sedimentation rate (ESR) – blood test to determine the rate at which RBCs settle in a long, narrow tube; the distance the RBCs settle in 1 hour is the optimal rate

hematocrit (Hct) – blood test performed on whole blood to determine the percentage of red blood cells in the total blood volume

hemoglobin (Hb, Hgb) – blood test to determine the amount of iron-containing pigment of the RBCs

partial thromboplastin time (PTT) – test performed on blood plasma to determine how long it takes for fibrin clots to form

platelet count – test performed on whole blood to determine the number of thrombocytes present

prothrombin time (PT or pro time) – test performed on blood plasma to determine the time needed for oxalated plasma to clot

red blood cell morphology – test performed to determine the shape or form of individual red cells; useful in diagnosing sickle-cell anemia

red blood (cell) count (RBC) – test performed on whole blood to determine the number of erythrocytes present

smear – material spread thinly over a microscopic slide (pathology) or over the medium in a Petri dish for culture (microbiology)

white blood cell differential – blood test used to determine the number of different types of leukocytes (immature and mature forms)

white blood (cell) count (WBC) – blood test to determine the number of leukocytes present; an increase in the WBCs indicates infection and/or inflammation; a decrease in WBCs indicates aplastic anemia, pernicious anemia, or malaria

Surgical Procedures Used in Treatment of Cancer

biopsy – a sample of tissue is removed from a patient and submitted for pathologic examination

punch biopsy – a cylindrical instrument is used to obtain a plug of tissue for pathologic examination

curettage – a surgical scraping

excisional biopsy – surgical removal of an entire tumor, lesion, or diseased organ from a patient

fine-needle aspiration – technique used to remove cells by suction from certain structures such as the prostate, subcutaneous lymph nodes, other neck masses, or breast masses

incisional biopsy – refers to the surgical removal of part of a tumor, lesion, or diseased organ for pathologic study

needle biopsy – a needle is passed through the skin directly into the organ to be studied, and an inner cutting needle slices and removes a core of tissue

shave biopsy – a thin layer of skin consisting mostly or entirely of epidermis is removed with a blade held approximately parallel to the surface

curative surgery – removal of the primary site of malignancy and any lymph nodes to which the neoplasm has extended; such surgery may be all that is required to rid the patient of cancer.

palliative surgery – surgery that attempts to relieve the complications of cancer (e.g., obstruction of the gastrointestinal tract or pain produced by tumor extension into surrounding nerves)

preventive or prophylactic surgery – removal of lesions which, if left in the body, are likely to develop into cancer

surgery combined with radiation, chemotherapy, or immunotherapy – combination treatment required to halt the spread of a malignancy

Further Treatment Modalities

Oncology treatment paradigms have been evolving fairly rapidly over the last 10 years. Current methods of therapy are referred to as "targeted therapy" and consist of drugs designed to act against specific proteins on the surface of tumor cells or by blocking the growth of cancers by interfering with specific targeted molecules needed for cancer growth. These drugs fall into various categories including:

1. **Monoclonal antibodies**—Artificially designed antibodies to specific protein markers. They currently include:

   - Rituxan (generic rituximab) – targets CD20 found on B cells. It is used in non Hodgkin lymphoma.

   - Herceptin (generic trastuzumab) – targets the Her2/neu (also known as ErbB2) receptor expressed in some types of breast cancer.

   - Erbitux (generic cetuximab) – targets EGFR, the epidermal growth factor receptor. It is used in the treatment of colon cancer and non-small cell lung cancer. *NB*: In adenocarcinoma of the colon, this drug must be used with tumors that do not possess the KRAS mutation in order to be effective.

   - Avastin (generic bevacizumab) – targets circulating VEGF ligand-vascular endothelial growth factor. It is approved for use in the treatment of colon cancer, breast cancer (the FDA pulled this recommendation, but the data supporting use is still valid), non-small cell lung cancer, and is investigational in the treatment of sarcoma. Its use for the treatment of brain tumors has been recommended as well.

   - Campath (generic alemtuzumab) – targets CD52 for treatment of B-cell chronic lymphocytic leukemia (B-CLL).

   - Arzerra (generic ofatumumab) – targets CD20 as well and is indicated for the treatment of patients with chronic lymphocytic leukemia (CLL) refractory to fludarabine and alemtuzumab.

   - Zevalin (generic ibritumomab) – targets CD20 and is radiolabeled with Yytrium for treatment of lymphoma.

   - Bexxar (generic tositumomab) – targets CD20 and is radiolabeled with Iodine 131 for treatment of lymphoma.

   - Vectibix (generic panitumumab) – targets EGFR and is approved for the treatment of colorectal cancer.

   - Adcetris (generic brentuximab) – targets CD30 and is indicated for 3rd line therapy in Hodgkin disease. First major advance in Hodgkin disease therapy in over 30 years.

   - Mylotarg (generic gemtuzumab ozogamicin) – targets CD33 and is indicated for the treatment of acute myeloid leukemia.

   - Yervoy (generic ipilimumab) – targets CTLA-4 and is approved for front-line therapy in metastatic melanoma.

2. **Small molecule targeted drugs**. They currently include:

   - Gleevec (generic imatinib mesylate) – targets BCR-ABL tyrosine kinase inhibitor and is approved for chronic myelogenous leukemia and gastrointestinal stromal tumor (GIST).

   - Tarceva (generic erlotinib) – inhibits epidermal growth factor receptor and is approved in metastatic non-small cell lung cancer, pancreatic cancer, and gastric cancer.

   - Velcade (generic bortezomib) – an apoptosis-inducing proteasome inhibitor approved to treat multiple myeloma and mantle cell lymphoma.

   - Sprycel (generic dasatinib) – targets BCR-ABL tyrosine kinase inhibitor and is approved for chronic myelogenous leukemia in Gleevec failures.

   - Tasigna (generic nilotinib) – targets BCR-ABL tyrosine kinase inhibitor and is approved for chronic myelogenous leukemia in Gleevec failures.

These are just the FDA approved and available drugs at the time of publication of this manual; the list of agents undergoing clinical trials is actually larger than this entire list. The compendia of drugs are growing fairly quickly and should continue to do so for the foreseeable future. *NB:* Several web resources are available to help keep current in-between revisions of this manual.

Thanatology

Thanatology is the medicolegal study of death and conditions affecting dead bodies. In this field the mechanisms and forensic aspects of death, such as bodily changes that are associated with death and the post-mortem period, are explored. The study also includes the wider social aspects related to death. In a college or university, it is an interdisciplinary study, a section of forensic sciences. People who take a course in thanatology study the biology of death and what happens physically to people at the moment of dying and after death; the psychological principles and therapeutic drugs involved; also medical ethics, especially the issue of euthanasia (right to die).

Thanatologists study, teach, and conduct research into cultural patterns, attitudes, anthropology, sociology, and the psychology of death and dying. Thanatologists do not provide medical care. Thanatology is not the same subject as palliative care, which is a medical specialty covering pain and symptom management in dying patients. Thanatology also differs from non-specific grief support, a general service that many psychologists, clergy, and healthcare personnel may provide. While many care providers may provide grief support from time to time, not all have received special training in thanatology.

Supportive Web Sites

http://www.nccn.org	The National Comprehensive Cancer Network web site. The NCCN Compendium is now recognized by the Centers for Medicare and Medicaid Services (CMS) and United Healthcare as the authoritative reference for oncology coverage policy. This site is very current with regard to the standard of care.
http://www.cancer.gov	The National Cancer Institute web site that has excellent information on standard of care as well as current research protocols.
http://www.asco.org	The American Society of Clinical Oncology web site that has comprehensive resources for cancer care, but membership is required.
http://www.uptodate.com	The website for UpToDate online, which is an excellent peer-reviewed evidence-based knowledge system authored by physicians to help clinicians make the right decisions at the point of care. All UpToDate content is written and edited by a global community of 4800 physicians, world-renowned experts in their specialties. Supported by UpToDate's 45 in-house physician editors, these authors follow a rigorous editorial process, continually reviewing the content to ensure it is of the highest quality and based on the latest evidence.
http://www.oncolink.org/types/index2.cfm	Provides an alphabetical list of cancer types; click on type of interest to read detailed information about the particular cancer

http://cancer.med.upenn.edu/	Click on "Types of Cancer" or "Treatment Options" for helpful information.
http://content.health.msn.com/	Search on "cancer" or "oncology" for other links of interest.
http://www.cancer.gov	Click on "Clinical Trials," "Developments," "Newly Approved Cancer Treatments," and other links of interest.
http://www.canceradvocacy.org/	Click on "Resources," then on "Glossary" for a list of terms.
http://www.cancerkids.org/	Use this site's Search function for any cancer-related term.

Index of Hematology/Oncology Reports

Exercise#	Patient Name	Type of Report/Procedure
TE#1	Doris Elizabeth Moore	Hematology/Oncology Followup Letter
TE#2	Hans Helland	Hematology/Oncology Followup Letter
TE#3	Julia Paternoster	Consultation, anemia
TE#4	Samuel Tyler Peace	Postop Followup HPIP Note
TE#5	Janet L. Clark	Radiology Oncology 3-D Simulation
TE#6	Janet L. Clark	Radiology Oncology Progress Note
TE#7	Janet L. Clark	Radiology Oncology Progress Note
TE#8	Janet L. Clark	Radiology Oncology Progress Note
TE#9	Janet L. Clark	Radiology Oncology Progress Note
TE#10	Janet L. Clark	Radiation Oncology Treatment Summary
TE#11	Jonathan Olivier	Death Summary
TE#12	Nicholas Youngblood	Memorandum regarding chemotherapy

CHAPTER 8

NEUROLOGY/
NEUROSURGERY

Introduction

Neurology, neurosurgery, and *neuroradiology* are the medical specialties concerned with diagnosis and treatment of disorders of the brain, spinal cord, and peripheral nerves. The nervous system, which comprises the complicated communication network of the body, is the mechanism for the exchange of messages between the brain and more than 10 billion nerve cells. This interaction is what makes a human body into an intelligent, functioning individual.

Anatomically and functionally the *nervous system* is divided into the brain, spinal cord, and nerves. The *brain* (encephalon) and the *spinal cord* (medulla spinalis) make up the *central nervous system* (*CNS*). The *peripheral nervous system* (*PNS*) is composed of a series of nerves that extend from the central nervous system to all portions of the body; the PNS coordinates all other body systems so that they work together as a unit.

Neurologists diagnose and treat diseases affecting the brain, spinal cord, peripheral nerves, and muscles. Disordered thought processes or emotions are treated by psychiatrists, although the two specialties overlap, particularly in relation to dementia or psychosomatic symptoms.

Contemporary neurologists interact closely with related specialists. Neurosurgeons treat tumors and subarachnoid hemorrhages; neuroradiologists image structural diseases of the brain and spinal cord; neurophysiologists investigate seizures using electroencephalography and diseases of nerve and muscle using nerve conduction studies and electromyography.

Headaches, strokes, epilepsy, Parkinson disease, multiple sclerosis, and *sleep disorders* are common maladies treated by the neurologist. Neurological disorders may be caused by organic injury, congenital defects, or diseases such as infections. Diagnosis in neurology is founded on clinical principles, attending closely to the patient's history and to careful physical examination.

The related specialty of neurosurgery treats the surgical aspects of nervous system disease and disorder. Diskectomy, spinal fusion, and craniotomy for tumor or trauma are the procedures most commonly performed by neurosurgeons.

Neuroradiology is an area of expertise that uses various procedures to diagnose neurological abnormalities. Interventional radiologists also treat abnormalities. X-ray, ultrasound, nuclear studies, and magnetic resonance imaging are utilized to diagnose neurological disorders. As technology advances, other subspecialties will inevitably arise.

Critical Thinking Exercise

?

You are speaking to a Health Documentation Specialty (HDS) class, and a student asks what role a transcriptionist plays in a facility that uses a voice-activated dictation system. How would you respond?

Neurology/Neurosurgery Abbreviations

The abbreviations, acronyms, and terms in the following abbreviations and terminology sections are often dictated in this specialty. We offer abbreviated definitions here. Please see an unabridged medical dictionary or the suggested web sites in this chapter for more information on each term.

AD	Alzheimer disease		**CMG**	cystometrogram
ADLs	activities of daily living		**CNS**	central nervous system
AJ	ankle jerk		**CP**	cerebral palsy
ALS	amyotrophic lateral sclerosis		**CPAP**	continuous positive airway pressure
ANS	autonomic nervous system		**CSF**	cerebrospinal fluid
APLD	automated percutaneous lumbar diskectomy		**CVA**	cerebrovascular accident
			CVP	central venous pressure
AVM	arteriovenous malformation		**DBS**	deep brain stimulation
BAER	brainstem auditory-evoked response		**DCS**	dorsal cord stimulation
BPV	benign positional vertigo		**DICOM**	Digital Imaging and Communications in Medicine (teleradiology)
CAE	carotid artery endarterectomy			
CASA	Center on Addiction and Substance Abuse		**DT**	delirium tremens
CAT/CT	computerized axial tomography		**DTP**	distal tingling on percussion
CBS	chronic brain syndrome		**DTR**	deep tendon reflexes
CIDP	chronic inflammatory demyelinating polyneuropathy		**EEG**	electroencephalogram

EMG	electromyogram
ENG	electronystagmograph
EST	electric shock therapy
GBM	glioblastoma multiforme
GBS	Guillain-Barré syndrome
GCS	Glasgow coma scale
GSW	gunshot wound
GTCS	generalized tonic-clonic seizure (grand mal seizure)
HDS	herniated disk syndrome
HNP	herniated nucleus pulposus
ICP	intracranial pressure
IGS	image-guided surgery
IMV	intermittent mandatory ventilation
IVC	intraventricular catheter
IVIG	intravenous immunoglobulin
LGB	Landry-Guillain-Barré (syndrome)
LOA	left occiput anterior
LOP	left occiput posterior
LP	lumbar puncture (see page 128)
MD	muscular dystrophy
MEG	magnetoencephalography
MMSE	mini mental status exam
MRA	magnetic resonance arteriogram
MRI	magnetic resonance imaging
MS	multiple sclerosis
MSI	magnetic source imaging

MSLT	mean (or multiple) sleep latency test
MVA	motor vehicle accident
MVV	maximal voluntary ventilation
NCV	nerve conduction velocity
NIHSS	National Institute of Health Stroke Scale
OBS	organic brain syndrome
PDD	primary degenerative dementia
PEG	pneumoencephalography
PET	positron emission tomography
PMS	petit mal seizure
PNS	peripheral nervous system
PSG	polysomnography
RIND	reversible, ischemic neurological deficit
RNA	ribonucleic acid
ROM	range of motion
RPR	rapid plasma reagin
SAH	subarachnoid hemorrhage
SBX	stereotactic brain biopsy
SSEP	somatosensory-evoked potential
TEE	transesophageal echocardiogram
TENS	transcutaneous electrical nerve stimulation
TIA	transient ischemic attack
TNS	transcutaneous nerve stimulation
TPA	tissue plasminogen activator
TS	trauma score

Anatomic Illustrations

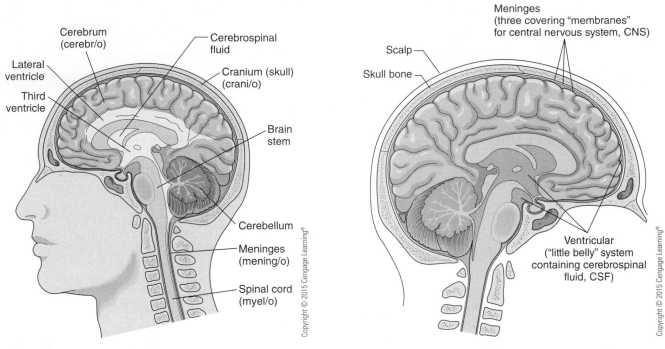

FIGURE 8-1 Cross-section of the brain

FIGURE 8-2 The meninges and ventricles

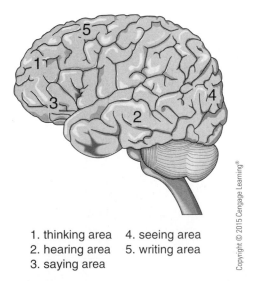

1. thinking area   4. seeing area
2. hearing area   5. writing area
3. saying area

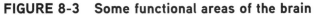

FIGURE 8-3 Some functional areas of the brain

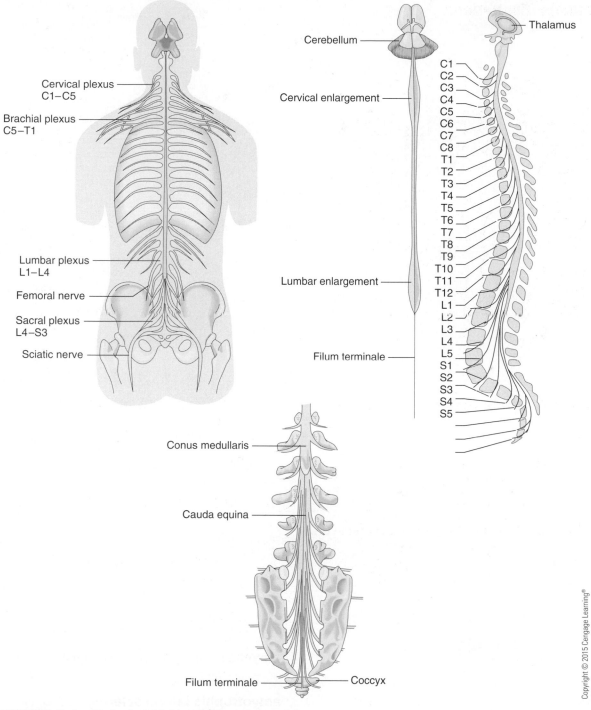

Cervical plexus
C1–C5

Brachial plexus
C5–T1

Lumbar plexus
L1–L4

Femoral nerve

Sacral plexus
L4–S3

Sciatic nerve

Cerebellum

Cervical enlargement

Lumbar enlargement

Filum terminale

Thalamus

C1
C2
C3
C4
C5
C6
C7
C8
T1
T2
T3
T4
T5
T6
T7
T8
T9
T10
T11
T12
L1
L2
L3
L4
L5
S1
S2
S3
S4
S5

Conus medullaris

Cauda equina

Filum terminale   Coccyx

FIGURE 8-4   Spinal cord (myel/o) and nerves

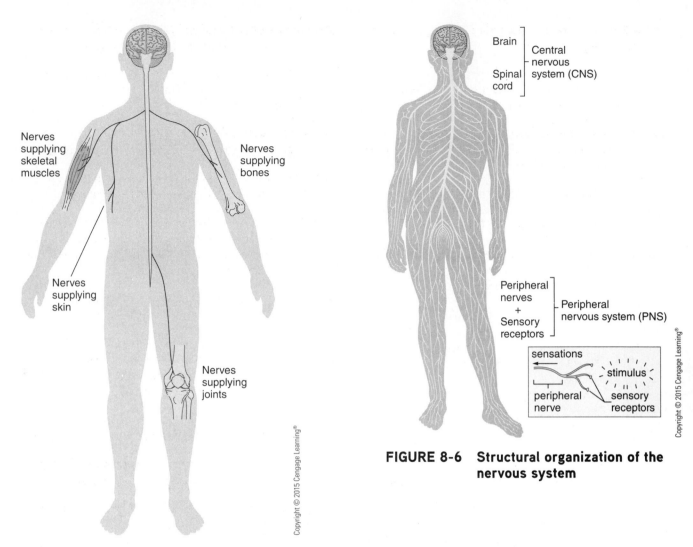

FIGURE 8-6 Structural organization of the nervous system

FIGURE 8-5 The somatic nervous system (SNS)

Neurology/Neurosurgery Terminology

A

agrammatism (ā-gram'-uh-tizm") – inability to speak grammatically because of brain injury or disease

akinesia (ā"-kih-nē'-zē-uh) – absence or poverty of movements; the temporary paralysis of a muscle by the injection of procaine

Alzheimer disease (altz'-hī-mer) – progressive degeneration of the brain that causes impairment of memory and dementia manifested by confusion and ongoing deterioration of judgment; death may occur in 5 to 10 years (syn. dementia)

amyelia (ā"-mī-ē'-lē-uh) – congenital absence of spinal cord

amyotrophic lateral sclerosis (ALS) (ā"-mī-ō-trō'-fik skleh-rō'-sis) – degeneration involving the principal pyramidal tracts of the brain and spinal cord and the anterior horn cells in the spinal cord; results in loss of motor function; death usually occurs because of pharyngeal muscle failure (also known as Lou Gehrig disease)

anencephalia (an"-en-seh-fā'-lē-uh) – congenital absence of the cranial vault with cerebral hemispheres completely missing or reduced to small masses attached to the base of the skull

aphasia (ă-fă'-zē-uh) – loss of the power of speech due to a central lesion

apoptosis (ā"-pō-tō'-sis) – "cell suicide"; condition in which cells shrivel rather than swell, with only minimal damage to surrounding cells

arteriovenous malformation (AVM) (ar-tē"-rē-ō-vē'-nus malfŏr-mā'-shun) – an abnormal connection of veins to arteries

astereognosis (ā-stăr"-ē-ahg-nō'-sis) – loss of power to recognize objects or to appreciate their form by touching or feeling them

astrocytoma (as"tro-si-to'mə) – a tumor composed of astrocytes; the most common type of primary brain tumor, it is found throughout the central nervous system

aura (aw'-ruh) – a subjective sensation or motor phenomenon that precedes and marks the onset of a paroxysmal attack, such as a seizure or migraine headache

B

Biernacki sign (bī-er-naht'-skē) – analgesia of the ulnar nerve in paralytic dementia and tabes dorsalis

Brantigan cage (bran'-tih-gun) – internal fixation device used after lumbar spinal fusion

Brown-Sequard syndrome (brown'-sah-kar') – a syndrome due to damage of one-half of the spinal cord

Brudzinski sign (brood-zin'-skē) – a physical sign that suggests the presence of meningitis

C

cauda equina (kaw'-duh) (ē'-kwih-nuh) – "horse's tail"; the group of peripheral nerves that exit the spinal column below the end of the spinal cord

cephalalgia (sef"-ul-al'-jē-uh) – pain in the head; headache

cerebellum (sār"-eh-bel'-um) – the second largest portion of the brain; it is concerned with the coordination of movements and balance

cerebral dysrhythmia (sir'-ē-brul dis-rith'-mē-uh) – irregularity in the electrical impulses given off by the brain

cerebromeningitis (sir"-ē-brō-men"-in-jī'-tis) – inflammation of the brain and meninges

cerebrum (sir'-ē-brum) – the largest and uppermost portion of the brain; divided into two cerebral hemispheres

Charcot-Marie-Tooth disease (shar-kō') – progressive neuropathic (peroneal) muscular atrophy

chondrosarcoma (kon"dro-sahr-ko'mə) – a malignant bone cancer that affects mainly cartilage

cisterna (sis-ter'-nuh) – a closed space serving as a reservoir for lymph or other body fluid, especially one of the enlarged subarachnoid spaces containing cerebrospinal fluid

clonic (klah'-nik) – spasm in which rigidity and relaxation alternate in rapid succession

conus medullaris (ko'-nus med'-yoo-lar"-ıs) – medullary cone; the cone-shaped lower end of the spinal cord at the level of the upper lumbar vertebrae; the end of the spinal cord

cordectomy (kor-dek'-tuh-mē) – ablative destruction of a portion of the spinal cord

craniocele (krā'-nē-ō-sēl") – a protrusion of any part of the cranial contents through a defect in the skull

cranioclast (krā'-nē-ō-klast") – an instrument for performing craniotomy

craniotomy (krā"-nē-ot'-uh-mē) – surgical procedure on the cranium

cryptococcosis (krip"-tō-kok-ō'-sis) – infection by the Cryptococcus species; it may involve the skin, lungs, or other organs but has a predilection for the brain and meninges

D

decerebrate (dē-sār'-eh-brāt) – to eliminate cerebral function by transecting the brain stem between the anterior colliculi and the vestibular nuclei or by ligating the common carotid arteries and the basilar artery at the center of the pons

demyelinate (dē-mī'-eh-lin-āt) – to destroy or remove the myelin sheath of a nerve or nerves

diastematomyelia (dī"-uh-stē"-ah-tō-mī-ē'-lē-uh) – a congenital defect, often associated with spina bifida, in which the spinal cord is split into halves by a bony spicule of fibrous band, each half being surrounded by a dural sac

diencephalon (dī"-en-sef'-uh-lahn) – the inner brain, thalamus, and hypothalamus

diplegia (dī-plē'-jē-uh) – paralysis affecting like parts on both sides of the body; bilateral paralysis

dura mater (doo'-ruh mā'-tur) – the outermost, toughest, and most fibrous of the three membranes (meninges) covering the brain and spinal cord

dysautonomia (dis"-aw-tō-nō'-mē-uh) – a disorder of the autonomic nervous system (ANS) function

dystonia (dis-tō'-nē-uh) – a neurologic muscle disorder characterized by involuntary muscle spasms

electromyography (ē-lek"-trō-mī-og'-ruh-fē) – the recording and study of the intrinsic electrical properties of skeletal muscle

encephalitis (en"-sef-uh-lī'-tis) – inflammation of the brain

encephalocele (en-sef'-uh-lō-sēl") – a herniation of a part of the brain through any opening in the skull

encephalomalacia (en-sef"-uh-lō-muh-lā'-shē-uh) – softening of the brain

encephalomyeloradiculitis (en-sef"-uh-lō-mī"-eh-lō-rah-dik"-yoo-lī'-tis) – inflammation of the brain, spinal cord, and spinal nerve roots

encephalopathy (en-sef"-uh-lop'-uh-thē) – any degenerative disease of the brain

epencephalon (ep"-en-sef '-uh-lahn) – cerebellum; metencephalon

ependymitis (ē-pen"-dih-mī'-tis) – inflammation of the ependyma, which is the lining membrane of the ventricles of the brain and of the central canal of the spinal cord

epileptologist (ep"-ih-lep-tahl'-uh-jist) – a practitioner who specializes in the diagnosis and treatment of epilepsy

fasciculation (fuh-sik"-yoo-lā'-shun) – a small, local contraction of muscles representing a spontaneous discharge of a number of fibers innervated by a single motor nerve filament

Gamma Knife™ – a minimally invasive radiosurgical system used in the treatment of benign and malignant intracranial neoplasms and arteriovenous malformations (AVMs); a common method of radiosurgery

glioblastoma multiforme (glē"-ō-blas-tō'-muh mul'-tih-form) – a glioma (neoplasm) consisting of undifferentiated anaplastic cells of astrocytic origin; these neoplasms grow rapidly, invade extensively, and occur most frequently in the cerebrum of adults

glioma (glē-ō'-muh) – any neoplasm derived from one of the various types of cells that form the interstitial tissue of the brain, spinal cord, pineal gland, posterior pituitary gland, and retina

grand mal (gran mahl) – generalized tonic/clonic seizure, as seen in epilepsy; a sudden loss of consciousness immediately followed by generalized convulsions

Guillain-Barré syndrome (gē-yayn'-bar-rā') – a rare disease of the nervous system involving peripheral nerves, nerve roots, and spinal cord

hemangioblastoma (hē-man"-jē-ō-blas-tō'-muh) – a capillary hemangioma of the brain, consisting of proliferated blood vessel cells or angioblasts

hemilaminectomy (hem"-ē-lā"-ih-nek'-tuh-mē) – removal of the vertebral laminae on only one side

hemiparesis (hē"-ē-pah'-rē-sis) – muscular weakness affecting one side of the body

hypersomnia (hī"-per-sahm'-nē-uh) – excessive sleep with uncontrollable drowsiness

hypopnea (hī"-pō-nē'-uh) – abnormal decrease in the rate and depth of the respiratory movements

hypothalamus (hī"-pō-thal'-uh-mus) – the portion of the diencephalon that forms the floor and part of the lateral wall of the third ventricle

kernicterus (ker-nik'-ter-us) – a condition with severe neurologic symptoms associated with high levels of bilirubin in the blood, as seen in liver failure

Kernig sign (ker'-nig) – a symptom of meningitis evidenced by reflex contraction and pain in the hamstring muscles when the patient attempts to extend the leg after flexing the thigh upon the abdomen

kinesioneurosis (kih-nē"-sē-ō-noo-rō'-sis) – a functional nervous disorder characterized by motor disturbances, such as spasms or tics

kyphoplasty (kī'-fō-plas"-tē) – injection of bone cement into a compressed vertebra, restoring its height

lateropulsion (lat"-er-ō-pul'-shun) – an involuntary movement of the body or turning of the gait toward one side

leptomeninges (lep"-tō-meh-nin'-jēz) – the pia-arachnoid, a combined delicate web-like membrane that ultimately covers the brain; also called the pia mater

leptomeningitis (lep"-tō-men"-in-jī'-tis) – inflammation of the pia and arachnoid of the brain or spinal cord

linear accelerator (lin'-ee-ar ak-se'-lə-rā-tər) – equipment used in stereotactic radiosurgery to deliver a concentrated dose of radiation to a predetermined target, using x-rays

macrocrania (mak"-rō-krā'-nē-uh) – abnormal increase in the size of the skull, the facial area being disproportionately small in comparison

Magendie foramen (mah-jen'-dē fōr-a'-men) – an opening in the lower portion of the roof of the 4th ventricle through which the cerebrospinal fluid communicates with the subarachnoid space

magnetoencephalography (MEG) (mag-nē"-tō-en-sef'uh-lah'-gruh-fē) – the recording of magnetic signals proportional to electroencephalographic waves emanating from electrical activity in the brain

medulla oblongata (meh-doo'-luh ahb-long-gah'-tuh) – the end of the brainstem that transitions into the spinal cord

meninges (meh-nin'-jēz) – the covering membranes of the brain and spinal cord

meningioma (me-nin"-jē-ō'-mah) – a hard, slow-growing, usually vascular tumor that arises from the meninges or covering membranes of the brain

meningoencephalitis (me-ning"-gō-en-sef"-uh-lī'-tis) – inflammation of the brain and meninges

meningomyelocele (me-ning"-gō-mī'-eh-lō-sēl") – protrusion of a part of the meninges and substance of the spinal cord through a defect in the vertebral column

MicroLYSIS™ (mī"-krō-lī'-sis) – ultrasound-enhanced drug delivery system that delivers thrombolytic drugs directly into the area of a brain clot

milliampere (mA) (mil"e-am'pēr) – a measurement used in radiology (1/1000th of an ampere)

millijoule (mJ) (mil'-ih-jool) – a measurement used in YAG laser and argon laser applications (1/1000th of a joule)

myelomalacia (mī"-eh-lō-muh-lā'-shē-uh) – morbid softening of the spinal cord

narcolepsy (nar'-kō-lep"-sē) – a condition marked by an uncontrollable desire for sleep or by sudden attacks of sleep occurring at intervals

neurectomy (noo-rek'-tuh-mē) – surgical excision of a nerve

neurilemma (noo"-rih-lē'-uh) – the delicate membranous sheath (covering) of a peripheral nerve fiber

neurodegeneration (noo'-rō-dē-jen"-er-ā'-shun) – pertaining to the deterioration of nervous tissue

neurofibromatosis (noo"-rō-fī"-brō-muh-tō'-sis) – an inherited condition characterized by developmental changes in the nervous system, muscles, bones, and skin; marked superficially by the formation of multiple pedunculated soft tumors (neurofibromas) distributed over the entire body and associated with areas of pigmentation

neurogenic (noor"o-jen'ik) – originating in the nervous system or from a lesion in the nervous system

neurogenetics (noo"-rō-jeh-net'-iks) – pertaining to the development of nervous tissue

neuromatous (noo-rahm'-uh-tus) – affected with or of the nature of a tumor or new growth largely made up of nerve cells and nerve fibers

neuronopathy (noor"on-op'ǝ-the) – polyneuropathy involving destruction of the cell bodies of neurons

neuro-ophthalmologist (noo"-rō-of"-thuhl-mahl"-uhjist) – a physician who diagnoses and treats patients suffering from optic nerve disorders, problems with eye and lid movement (double vision, lid spasm, or droop), and unexplained visual loss

neuro-otologist (noo"-rō-ō-tahl'-uh-jist) – a physician who works with patients who have problems that cause vertigo and balance dysfunction, including labyrinthitis, benign positional vertigo, and Ménière disease

nuclear imaging (PET and SPECT) (noo"-klee-ar) – imaging techniques that employ small amounts of radioactive isotopes (radionuclides) to measure cellular and/or tissue metabolism

nystagmus (nis-tag'-mus) – involuntary rhythmic oscillation of the eyeballs, either like a pendulum or with a slow and fast component

obstructive sleep apnea (ap'-nē-uh) – a condition characterized by a particular snoring pattern, which is interrupted by pauses and then gasps; this includes periodic cessation of breathing during sleep

oligodendroglia (ol"-ih-gō-den-drahg'-lē-uh) – a glial cell of ectodermal origin that forms part of the support structure of the central nervous system

pacchionian (pak"-ē-ō'-nē-un) – smooth granular structures found in the meninges of the brain

pallidotomy (pah"-lih-dah'-tuh-mē) – stereotactic surgery in which lesions are produced in the globus pallidus for treatment of extrapyramidal syndromes

paramyotonia (pār"-uh-mī"-ō-tō'-nē uh) – a disease marked by tonic spasms due to disorder of muscular tonicity, especially a hereditary and congenital affection

paresthesias (pār"-es-thē'-zē-uhz) – spontaneous abnormal, usually nonpainful sensations, as in burning or pricking, that may be due to lesions of both the central and peripheral nervous systems

parieto-occipital (puh-rī"-eh-tō-ok-sip'-ih-tul) – pertaining to the parietal and occipital bones or lobes

petit mal (peh-tē mahl') – "absence seizures" that usually last for only a few seconds

pia mater (pē'-uh mā'-tur) – the innermost of the three membranes (meninges) covering the brain and spinal cord

plasmapheresis (plaz"mǝ-fǝ-re'sis) – the removal of plasma from withdrawn blood, with retransfusion of the formed elements into the donor

pleocytosis (plē"-ō-sī-tō'-sis) – presence of a greater-than-normal number of cells in the cerebrospinal fluid

plexopathy (plek-sop'ǝ-the) – any disorder of a network of lymphatic vessels, nerves, or veins

pneumocephalus (noo"-mō-sef '-uh-lus) – air within the skull

polyneuropathy (pahl"-ē-noo-rahp'-uh-thē) – a disease that involves multiple nerves

polysomnogram (pahl"-ē-sahm'-nuh-grā) – test conducted to evaluate sleep apnea syndrome

postictal (pōst-ik'-tul) – following a seizure, e.g., epileptic

precuneus (prē-kyoo'-nē-us) – a small, square-shaped convolution on the medial surface of the parietal lobe of the cerebrum

proprioception (prō"-prē-ō-sep'-shun) – the sensory system mechanism concerned with movement of the body, its balance, posture, and coordination

quadriplegia (kwah"-drih-plē'-jē-uh) – paralysis of all four limbs (syn. tetraplegia)

radiculitis (rah-dik"-yoo-lī'-tus) – inflammation of the root of a spinal nerve, especially of the portion of the root lying between the spinal cord and the intervertebral canal

radiculopathy (rah-dik"-yoo-lop'-uh-thē) – disease of the nerve roots

satellitosis (sat"-eh-lī-tō'-sis) – accumulation of neuroglial cells around neurons; seen whenever neurons are damaged

Schilder disease (shil'-der) – a rare, progressive demyelinating disorder that usually begins in childhood

schwannoma (shwon-nō'-muh) – a neoplasm of a peripheral nerve sheath

sella turcica (sel'-uh tur'-sih-kuh) – a bony shelf in approximately the central portion of the base of the skull that houses the pituitary gland

stereognosis (stār"-ē-ahg-nō'-sis) – the faculty of perceiving and understanding the form and nature of objects by the sense of touch

stereotactic (or stereotaxic) radiosurgery (steh'-rē -ō - tak"-tik [steh'-rē-ō-taks"-ik]) – the very precise delivery of radiation to a brain tumor without harm to the surrounding normal brain; to achieve this precision, special tools are used to pinpoint the location of the brain tumor: the stereotactic frame and the CT or MRI scan—a computerized system for calculating the radiation dose to the brain tumor and a precise system for delivering the radiation to the brain tumor

Sturge-Weber syndrome (encephalotrigeminal angiomatosis) (sturj-web'-er [en-sef"-uh-lō'-trī-jē'-ih-nul] an"-je-ō-muh-tō'-sis) – a congenital disorder characterized by a vascular facial birthmark and neurological abnormalities

subarachnoid (sub"-uh-rak'-noyd) – underneath the arachnoid membrane

synkinesis (sin"-kih-nē'-sis) – an involuntary movement accompanied by a voluntary one

syringobulbia (sih-ring"-gō-bul'-bē-uh) – the presence of cavities in the medulla oblongata

syringomyelia (sih-ring"-gō-mī-ē'-lē-uh) – the presence of abnormal cavities filled with liquid in the spinal cord

teratoma (tar"-uh-tō'-muh) – a true neoplasm made up of a number of different types of tissue, none of which is native to the area in which it occurs

tetraplegia (teh"-truh-plē'-jē-uh) – quadriplegia

thalamus (thal'-uh-mus) – a structure within the diencephalon that serves as the main relay center for sensory impulses

tic douloureux (tihk doo-loo-roo') – trigeminal neuralgia; a disorder of cranial nerve V, the trigeminal nerve

transverse myelitis (tranz-vurss mī"-ē-lī'-tis) – a neurological disorder caused by inflammation across both sides of one level (segment) of the spinal cord

trigeminal neuralgia (trī-jē'-ih-nul noor-al'-jē-uh) – severe, paroxysmal bursts of pain in one or more branches of the trigeminal nerve; see tic douloureux

trismus (trihz'-mus) – persistent contraction of the masseter muscles due to failure of central inhibition; often the initial manifestation of generalized tetanus (lockjaw)

uncovertebral (ung"ko-vur'tə-brəl) – pertaining to or affecting the uncinate processes of a vertebra

V

vagotonia (vā"-gō-tō'-nē-uh) – hyperexcitability of the vagus nerve; a condition in which the vagus nerve dominates in the general functioning of the body organs

ventriculocisternostomy (ven-trik"-yoo-lō-sis"-ternahss'-tuh-mē) – surgical establishment of a communication between the 3rd ventricle of the brain and the cisterna magna for flow of cerebrospinal fluid in hydrocephalus

wallerian degeneration (wah-ler'-ē-un) – degenerative changes in the distal segment of a peripheral nerve fiber when its continuity with its cell body is interrupted by a focal lesion

Transcription Tips

You will find it easier to transcribe neurology/neurosurgery dictation if you are familiar with the names and locations of the major organs and parts of the nervous system; combining forms, prefixes, and suffixes; and specialized terminology used in the field of neurology/neurosurgery. Familiarity with some of the communication disorders will also help.

The nervous system consists of:

- Three anatomic divisions:
    1. Central nervous system
    2. Autonomic nervous system
    3. Peripheral nervous system

- Four physiologic divisions:
    1. Sensory (afferent) system
    2. Motor (efferent) system, including the pyramidal and extrapyramidal divisions
    3. Autonomic nervous system, including the sympathetic and parasympathetic divisions
    4. Reticular activating system

Glossary of Selected Nervous System Terms

amnesia – loss of memory

analgesia – inability to feel pain

anesthesia – loss of feeling

ataxia – lack of muscular coordination

autonomic nervous system – that part of the nervous system that cannot be controlled, governing the heart, smooth muscle, and glands

central nervous system – the system concerned with the brain and spinal cord

cerebral hemorrhage – one type of stroke

cerebrospinal fluid – the protective fluid contained within the brain and spinal cord

coma – unconsciousness from which a patient cannot be awakened

cord – a stringlike structure; the portion of the central nervous system contained in the spinal canal

epilepsy – a deviation of the brain waves that may result in convulsions or motor sensory disturbances

foramen magnum – a passageway through the occipital bone for the spinal cord

frontal lobe – the foremost lobe of each cerebral hemisphere

hemiplegia – paralysis of one side of the body

hemisphere – either half of the brain, left or right

motor neuron – a nerve cell concerned with movement

neuron – nerve cell

occipital lobe – the posterior lobe of the cerebral hemisphere

palsy – paralysis

paraplegic – paralysis of the lower half of the body

parietal lobe – the lobe of the cerebral hemisphere located beneath the parietal bone

sensory neuron – any neuron concerned with sensory function

spinal cord – the nervous tissue within the vertebral canal

temporal lobe – the lobe of the cerebral hemisphere located behind the temporal bone

The 12 Cranial Nerves (alphabetically) with Corresponding Roman Numerals

abducens (eyeball muscle, lateral)	Cranial nerve VI
acoustic (ears)	Cranial nerve VII
facial (face, scalp, tears, salivary)	Cranial nerve VII
glossopharyngeal (taste, swallowing)	Cranial nerve IX
hypoglossal (tongue movements)	Cranial nerve XII
oculomotor (eyes, eyelids)	Cranial nerve III
olfactory (smell)	Cranial nerve I
optic (vision)	Cranial nerve II
spinal accessory (head/shoulders)	Cranial nerve XI
trigeminal (jaw, top of head)	Cranial nerve V
trochlear (eyeball muscle, superior)	Cranial nerve IV
vagus (pharynx, larynx, voice)	Cranial nerve X

Common Communication Disorders

anomia
aphasia

- Broca aphasia
- global aphasia
- Wernicke aphasia

apraxia
dysarthria
perseveration

Lumbar Puncture (LP)

When spinal fluid needs to be examined microscopically, the fluid is obtained via lumbar puncture, otherwise known as a spinal tap. While the patient lies on his or her side with the back slightly rounded and knees flexed toward the abdomen, a puncture is made into the subarachnoid space of the lumbar region at L3-4. Spinal fluid is obtained for either diagnostic or therapeutic purposes. This fluid can be sent to the laboratory where it is examined for color, pressure, protein level, chloride, glucose, lymphocytes, etc. It may be cultured for the presence of bacteria, parasites, or a virus. When necessary, the fluid is removed to release pressure on the spine.

An LP is considered a surgical procedure. Specialties qualified to perform the procedure include Neurosurgery, Pathology, and Orthopedic Surgery.

Supportive Web Sites

http://www.neurosurgery.com	Click on "conditions" or "procedures" for informative material.
http://www.hopkinsmedicine.org/	Search for "radiosurgery," then click on sites of interest for valuable information.
http://www.hopkinsmedicine.org/neurology_neurosurgery/specialty_areas/brain_tumor/treatment/radiation-therapy.html	Click on "diseases and conditions" for a list of specific types of brain tumors and related conditions.
http://www.ninds.nih.gov/	Click on "Disorders A-Z" for helpful links to other information.
http://www.nlm.nih.gov/	Click on "MEDLINEplus," then search for "neurology" or "neurosurgery."
http://www.radionics.com	Click on links of interest.

Index of Neurology/Neurosurgery Reports

CHAPTER 9
OBSTETRICS/GYNECOLOGY (OB/GYN)

Introduction

An **obstetrician** is a physician who has successfully completed specialized education and training in the management of pregnancy, labor, and the time period directly following childbirth.

A **gynecologist** is a physician who has successfully completed specialized education and training in the health of the female reproductive system, including the diagnosis and treatment of disorders and diseases.

Typically, the education and training for both fields occurs concurrently. Thus, an **obstetrician/gynecologist** (OB/GYN) is a physician specialist who provides medical and surgical care to women and has particular expertise in pregnancy, childbirth, and disorders of the reproductive system. This includes preventative care, prenatal care, detection of sexually transmitted diseases, Pap test screening, and family planning.

Ovaries, fallopian tubes, uterus, vagina, vulva, and *breasts* comprise the female reproductive system. Activity of the ovaries (the primary sex organs) is regulated by the anterior lobe of the *pituitary gland.*

The ovaries produce *ova* and *hormones.* The fallopian tubes convey the ovum from the ovary to the uterus and sperm from the uterus toward each ovary.

The uterus has an upper portion, a central area (called the *isthmus*), and the *cervix,* or lower portion. Within the uterus, the wall is made of three layers—the *peritoneum,* or outer layer; the *myometrium,* or middle layer; and the *endometrium,* or inner layer.

Because the uterus is supported by ligaments that affect its position, it may become malpositioned due to weakness of one or more of the ligaments. Four terms describing such abnormal positions are *anteflexion, retroflexion, anteversion,* and *retroversion.*

The vagina is the organ of copulation and receives the semen from the male penis. It also serves as the passageway for the bloody discharge during *menstruation* and the birth of a fetus.

The *vulva* is composed of the *mons pubis, labia majora, labia minora, vestibule,* and *clitoris,* which make up the external female genitalia. The breasts are the mammary glands that produce milk for newborns.

Anyone working as a physician's assistant or as a healthcare documentation specialist for a gynecologist or obstetrician should have a basic understanding of the female anatomy and the processes of pregnancy, childbirth, and its aftermath.

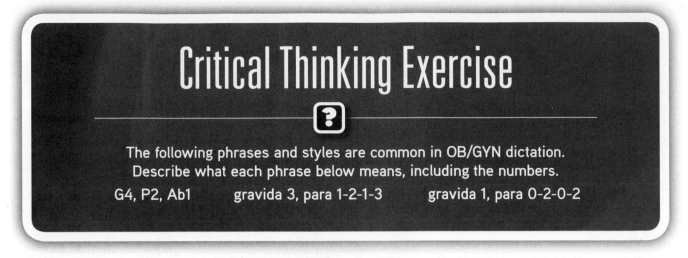

Critical Thinking Exercise

The following phrases and styles are common in OB/GYN dictation. Describe what each phrase below means, including the numbers.

G4, P2, Ab1   gravida 3, para 1-2-1-3   gravida 1, para 0-2-0-2

Obstetrics/Gynecology Abbreviations

The abbreviations, acronyms, and terms in the following abbreviations and terminology sections are often dictated in this specialty. We offer abbreviated definitions here. Please see an unabridged medical dictionary or the suggested web sites in this chapter for more information on each term.

AB	abortion*	**DUB**	dysfunctional uterine bleeding
AFP	alpha-fetoprotein	**EBL**	estimated blood loss
AH	abdominal hysterectomy	**ECC**	endocervical curettage
amnio	amniocentesis	**EDC**	expected (or estimated) date of confinement
AROM	artificial rupture of membrane	**EDD**	estimated day of delivery
BBT	basal body temperature	**EMB**	endometrial biopsy
BOW	bag of waters (BOW rupture)	**ERT**	estrogen replacement therapy
B&S	Bartholin and Skene (glands)	**FHT**	fetal heart tone
BUS	Bartholin gland, urethra, and Skene (glands)	**FSH**	follicle-stimulating hormone
CPD	cephalopelvic disproportion	**FT**	full term
CS, C-section	cesarean section	**G**	gravid (pregnant)
Cx	cervix	**GIFT**	gamete intrafallopian transfer
D&C	dilatation and curettage	**GPA**	gravida, para, abortio
DES	diethylstilbestrol (estrogen)	**HCG/hCG**	human chorionic gonadotropin

* In medicine, abortion can refer to a process that is either spontaneous (occurring from natural causes) or one that is artificially or therapeutically induced.

HELLP	hemolysis, elevated liver enzymes, and low platelet count (a syndrome)	**PDS**	polydioxanone suture
HRT	human replacement therapy	**PG**	pregnant
HSG	hysterosalpingography or hysterosalpingogram	**PID**	pelvic inflammatory disease
		PMP	previous menstrual period
IUD	intrauterine device	**PMS**	premenstrual syndrome
IVF	in vitro fertilization	**POC**	products of conception
IUP	intrauterine pregnancy	**PUD**	pregnancy undelivered
IVPB	intravenous piggyback	**Rh neg.**	Rhesus factor negative
LASH	laparoscopic supracervical hysterectomy	**Rh pos.**	Rhesus factor positive
LAVH	laparoscopic-assisted vaginal hysterectomy	**SAB**	spontaneous abortion
LEEP	loop electrosurgical excision procedure	**SNS**	sacral nerve stimulation
LMP	last menstrual period	**SROM**	spontaneous rupture of membranes
LNMP	last normal menstrual period	**TAH-BSO**	total abdominal hysterectomy with bilateral salpingo-oophorectomies
L/S	lecithin/sphingomyelin ratio (a test on amniotic fluid to determine the maturity of the fetal lungs)	**TOT**	transobturator tape
		TSS	toxic shock syndrome
multip	multipara; multiparous	**TVT**	tension-free vaginal tape (transvaginal tape)
NB	newborn		
NSVD	normal spontaneous vaginal delivery	**UC**	uterine contractions
OCPs	oral contraceptive pills	**UV**	uterovesical
para 3-1-1-3	3 full-term deliveries, 1 premature delivery, 1 abortion or miscarriage, and 3 living children	**VBAC**	vaginal birth after cesarean
		VTOP	voluntary termination of pregnancy
Pap smear	Papanicolaou smear		

Anatomic Illustrations

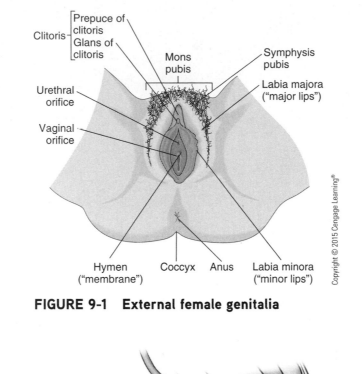

FIGURE 9-1   External female genitalia

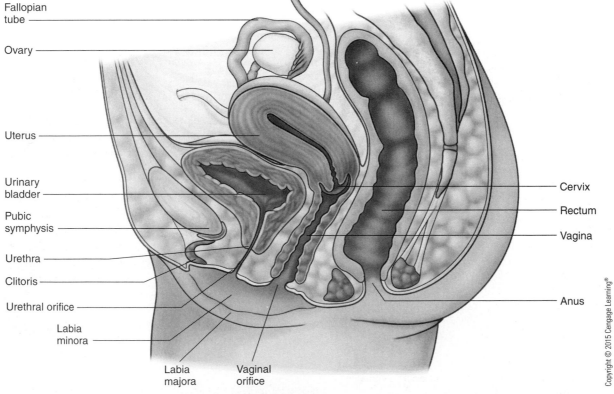

FIGURE 9-2   Structures of the female reproductive system shown in a lateral cross-section

procidentia (prō"-sih-den'-shē-uh) – condition present when the uterus falls to the degree that the cervix protrudes from the vagina

progesterone (prō-jes'-ter-ōn) – a female hormone that prepares the uterus for the reception and development of the fertilized ovum by inducing secretion in the proliferated glands

pruritus (proo-ri'təs) – itching

pruritus vulvae (proo-ri'təs vul'və) – itching of the external female genitalia

pseudocyesis (soo"-dō-sī-ē'-sis) – a false pregnancy

pudendal (pu-den'-dul) – pertaining to the female genitalia

pudendal block – local anesthesia produced by blocking the pudendal nerves near the spinal processes of the ischium; used in obstetrics

pyometritis (pī"-ō-me-trī'-tis) – purulent inflammation of the uterus

retroflexion (reh"-trō-flek'-shun) – the bending backward of the body of the uterus toward the cervix

Retzius space (ret'-zē-us) – space in lower portion of abdomen between bladder and pubic bones and bounded superiorly by peritoneum

salpingectomy (sal"-pin-jek'-tuh-mē) – surgical removal of the uterine tube

salpingitis (sal"-pin-jī'-tus) – inflammation of the uterine tube

salpingo (sal-ping'-gō) – a combining form denoting relationship to a tube, specifically to the uterine or to the auditory tube

salpingo-oophorectomy (sal-ping"-gō-ō"-ō-fōr-ek'-tuh-mē) – surgical removal of a uterine tube and ovary

secundines (sek'-un-dī nz) – the afterbirth

sacral nerve stimulation (SNS) – a procedure in which an electrical stimulator is inserted under the skin above the buttocks; this stimulator is attached to electrodes that send pulses to a nerve in the sacrum, which plays a role in urinary bladder storage and emptying

Stein-Leventhal syndrome (stīn-lev'-en-thahl) – a clinical symptom complex characterized by secondary amenorrhea and anovulation (hence sterility); regularly associated with bilateral polycystic ovaries

subinvolution (sub"-in-vō-loo'-shun) – failure of a part to return to its normal size and condition after enlargement due to functional activity

suprapubic (soo"-pruh-pyoo'-bik) – situated or performed above the pubic arch

symphysis pubis (sim'-fih-sis) – the joint formed by union of the bodies of the pubic bones in the median plane by a thick mass of fibrocartilage

tenaculum (tē-nak'-yoo-lum) – a hook-like instrument for seizing and holding tissues

tension-free vaginal tape (TVT) – used at surgery to provide support for a drooping urethra, designed to prevent accidental release of urine

tocolysis (tō-kahl'-ī-sis) – inhibition of uterine contractions

toxemia (tok-sē'-mē-uh) – the clinical syndrome caused by toxic substances in the blood; a lay term referring to hypertensive disorders of pregnancy

transobturator tape (TOT) – surgical procedure employed to relieve stress incontinence; similar to TVT surgery

Trichomonas (trih-kō"-mō'-nus) – parasitic protozoa that cause urogenital infection; sometimes dictated "trich"

U

ultrasound (ul'-trah-sownd) – mechanical radiant energy with a frequency greater than 20,000 cycles per second

uterine prolapse (yoo"-ter-in proh"-laps) – protrusion of the uterus through the vaginal orifice

utero-ovarian (yoo"-ter-ō-ō-vār'-ē-un) – pertaining to the uterus and ovary

uterosacral ligament (yoo"-ter-ō-sā'-krul) – a part of the thickening of the visceral pelvic fascia beside the cervix and vagina, passing posteriorly in the rectouterine fold to attach to the front of the sacrum

uterovesical (yoo"-ter-ō-vess'-ih-kul) – pertaining to the uterus and bladder

vaginismus (vaj"ĭ-niz'məs) – painful spasm of the vagina due to involuntary contraction of the vaginal musculature, usually severe enough to prevent intercourse

vesicouterine (ves"-ih-kō-yoo'-ter-in) – pertaining to or communicating with the urinary bladder and the uterus

vesicovaginal (ves"-ih-kō-vaj'-ih-nul) – pertaining to the urinary bladder and vagina

vulva (vul'-vuh) – the external aspect of the female genitalia

vulvectomy (vul-vek'-tuh-mē) – surgical excision of the vulva

zygote (zī'-gōt) – the fertilized ovum

Transcription Tips

When transcribing obstetrics/gynecology dictation, become familiar with the organs of the female reproductive system, their locations, and their functions.

The female reproductive organs comprise the vulva, including the labia majora, the labia minora, and clitoris; the vagina; the uterus; two fallopian tubes; and two ovaries. The purpose of these organs is to produce ova, to nurture them after fertilization during their nine-month development period, and then to give birth with the proper delivery of the child and then the placenta. This part of the genitourinary system also secretes certain hormones for the maintenance of secondary sexual characteristics in the female.

Terms Used in Reference to Pregnancy

abort – the expulsion of an embryo or fetus before it is viable (syn. miscarry)

abortus – any or all products of conception

gravid – pregnant

gravida – a pregnant woman

multipara – a woman who has given birth at least twice to an infant, live born or not, weighing 500 g or more and having an estimated length of gestation of at least 20 weeks

nullipara – a woman who has not borne a child

para – a woman who has given birth to one or more infants

parity – the condition of having given birth, alive or dead

parturient – relating to or in the process of childbirth

placenta – fetomaternal organ of metabolic interchange between the embryo and mother; no direct mixing of fetal and maternal blood occurs, but the placental membrane allows the fetus to absorb nutrition, oxygen, and some harmful substances (like viruses) into the fetal blood along with the release of carbon dioxide and waste

primipara – a woman who has given birth for the first time

Supportive Web Sites

http://www.totalwomanhealth.com/glossary.php	Presents a glossary of OB/GYN terms.
http://www.medicaltranscription.com/ob-gyn-words.html	Contains an extensive list of OB/GYN terms, no definitions.
http://emedicine.medscape.com/obstetrics_gynecology	Contains links that can be accessed to read articles of various topics relating to OB/GYN.
http://www.wilkersonobgyn.com/gynoprocedures.html	Lists surgical procedures.
http://www.medsolution.com/content/surgery_urogen-TVT.asp	Provides a detailed description of the TVT procedure.
http://www.miklosandmoore.com/TOT.php#	Gives detailed description of the TOT procedure; click on "procedures" for links to different GYN procedures.
http://www.davincihysterectomy.com/hysterectomy-options/index.aspx	Information on this link concerns the different types of hysterectomies with a comparison to the da Vinci system.
http://www.mayoclinic.com	Under "Health information" click on "diseases & conditions"; then select the initial letter of a disease or condition in which you are interested.

Index of Obstetrics/Gynecology Reports

Exercise#	Patient Name	Type of Report/Procedure
TE#1	Jane Philbin	Unilateral left mammogram
TE#2	Brittney Davidson	OB: Preop H&P exam
TE#3	Brittney Davidson	OB: C-section delivery
TE#4	Kinsey R. Yerrington	Memorandum: Mammography results
TE#5	Merci Fernandez	Preop Consultation: Right breast lump
TE#6	Marianna Aponte	Preop H&P: Ovarian mass and metrorrhagia
TE#7	Susan Orlando	Discharge Summary: Colporrhaphy and perineorrhaphy
TE#8	Penelope Monroe	GYN: Excisional biopsy, right breast
TE#9	Teresa Haniskova	GYN: Port-A-Catheter placement
TE#10	Nell R. Lee	Lap-assisted vaginal hysterectomy with BSO and midurethral sling
TE#11	Angela M. Roseberry	da Vinci robotic-assisted hysterectomy with BSO
TE#12	Peggy A. Fraser	da Vinci robotic-assisted surgical procedures

CHAPTER 10

ORTHOPEDICS/ORTHOPEDIC SURGERY

Introduction

Orthopedics is the branch of medicine concerned with the preservation and restoration of the function of the *musculoskeletal system* and the treatment of muscular and skeletal diseases such as *poliomyelitis* and *muscular dystrophy.* Disorders of vertebral *disks, fractures, joint injuries,* correction of *deformities,* and diseases such as *arthritis* are also concerns of orthopedics.

The human body is made up of about 40 percent to 50 percent muscle and 206 bones. In the body, bones perform three major functions: They form the support framework, provide protection for internal organs, and make movement possible with the help of muscles. Bones are made up of approximately 50 percent water and 50 percent solid matter called *osseous tissue.*

Bones are classified into long, short, flat, irregular, and sesamoid. Features found in all bones include compact bone, periosteum, epiphysis, diaphysis, endosteum, medullary canal, and cancellous or spongy bone.

The *vertebral column* is made up of 26 separate bones called vertebrae, grouped in five segments from the base of the skull to the tailbone. The *spinal column* consists of 7 cervical, 12 thoracic, and 5 lumbar vertebrae. The *sacrum* is one fused vertebra, and the *coccyx,* or tailbone, is the last bone in the vertebral column. When the vertebral column is not aligned properly, 3 curvatures may occur—*scoliosis, lordosis,* and *kyphosis.*

A very serious bone abnormality, *osteoporosis,* is caused by a decrease in bone mass. This serious condition affects more than 25 million Americans. More women than men are affected by this disease process.

The muscles are connected to the bones, ligaments, cartilage, and skin either directly or through the intervention of fibrous structures called *tendons* or *fascia,* sometimes called *aponeuroses.*

Common operative procedures performed by orthopedists are hip replacements; knee replacements; open reductions and internal fixations (ORIFs); arthroscopy of the knee, shoulder, and joints (e.g., ankle, elbow, wrist); and amputations. *Arthroscopies* are some of the most common orthopedic procedures performed today. Orthopedic surgeons are now able to perform ligament reconstructions, meniscal repairs, and tendon repairs with the aid of an arthroscope.

Critical Thinking Exercise

A healthcare documentation specialist gives notice to the rather shaky transcription firm for which he has been working. They reply by demanding the company-owned laptop before giving him his final check. What to do? Give back the laptop and risk never getting paid? Keep the only collateral he has, demanding his final check be paid before turning over the equipment? Consult a lawyer?

Orthopedics/Orthopedic Surgery Abbreviations

The abbreviations, acronyms, and terms in the following abbreviations and terminology sections are often dictated in this specialty. We offer abbreviated definitions here. Please see an unabridged medical dictionary or the suggested web sites in this chapter for more information on each term.

ABDs	a type of plain gauze dressing	**CRNA**	certified registered nurse anesthetist
AC	acromioclavicular	**CTR**	carpal tunnel release
ACL	anterior cruciate ligament	**CVA**	costovertebral angle
AO	anterior oblique	**DI**	dorsal interossei
AP	anteroposterior	**DIPJ**	distal interphalangeal joint
APB	abductor pollicis brevis (tendon)	**DJD**	degenerative joint disease
AVN	avascular necrosis	**DP**	dorsalis pedis
C1	cervical vertebra, first	**DTR**	deep tendon reflex
C2	cervical vertebra, second	**DVT**	deep venous thrombosis
C3	cervical vertebra, third	**EPL**	extensor pollicis longus (tendon)
CAM	controlled ankle motion (a boot or walker used in patients with severe ankle injuries)	**Fx**	fracture
		FROM	full range of motion
CDH	congenital dislocation of hip	**FWB**	full weightbearing
CPM	continuous passive motion	**HD**	hip disarticulation
CPPD	calcium pyrophosphate deposition disease		

HNP	herniated nucleus pulposus
I&D	incision and drainage
IDK	internal derangement of the knee
IM	intramuscular
INR	international normalized ratio
IP	interphalangeal
IPJ	interphalangeal joint
IT	iliotibial
KB	knee bearing
KD	knee disarticulation
KJ	knee jerk
L1	lumbar vertebra, first
L2	lumbar vertebra, second
L3	lumbar vertebra, third
LAC	long arm cast
LLC	long leg cast
LLCC	long leg cylinder cast
LOM	limitation or loss of motion
MCP	metacarpophalangeal
MPJ	metacarpophalangeal joint
MS	musculoskeletal
NWB	nonweightbearing
OA	osteoarthritis
OATS	osteochondral autograft transfer system (surgical procedure)
ORIF	open reduction, internal fixation
PCL	posterior cruciate ligament

PEMFS	pulsing electromagnetic fields
PIPJ	proximal interphalangeal joint
PMR	physical medicine and rehabilitation
PWB	partial weight bearing
RA	rheumatoid arthritis
RF	radiofrequency
ROM	range of motion
RUE	right upper extremity
SAC	short arm cast
SACH foot	solid ankle, cushioned heel (type of prosthetic foot that allows flexion, extension, inversion, and eversion)
SCFE	slipped capital femoral epiphysis
SD	shoulder disarticulation
SERF	Severity of Exacerbation and Risk Factors
SLAP lesion	superior labral anteroposterior (shoulder) lesion
SLC	short leg cast
SLR	straight leg raising
T1	thoracic vertebra, first
T2	thoracic vertebra, second
T3	thoracic vertebra, third
TENS	transcutaneous electrical nerve stimulation (unit)
THR	total hip replacement
TJ	triceps jerk
Tx	traction

Anatomic Illustrations

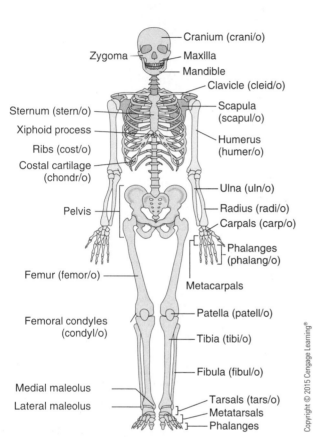

FIGURE 10-1   Skeletal system

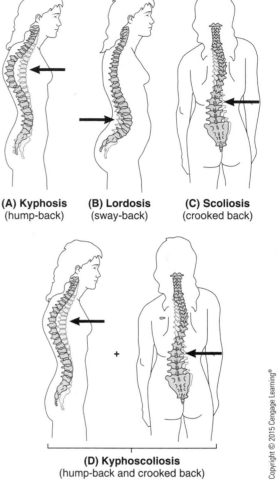

(A) Kyphosis (hump-back)   **(B) Lordosis** (sway-back)   **(C) Scoliosis** (crooked back)

(D) Kyphoscoliosis (hump-back and crooked back)

FIGURE 10-2   Abnormal curvatures of the vertebral column

Orthopedics/Orthopedic Surgery Terminology

A

acetabulum (as"-eh-tab'-yoo-lum) – a cup-shaped bony recess in the ilium that holds the head of the femur

achondroplasia (ā-kon"-drō-plā'-zē-uh) – a hereditary, congenital disturbance of epiphyseal chondroblastic growth and maturation, causing inadequate enchondral bone formation and resulting in a peculiar form of dwarfism with short limbs, normal trunk, small face, normal vault, lordosis, and trident hand

acromion process (ə-krō'me-ən) – the outer end of the spine of the scapula that protects the glenoid cavity; forms the outer edge of the shoulder, and articulates with the clavicle

AlloAnchor RC™ (al'-ō-ang'-ker) – a graft of tissue (allograft) machined from cortical bone and used in soft tissue reattachment for rotator cuff repair

amphiarthrosis (am"fe-ahr-thro'sis) – a type of articulation between bony surfaces that permits limited motion and is connected by ligaments or elastic cartilage, such as that between the vertebrae

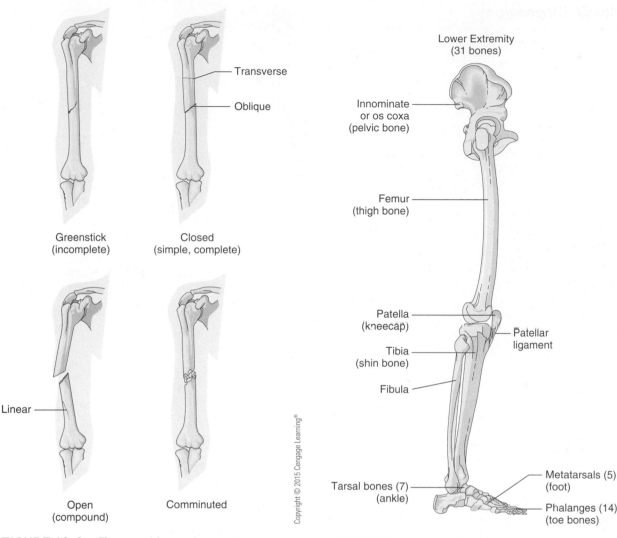

FIGURE 10-3   Types of bone fractures

Transverse

Oblique

Greenstick
(incomplete)

Closed
(simple, complete)

Linear

Open
(compound)

Comminuted

Lower Extremity
(31 bones)

Innominate
or os coxa
(pelvic bone)

Femur
(thigh bone)

Patella
(kneecap)

Patellar
ligament

Tibia
(shin bone)

Fibula

Tarsal bones (7)
(ankle)

Metatarsals (5)
(foot)

Phalanges (14)
(toe bones)

FIGURE 10-4   Lower extremity (31 bones)

ankylosis (ang"kə-lo'sis) – stiffness or fixation of a joint by disease or surgery

antalgic gait (ant-al'-jik) – a limp characteristic of recovered cases of coxalgia, noted by avoidance of weightbearing on the affected side

aponeurosis (ā"-pō-nyoo-rō'-sis) – the end of a muscle where it becomes a tendon; the tendon attaches the muscle to bone

arthroclasia (ar"-thrō-klā'-zē-uh) – the surgical breaking down of an ankylosis in order to secure free movement in a joint

arthrodesis (ar"-thrō-dē'-sis) – the surgical fixation of a joint by a procedure designed to accomplish fusion of the joint surfaces by promoting the proliferation of bone cells

arthrogryposis (ar"-thrō-grī-pō'-sis) – persistent flexure or contracture of a joint

astragalus (uh-strag'-uh-lus) – the ankle bone (talus)

Austin Moore prosthesis (prahs-thē'-sis) – artificial device used for hip fractures

boutonnière injury (bü-tən-ir) – deformity of finger characterized by flexion of the proximal interphalangeal joint and hyperextension of the distal joint; also called buttonhole deformity

brachiocrural (bra"ke-o-kroo'rəl) – pertaining to the arm and leg

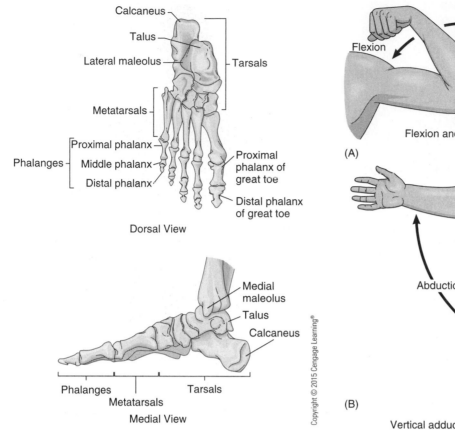

Calcaneus

Talus

Lateral maleolus

Tarsals

Metatarsals

Phalanges
Proximal phalanx
Middle phalanx
Distal phalanx

Proximal phalanx of great toe

Distal phalanx of great toe

Dorsal View

Medial maleolus

Talus

Calcaneus

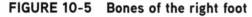

Phalanges   Tarsals

Metatarsals

Medial View

FIGURE 10-5   Bones of the right foot

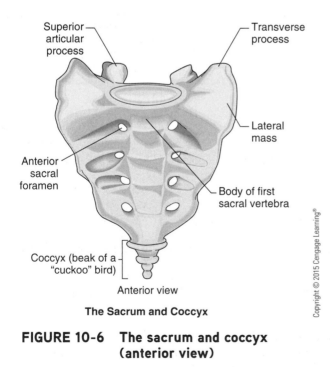

Superior articular process

Transverse process

Lateral mass

Anterior sacral foramen

Body of first sacral vertebra

Coccyx (beak of a "cuckoo" bird)

Anterior view

The Sacrum and Coccyx

FIGURE 10-6   The sacrum and coccyx (anterior view)

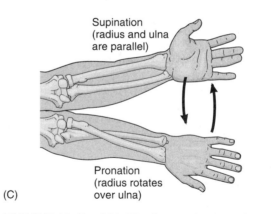

Flexion   Extension

Flexion and extension of forearm

(A)

Adduction

Abduction

(B)

Vertical adduction and abduction of arm

Supination (radius and ulna are parallel)

Pronation (radius rotates over ulna)

(C)

FIGURE 10-7   (A) Flexion and extension of the forearm; (B) Vertical adduction and abduction of the arm; (C) Pronation and supination of the hand

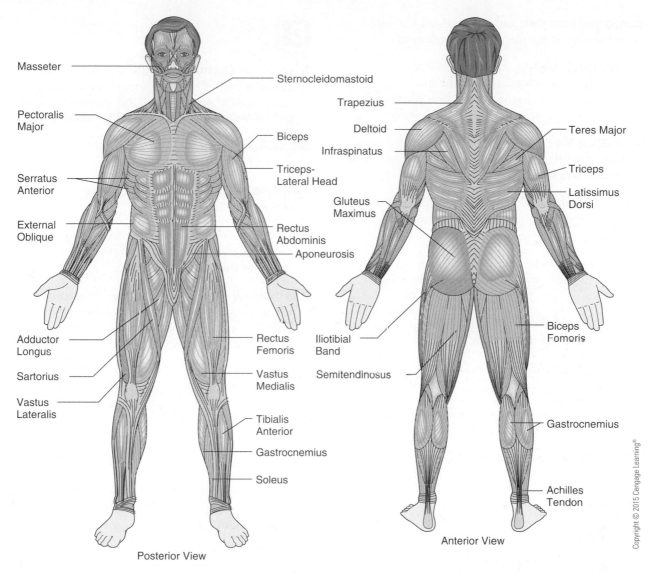

Masseter
Pectoralis Major
Serratus Anterior
External Oblique
Adductor Longus
Sartorius
Vastus Lateralis
Sternocleidomastoid
Biceps
Triceps-Lateral Head
Rectus Abdominis
Aponeurosis
Rectus Femoris
Vastus Medialis
Tibialis Anterior
Gastrocnemius
Soleus

Posterior View

Trapezius
Deltoid
Infraspinatus
Gluteus Maximus
Iliotibial Band
Semitendinosus
Teres Major
Triceps
Latissimus Dorsi
Biceps Femoris
Gastrocnemius
Achilles Tendon

Anterior View

Copyright © 2015 Cengage Learning®

FIGURE 10-8 Posterior and anterior views of the muscles

bursa (pl. bursae) (ber'-suh [ber'-see]) – a sac or sac-like cavity filled with a viscid fluid and situated at places in the tissues at which friction would otherwise develop

bursectomy (bər-sek'tə-me) – surgical excision of a bursa

C

C-arm fluoroscopy (floo"-ur-os'-kuh-pē) – x-ray equipment that can be rotated over or under a patient without moving the patient; provides a constant view of the bone

calcaneoapophysitis (kal-ka'-nē-ō-uh-pof"-ih-zī'-tis) – a diseased condition of the posterior part of the calcaneus marked by pain at the point of insertion of the Achilles tendon with swelling of the soft parts

callus (kal-əs) – noun; a composite mass of tissue that forms at a fracture site to establish continuity between the bone ends (syn. callosity)

callous (kal-əs) – adj.; relating to a callus, as in callous formation

calvaria (kal-vā'-rē-uh) – the dome-like superior portion of the cranium

capitellum (kap"-ih-tel'-um) – an eminence on the distal end of the lateral epicondyle of the humerus for articulation with the head of the radius

capsuloplasty (kap'-syoo-lō-plas"-tē) – rearrangement or reshaping of a capsule; a plastic operation on a joint capsule

carpometacarpal (kar"-pō-met"-uh-kar'-pul) – pertaining to the carpus and metacarpus

chemonucleolysis (kē"-mō-noo'-klē-ō-lī'-sis) – the enzymatic dissolution of the nucleus pulpous by injection of chymopapain; procedure used in the treatment of intervertebral disk lesions

chondrolysis (kahn-drahl'-ih-sis) – the degeneration of cartilage cells that occurs in the process of intracartilaginous ossification

chondromalacia (kahn"-drō-muh-lā'-shēē-uh) – softening of the articular cartilage, most frequently in the patella

chymopapain (kī"-mō-puh-pā'-in) – an enzyme from the latex of a tree chiefly found in the tropics

coarctation splint (ko"ahrk-ta'shən) – pressed together, made tight, restrained

coccydynia (kok"-sē-dī'-nē-uh) – pain in the coccyx and neighboring region (syn. coccygodynia)

coccyx (kok'-siks) – the terminal bony complex of the caudal end of the vertebral column composed of three to five fused bones

condyle (kahn'-dīl) – a rounded projection on a bone

coracoacromial (kor"-uh-kō-ā-krō'-mē-ul) – pertaining to the coracoid and acromion processes

coracoclavicular (kor"-uh-kō-klah-vik'-yoo-lur) – pertaining to the coracoid process and the clavicle

coracoclavicular ligament (klə-,vik'-yə-lər- [OR -kla-,vik'-yə-lər]) – a ligament that joins the clavicle and the coracoid

CorIS Interference Screw™ (kōr'-iss in"-ter-fẽr'-ens) – a device machined from allograft cortical bone and designed to reattach soft tissue grafts to bone in the knee

costovertebral (kos"-tō-ver'-tē-bral) – pertaining to a rib and a vertebra

coxalgia (koks-al'-jē-uh) – hip-joint disease; pain in the hip

crepitation (krep"-ih-tā'-shun) – the noise made by the rubbing together of the ends of a fractured bone

de Quervain tenosynovitis (duh-kwor'-van ten"-ō-sin"-ō-vī'-tis) – inflammation caused by narrowness of common tendon sheath of abductor pollicis longus and extensor pollicis brevis

deossification (dē-ahs"-ih-fih-kā'-shun) – loss of or removal of the mineral elements of bone

diathesis (dī-af'-ih-sis) – the long, narrow shaft of the bone

diarthroses (di"ahr-thro'sēz) – any of several types of bone articulation permitting free motion in a joint, as that of the shoulder or hip

diastasis (dī-as'-tuh-sis) – a form of dislocation in which there is separation of two bones normally attached to each other without the existence of a true joint, as in separation of the pubic symphysis

diskectomy (dis-kek'-tuh-mē) – surgical removal of a herniated intervertebral disk (**NB**: *disk* is used in every specialty except ophthalmology, in which *disc* is used)

diskogram (dis'-kō-gram) – an x-ray of the intervertebral disk

Dupuytren contracture (doo-pwē-truhn) – shortening, thickening, and fibrosis of the palmar fascia, producing a flexion deformity of a finger

enarthrosis (en"-ar-thrō'-sis) – a joint in which the globular head of one bone is received into a socket in another, as in the hip joint

en bloc resection (awn blahk' rē-sek'-shun) – process whereby a malignant tumor is surgically removed in a lump or whole, sometimes along with a large area of surrounding tissue or lymph nodes

enchondromatosis (en-kahn"-drō-muh-tō'-sis) – a condition characterized by hamartomatous proliferation of cartilage cells within the metaphysis of several bones causing thinning of the overlying cortex and distortion of the growth in length

epicondyle (ep"ĭ-kon'dīl) – an eminence upon a bone above its condyle

epidurogram (ep"ĭ-doo'-ro-gram) – record of an x-ray of the spine

epiduroscopy (ep"ĭ-doo'-ros'kə-pe) – insertion of an endoscope into the epidural space, usually in the lumbar region, for the administration of drugs or radiologic visualization

epiphyseal (ep"-ī-fiz'-ē-ul) – adj.; pertaining to or of the nature of an epiphysis

epiphysis (ē-pih'-fih-sis) – noun; the knob-like end of a long bone

exarticulation (eks"-ar-tik-yoo-lā'-shun) – amputation at a joint; removal of a portion of a joint

exostosis (pl. exostoses) (eks"-ō-stō'-sis [eks"-ō-stō'-seez]) – a benign bony growth projecting outward from the surface of a bone, characteristically capped by cartilage

fasciculation (fah-sik"-yoo-lā'-shun) – the formation of small bundles of nerves, muscles, or tendon fibers

fasciotomy (fash"-ē-ot'-uh-mē) – a surgical incision or transection of fascia

genu valgum (jē'-noo val'-gum) – a deformity in which the knees are abnormally close together and the space between the ankles is increased; known also as knock-knee

glenohumeral (glē"-nō-hyoo'-mer-ul) – pertaining to the glenoid cavity and to the humerus

H

hallux (hal'-uks) – the great toe, or first digit of the foot

hallux valgus (hal'-uks val'-gus) – everted foot; displacement of the great toe toward the other toes

hallux varus (hal'-uks vā'-rus) – displacement of the great toe away from the other toes

HANA™ table (ha'-nuh) – a special operating table used in performing anterior approach hip replacement surgery; allows the surgeon to manipulate the patient's leg to allow for the movement of muscles versus cutting and detaching muscle around the hip joint; the HANA table also allows the surgeon to take x-rays during the procedure to ensure precise fit and placement of all components, resulting in less recovery time and a smaller incision

hematopoietic (hem"ə-to-poi-et'ik) – of, relating to, or involved in the formation of blood cells

heterotopic (het"ər-o-top'ik) – occurring in an abnormal place

humeroradial (hyoo"-mer-ō-rā'-dē-ul) – pertaining to the humerus and the radius

humeroscapular (hyoo"-mer-ō-skap'-yoo-lur) – pertaining to the humerus and the scapula

hydrarthrosis (hī"-drar-thrō'-sis) – an accumulation of watery fluid in the cavity of a joint

hyperbaric (hi"pər-bar'ik) – pertaining to pressure of ambient gases greater than one atmosphere; concerning solutions more dense than the diluent or medium; e.g., in spinal anesthesia a hyperbaric solution has a density greater than that of spinal fluid

hyperesthesia (hi"pər-es-the'zhə) – increased sensitivity, particularly a painful sensation from a normally painless touch stimulus

hypesthesia (hīp"es-the'zhə) – hypoesthesia; abnormally decreased sensitivity, particularly to touch

IDET procedure (i'-det) – intradiskal electrothermal therapy; a minimally invasive outpatient surgical procedure for treatment of patients with chronic low back pain caused by tears or small herniations of the lumbar disks

iliotibial (il"-ē-ō-tib'-ē-ul) – pertaining to or extending between the ilium and tibia

ilium (il'-ē -um) – the broad, flaring portion of the hip bone (*NB*: do not confuse this word with *ileum*, the third portion of the small intestine)

Ilizarov external fixation (ihl"-ih-zahr'-ahv) – used externally to hold broken bones in place until they have healed; there are many Ilizarov orthopedic devices and techniques

interosseous (in"-ter-os'-ē -us) – between bones

intertrochanteric (in"-ter-trō"-kan-tār'-ik) – situated in or pertaining to the space between the greater and the lesser trochanter

intramedullary (in"-truh-med'-yoo-lār"-ē) – within the spinal cord, marrow cavity of a bone, or within the medulla oblongata of the brain

ischium (is'-kē-um) – the inferior dorsal part of the hip bone

kyphoplasty (kī'-fō-plas"-tē) – the vertebroplasty procedure

kyphoscoliosis (kī"-fō-skō"-lē-ō'-sis) – backward and lateral curvature of the spinal column, as in vertebral osteochondrosis

kyphosis (kī-fō'-sis) – outward curvature of the upper portion of the spine; also known as hunchback

LactoSorb™ copolymer (lak'-tō-sōrb kō-pahl'-ē-mer) – resorbable bone material

laminectomy (lam"-ih-nek'-tuh-mē) – excision of the posterior arch of a vertebra

latissimus (lah-tis'-ih-mus) – a general term denoting a broad structure, as a muscle

malleolus (mah-lē'-ō-lus) – a rounded process, such as the protuberance on each side of the ankle joint

McMurray test (mak-mur'-ē) – rotation of the tibia on the femur to determine injury to meniscal structures

meniscectomy (men"-ih-sek'-tuh-mē) – surgical removal of the meniscus

meniscus (meh-nis'-kus) – a disk of fibrocartilage found in certain joints

metacarpophalangeal joint (met"ə-kahr"po-fə-lan'je-əl) – relating to or involving both the metacarpus and the phalanges

metaphysis (meh-taf'-ih-sis) – the wider part at the extremity of the shaft of a long bone, adjacent to the epiphyseal disk

methyl methacrylate bone cement (meth'-il meth-ak'-rih-lāt") – glue used to hold artificial prostheses in place (total hip, etc.)

myasthenia (mī"-as-thē'-nē-uh) – muscular debility

myelomeningocele (mī"-ē-lō-meh-ning'-gō-sēl) – hernial protrusion of the cord and its meninges through a defect in the vertebral canal

myesthesia (mī"-es-thē'-zē-uh) – muscle sensibility; consciousness of muscle contraction

myositis ossificans (mī"-ō-sī'-tis ah-sif'-ih-kanz) – a condition in which the healing lesion creates new bone formed in the muscle; may occur as the result of repeated injury or severe injury to a muscle

Navitrack™ system (nav'-ih–trak) – computer-assisted surgery system that provides real-time three-dimensional visualizaton for navigation during orthopedic surgery; used in total hip and knee replacements, anterior cruciate ligament procedures, and spinal surgeries

olecranon (ō-lek'-ruh-non) – the proximal bony projection of the ulna at the elbow; also known as the "funny bone"

ossification (ah"-sih-fih-kā'-shun) – the conversion of muscle into a bony substance

osteoarthrotomy (ah"-stē-ō-ar-throt'-uh-mē) – excision of an articular end of a bone

osteochondritis (ah"-stē-ō-kon-drī'-tis) – inflammation of both bone and cartilage

osteoclasia (ah"-stē-ō-klā'-zē-uh) – the absorption and destruction of bony tissue; surgical fracture of a bone done to correct a deformity

osteodystrophy (ah"-stē-ō-dis'-truh-fē) – defective bone formation

osteomyelitis (ah"-stē-ō-mī"-eh-lī'-tis) – inflammation of bone and bone marrow usually caused by a pus-forming bacteria

osteoporosis (ah"-stē-ō-pō-rō'-sis) – a disease characterized by an abnormal absorption of bone

osteonecrosis (os"te-o-nə-kro'sis) – the death of bone in mass, as distinguished from caries, which is the microscopic destruction of teeth

osteotomy (ah"-stē-ot'-uh-mē) – cutting or transecting bone

Paget disease (paj'-et) – a degenerative disease of bone, cause unknown, with associated inflammation and resultant deformity

patellofemoral (pah-tel"-ō-fem'-ur-ul) – relating to the patella and femur

perichondrium (pār"-ih-kahn'-drē-um) – the layer of dense fibrous connective tissue that surrounds all cartilage except the articular cartilage of synovial joints

periosteum (pār"-ē-os'-tē-um) – a tough fibrous membrane that covers the outside of the diaphysis

Perthes disease (per'-tēz) – osteonecrosis of the of the upper end of the femur (syn. Legg-Calvé-Perthes disease)

polydactylism (pol-ē-dak'-til-izm) – a developmental anomaly characterized by the presence of too many fingers on the hands or toes on the feet

polymyositis (pol"-ē-mī"-ō-sī'-tis) – inflammation of several or many muscles at once

porosis (pō-rō'-sis) – the formation of callus in the repair of a fractured bone

pseudoarthrosis (soo"-dō-ar-thrō'-sis) – a false joint

psoas (sō'-az) – a muscle in the back wall of the abdomen

Pulsavac™ lavage debridement system (pul'-suh-vak lah-vahzh' dā-brēd'-mawn) – system used to irrigate operative wounds with pulsation-type action

rachitis (rah-kī'-tis) – inflammatory disease of the vertebral column

rhabdomyoma (rab"-dō-mī-ō'-muh) – a benign tumor of striated muscle

RIO Robotic Arm Interactive Orthopedic System™ (ree'-o) – enables the surgeon to preoperatively plan the alignment and placement of knee resurfacing implants and to intraoperatively sculpt complex, anatomic, tissue-sparing and bone-conserving cuts accurately; utilized in the MAKOplasty™ procedure.

rongeur (raw-zhur') – an instrument used for cutting tissue, particularly bone

sarcolemma (sar"-kō-lem'-uh) – the delicate plasma membrane that surrounds every striated muscle fiber

scapulothoracic (skap"u-lo-thə-ras'ik) – of or relating to the scapula and the thorax

Scheuermann disease (kyphosis) (shoy'-er-mun dihzēz' kī-fō'-sis) – osteochondrosis of vertebral epiphyses in juveniles

sciatica (sī-at'-ih-kuh) – a syndrome characterized by pain radiating from the back into the buttock and into the lower extremity along its posterior or lateral aspect; also used to refer to pain anywhere along the course of the sciatic nerve

scoliosis (skō"-lē-ō'-sis) – a lateral or sideways curvature of the spinal column

sequestrectomy (sē"-kwes-trek'-tuh-mē) – surgical removal of dead bone

sequestrum (sē-kwes'-trum) – a piece of dead bone that has become separated from the healthy or living bone during the process of necrosis

sesamoid (ses'-uh-moyd) – denoting a small nodular bone embedded in a tendon or joint capsule

sphenoid (sfē'-noyd) – designating a very irregular wedge-shaped bone at the base of the skull

spina bifida (spī'-nuh bif'-ih-duh) – a developmental anomaly characterized by defective closure of the bony encasement of the spinal cord through which the cord and meninges may or may not protrude

spondylitis (spahn"-dih-lī'-tis) – inflammation of the vertebrae

spondylodesis (spahn"-dih- lō-deh'-sis) – the operation of fusing vertebrae

spondylolisthesis (spahn"-dih-lō-lis"-thē'-sis) – forward subluxation of the body of one of the lower lumbar vertebrae onto the vertebra below it or onto the sacrum

Stryker ADM™ hip cup (stri'kər) – this replacement component used in hip surgery allows the doctor to more closely match the implant to the patient's anatomy, providing for more natural movement.

Stryker SERFAS Energy Probe™ (stri'kər) – surgical equipment, a probe or wand

Stryker SERFAS Radiofrequency Ablation System™ (stri'kər) – surgical equipment used in anterior cruciate ligament (knee) repair

supracondylar (soo"-pruh-kahn'-dih-lur) – situated above a condyle or condyles

supraspinatus (soo"-pruh-spī-a'-tus) – a muscle in the back of the shoulder that helps make up the rotator cuff

supraspinous (soo"-pruh-spī'-nus) – situated above a spine or a spinous process

sural nerve (soo'-rul) – the nerve in the skin on the back of the leg and skin and joints on the lateral side of the heel and foot

Suretac™ system (shoor'-tak) – method for fracture fixation

symphysis joint (sim'-fih-sis) – permits slight movement

synarthrosis (sin"ahr-thro'sis) – a form of articulation in which the bones are rigidly joined by fibrous tissue

synchondrosis (sin"-kahn-drō'-sis) – a type of cartilaginous joint that is usually temporary; the intervening hyaline cartilage is ordinarily converted into bone before adulthood

syndactylia (sin"-dak-til'-ē-uh) – the most common congenital anomaly of the hand, marked by persistence of the webbing between adjacent digits so they are more or less completely attached

syndesmosis (sin"-des-mō'-sis) – a type of fibrous joint in which the intervening fibrous connective tissue forms as an interosseous membrane or ligament

synovium (sih-nō'-vē-um) – a synovial membrane; a membrane that secretes a transparent alkaline viscid fluid resembling the white of an egg

talipes (tal'-ih-pēz) – a congenital deformity of the foot, which is twisted out of shape or position

tendinitis (ten"-dih-ni'-tis) – inflammation of tendons and of tendon-muscle attachments

tendolysis (ten-dol'-ih-sis) – the operation of freeing a tendon from its adhesions

tenodesis (ten-od'-eh-sis) – tendon fixation; suturing the end of a tendon to a bone

tibiofibular (tib"-ē-ō-fib'-yoo-lur) – pertaining to the tibia and the fibula

torticollis (tor"-tih-kol'-is) – wryneck; a contracted state of the cervical muscles, producing twisting of the neck and an unnatural position of the head

tuberosity (too"bə-ros'ĭ-te) – a large bump on a bone usually serving for the attachment of muscles or ligaments

tuberous (too'bər-əs) – characterized by or being knobby or nodular lesions

Unna™ boot, Unna™ paste boot (oo'-nuh) – a dressing for varicose ulcers consisting of a paste applied to the entire leg, then covered with a spiral bandage, which is then given a coat of the paste

valgus (val'-gus) – bent outward, twisted; the term is an adjective and should be used only with the noun it describes, as talipes valgus, genu valgum, etc.

varus (vā'-rus) – bent inward; the term is an adjective and should be used only with the noun it describes, as talipes varus, genu varum, etc.

vertebra (ver'-teh-bruh) – any of the 33 bones of the spinal column

vertebroplasty (ver"-teh-brō-plass'-tē) – a nonsurgical method for the repair of back fractures caused by osteoporosis

Xia™ spinal system (zē'-uh) – a comprehensive system of implants and instruments for stabilization of the spine in the thoracic, lumbar, and sacral regions

xiphoid process (zī'-foyd) – the pointed bottom part of the sternum or breastbone

Transcription Tips

When transcribing orthopedics dictation, it is helpful to be familiar with the location and names of the major bones, joints, and muscles of the musculoskeletal system. Acquiring knowledge of the skeletal system and body movements will enhance the accuracy of your transcription skills. The following information is provided to help students learn this specialty, including supportive web sites.

Glossary of the Skeletal System

articulation – joint

brachial – pertaining to the arm

carpus – wrist

clavicle – collarbone

coccyx – tailbone

femur – thigh bone

fibula – calf bone

frontal bone – forehead

humerus – upper arm bone

ilium – upper hip bone

ischium – lower hip bone

malar – cheekbone

mandible – lower jawbone

maxilla – upper jawbone

metacarpus – the part of the skeleton between the wrist and the finger

metatarsus – the part of the skeleton between the ankle and the toes

occipital bone – the base of the skull

parietal bones – the two bones forming upper sides of the skull

patella – kneecap

periosteum – the membrane around the bones

phalanx – one of the bones of a finger or toe

radius – the bone of the forearm located on the thumb side

sacrum – the bone just below the lumbar vertebrae and above the coccyx

scapula – the shoulder blade

scoliosis – abnormal lateral curvature of the spine

sternum – the breast bone

symphysis pubis – the junction of the pubic bones

tarsus – the ankle

temporal bones – the two bones forming part of the lateral surfaces and base of the skull

tibia – the shin bone

ulna – the larger bone of the forearm located opposite the thumb side

vertebra – a bone of the spinal column

Whereas the skeletal system provides a frame for the body and the flexibility of the joints, the muscular system gives a new dimension to the mobility of the skeleton.

Glossary of the Muscular System

active movement – voluntary movement involving the contraction of muscles with energy supplied by the patient

ambulation – walking

antagonist – a muscle that opposes the action of another muscle

asthenia – weakness

contracture – a shortened or distorted muscle

deltoid – the triangular muscle that invests the shoulder

fascia – a band of tissue enveloping muscles and certain organs of the body

flaccid – limp

gastrocnemius – the calf muscle

gluteus – the buttock muscle

involuntary muscle – a muscle that is not controlled by the patient

ligament – a strong band of fibrous tissue that holds bones to bones or supports large organs

muscle – an organ that produces movement by contracting

myodiastasis – separation of a muscle

myoedema – swelling or edema of a muscle

myogelosis – hardening of a muscle

myotasis – stretching of muscle

passive movement – any movement involving the contraction of muscles with the energy to do so supplied from an outside source

pectoralis major and pectoralis minor – chest muscles

popliteus – muscle posterior to the knee

spasm – an involuntary contraction of a muscle

sphincter – a ring-like band of muscle fibers that closes a natural orifice

synergist – a muscle that acts together with another

tendon – a strong, fibrous band of tissue that attaches muscle to bone

tone, tonus – slight, continuous contraction of muscle

voluntary muscle – a muscle that is controlled by the patient

Glossary of Body Movements

abduction – drawing away from the midline (often dictated "a-b-duction")

adduction – drawing toward the midline (often dictated "a-d-duction")

circumduction – circular movement

extension – straightening

flexion – bending

hyperextension – extreme or excessive straightening

lateral rotation – turning away from the midline

medial rotation – turning toward the midline

pronation – the act of turning the palm or sole of the foot backward or downward

supination – the act of turning the palm or sole of the foot forward or upward

Classifications of Bone Fractures (Selected)

Colles – a break in the distal part of the radius

comminuted – a fracture where the bone is shattered into fragments

compound (or open) – a fracture where bone protrudes through the skin

compression – a fracture occurring in vertebrae, generally caused by falling on the tailbone

epiphyseal – occurs where the matrix is calcifying and chondrocytes are dying and fractures occur through this growth plate

greenstick – a fracture where one side of the bone is broken and the other side bent

Potts – a break in the ankle that affects both bones of the lower leg

simple (or closed) – the fracture where bone does not protrude through the skin

spiral – a fracture, caused by twisting stresses, that extends along the length of the bone

stress – micro-cracks that occur in the bone as a result of the body not producing enough bone

transverse – the fracture occurring when a shaft bone breaks across its long axis

Types of Joints

There are three general morphologic types of joints: fibrous, cartilaginous, and synovial.

- **amphiarthrosis (also called symphysis)** – form of cartilaginous joint in which union between two bones is effected by means of fibrocartilage
- **diarthrosis (synovial joint)** – permits free movement in many directions, such as in the hip, knee, wrist, foot, and elbow

- **synarthrosis** – an immovable union of rigid components, as in the skeletal system, including fibrous joints

Types of Splints (Selected)

acrylic
AirFlex carpal tunnel
airplane (also aeroplane)
aluminum bridge, fence, or finger-cot
anterior acute-flexion elbow
Aquaplast
baseball or baseball finger
birdcage
Brooke Army Hospital
buddy
Bunnell hand, finger, or knuckle-bender
calibrated clubfoot
Colles
Curry walking
Darco toe alignment
Denis Browne clubfoot or talipes hobble
dental
Denver nasal
DePuy open-thimble or rocking-leg
drop foot
elephant-ear clavicle
eZY WRAP
Flexisplint flexed-arm board
hand cock-up

Hirschtick utility shoulder
INRO surgical nail
Kanavel cock-up
Kirschner-wire
Magnuson abduction humerus
O'Donaghue knee or stirrup
Ortho Tech cock-up wrist
outrigger
Radstat wrist
Rolyan Gel Shell
Slattery-McGrouther dynamic flexion
synergistic wrist motion
T-finger
talipes hobble
Teare arm sling
Thumz'Up functional thumb
U-splint
utility shoulder
Velcro
von Rosen hip
Versi-Splint
wraparound
Xomed Silastic
Zim-Trac traction

Supportive Web Sites

http://www.chiroone.net/why_chiropractic/index.html	An interesting site where you can learn how each vertebra is connected to specific areas, organs and functions of your body.
http://orthoinfo.aaos.org/topic.cfm?topic=a00095	Select the link on the left for an extensive glossary of orthopedic terms; you can also access links to diseases and syndromes and many other orthopedics topics.
http://www.howmedica.com	Click on links to different kinds of orthopedic products.
http://www.mtdesk.com	Click on "sample reports" to see reports from different specialties.
http://orthopedics.about.com/od/orthopedicsinformation/a/companies.htm	Contains information on implants used in orthopedics.
http://www.surgery.com/guide/orthopedic-surgery/procedurescontains	Provides links to types of orthopedic surgical procedures.
http://www.mayoclinic.com	Under "Health information" click on "diseases & conditions"; then select the initial letter of a disease or condition in which you are interested.

Index of Orthopedics and Orthopedic Surgery Reports

Exercise#	Patient Name	Type of Report/Procedure
TE#1	Sandra M. Counselor	History and Physical: Multiple injuries
TE#2	Eric Alonso	HPIP Followup Note: Rash
TE#3	Pamela Jean Conrad	Preoperative H&P: Right knee injury
TE#4	Pamela Jean Conrad	Surgery: Arthroscopy, left knee
TE#5	Melissa Anne Bravo	Surgery: Foot surgery
TE#6	Jason C. Barnes	Surgery: I&D, osteomyelitis
TE#7	Matthew Johnson	Surgical Procedure: Lumbar puncture
TE#8	Kathryn H. Phoenix	Clinic Note: Evaluation of right shoulder
TE#9	Peter Dumas	Emergent Consultation: Reinjured broken arm

CHAPTER 11
ARTHRITIS/RHEUMATOLOGY

Introduction

Arthritis, defined as "inflammation of a joint," is a general term for various types of joint diseases. Three common types of arthritis include osteoarthritis, rheumatoid arthritis, and ankylosing spondylitis.

Osteoarthritis (OA) is a noninflammatory degenerative joint disease seen mainly in middle-aged to elderly persons. Aggravating factors include overuse of joints, obesity, or simply aging. The breakdown of cartilage, which is designed to cushion the ends of bones, causes the bones to rub together. This occurs commonly in the knees, hips, feet, and spine. OA is accompanied by pain, usually after prolonged activity, or stiffness, especially in the morning or with inactivity. OA is said to affect nearly 27 million Americans and 151 million people worldwide.

Rheumatoid arthritis (RA) is an autoimmune disease, which means that it is caused by a malfunction in the body's immune system that causes it to attack, break down cartilage, and damage the joints. RA is the most common type of inflammatory arthritis; chronic inflammation can lead to severe joint damage and deformities. Areas most commonly affected include hands, wrists, elbows, shoulders, knees, ankles, feet, jaw, and the spine. Research indicates that more than 1.3 million Americans are affected, about 75% of whom are women.

Ankylosing spondylitis (AS) is described as being an arthritis-related joint disease. Although the specific cause is unknown, genetics is thought to be involved in its development. This type of arthritis affects the spine and, if severe enough, can cause the spine to fuse, resulting in an unbending spine. AS is said to affect approximately 350,000 Americans, mostly men.

Rheumatology is the branch of medicine that deals with rheumatic disorders. These conditions are marked by inflammation, degeneration, or metabolic derangement of connective tissue structures of the body, especially the joints and related structures, including muscles, bursae, tendons, and fibrous tissue. These structures become afflicted with pain, stiffness, and eventually limitation of motion.

Critical Thinking Exercise

A person on public transportation has disfigured hands and fingers (see illustration on page 163). This person has trouble getting a token out of a pocket and into the machine. What other challenges might this person face? Could they live alone? Manage their ADLs? Shop and do laundry? Take medications properly? Hold down a job? What resources are available in your community?

Arthritis/Rheumatology Terminology and Abbreviations

The abbreviations, acronyms, and terms in the following list of terms and abbreviations are often dictated in this specialty. We offer abbreviated definitions here. Please see an unabridged medical dictionary or the suggested web sites in this chapter for more information on each term.

A

ADLs – activities of daily living

ANA – antinuclear antibodies; frequently found in rheumatoid arthritis, scleroderma, Sjögren syndrome, and mixed connective tissue disease

ankylosing spondylitis (ang"kə-lo'sing spon"də-li'tis) – abbreviated AS, this is a form of degenerative joint disease (DJD) that affects the spine; a systemic illness of unknown etiology affecting young persons predominantly; also called Marie-Strümpell syndrome

aphtha (af'thə) – (noun) a small ulcer on a mucous membrane; pl. aphthae

aphthous (af'thəs) – (adj.) characterized by or relating to aphthae or aphthosis

aphthous ulcer (af'thəs) – the ulcerous lesion on the mucous membrane seen in recurrent aphthous stomatitis

arthritis (pl. **arthritides**) (ahr-thri'tis [ahr-thri'ti-deez]) – inflammation of a joint; there are many subcategories of arthritis, ranging from acute spinal to juvenile onset to viral-associated arthritis

autoimmune (aw"to-ĭ-mūn') – characterized by a situation in which the body's own immune response system departs from normal operation and attacks the body, turning on itself

avascular necrosis (AVN) – coagulation necrosis or death of cells

B

Baker cyst (bā-kər sist) – a swelling behind the knee caused by escape of synovial fluid, which becomes enclosed in a membranous sac; also called popliteal cyst

Bouchard nodes (boo-shahr') – cartilaginous and bony enlargements of the proximal interphalangeal joints (PIP) of the fingers in degenerative joint disease

chondrocalcinosis (kon"dro-kal"sĭ-no'sis) – the presence of calcium salts, especially calcium pyrophosphate, in the cartilaginous structures of one or more joints

CMC – carpal metacarpal (joint)

connective tissue disease (kə-'nek-tiv) – a group of diseases of the connective tissue (muscle and cartilage) of unknown cause, including systemic lupus erythematosus (SLE), rheumatoid arthritis (RA), scleroderma, polymyositis, and dermatomyositis

costochondral (kos"to-kon'drəl) – pertaining to a rib and its cartilage

COX inhibitors ('käks- in-'hi-bə-tər) – cyclooxygenase inhibitors

CREST – calcinosis, Raynaud phenomena, esophagus disease, sclerodactyly, telangiectasia.

CTS – carpal tunnel syndrome

cytoprotection (si"to-pro-tek'shən) – enhancement of the ability of cells to resist injury; the protection of cells

dermatomyositis (dur"mə-to-mi"ə-si'tis) – a type of polymyositis with characteristic inflammatory skin changes, including an erythematous rash of the forehead, neck, trunk, and arms

DEXA – dual energy x-ray absorptiometry; a radiology scan to determine a person's bone mineral density; the results are used in the diagnosis of osteoporosis

DDD – degenerative disk disease

DISH – diffuse idiopathic skeletal hyperostosis

DJD – degenerative joint disease

DMARDs – disease-modifying antirheumatic drugs

epicondylitis (ep"ĭ-kon"də-li'tis) – inflammation of an epicondyle of the humerus (upper arm bone) or

of the tissues adjoining it, usually from an overuse injury

ESR – erythrocyte sedimentation rate, a nonspecific test that indicates inflammation anywhere in the body; often dictated "sed rate," the results may be elevated in certain types of rheumatism

facet (fas'ət [OR fə-set']) – also spelled facette; a small plane surface on a hard body, as on a bone; there are many facets in the human skeleton

fibromyalgia (fi"bro-mi-al'jə) – pain and stiffness in the muscles and joints; it can be either diffuse or have multiple trigger points (see trigger-point tenderness below)

FMS – fibromyalgia syndrome

gout (gowt) – an arthritic condition characterized by abnormally elevated levels of uric acid in the blood stream

glucosamine (gloo-kōs'ə-mēn) – the amino sugar derivative of glucose

glucosamine sulfate (sul'fāt) – the sulfate salt of glucosamine, prepared artificially as a nutritional supplement and as a popular remedy for osteoarthritis

Heberden nodes (he'bər-dən) – cartilaginous and bony enlargements of the distal interphalangeal joints of the fingers in degenerative joint disease

I

immune system (im-yoon) – a complex body system that protects us against infections and foreign substances; this system seeks out and kills invading microbes

IBS – irritable bowel syndrome

IP – interphalangeal (joint)

JH – joint hypermobility

joint – the place of union or junction between two or more bones of the skeleton

joint crepitus (krep'ĭ-təs) – the grating sensation caused by the rubbing together of the dry surfaces of joints; also called articular crepitus

JRA – juvenile rheumatoid arthritis; RA in a juvenile or child

juvenile idiopathic arthritis (id"e-o-path'ik) – a childhood disease of unknown etiology that causes inflamed, swollen joints

knee arthroplasty (ahr'thro-plas"te) – a surgical procedure that replaces the cartilage in an arthritically damaged knee joint with metal and plastic; it can be either a partial or a total replacement

MAKOplasty™ (ma" ko plas' tee) – a robotic-arm-assisted partial knee resurfacing procedure designed to relieve the pain caused by joint degeneration due to osteoarthritis (OA)

Marie-Strümpell disease (mah-rē'-strim'-pel) – rheumatoid spondylitis

MCP – metacarpophalangeal (joint)

MCTD – mixed connective tissue disease

MTX – methotrexate

node – (noun) a small mass of tissue in the form of a swelling, knot, or protuberance, either normal or pathological; i.e., gouty node

nodular – (adj.) marked with nodes

nodule – a small node or knot that can be detected by touch; i.e., rheumatoid nodule

NSAIDs – nonsteroidal anti-inflammatory drugs

osteoarthritis (os"te-o-ahr-thri'tis) – abbreviated OA, this is a form of chronic arthritis, typically with onset during middle or old age; "osteo" refers to bone

osteotomy (os"te-ot'ə-me) – the surgical cutting of a bone

periungual (per"e-ung'gwəl) – around the nail

PIP – proximal interphalangeal (joint)

PMR – polymyalgia rheumatica

polyarteritis (pol"e-ahr"tə-ri'tis) – multiple arterial and destructive arterial lesions; also polyarteritis nodosa (PAN)

polyarthritis (pol"e-ahr-thri'tis) – an inflammation of several joints together

polymyalgia rheumatica (pol"e-mi-al'jə ru ma' tee ka) – a rare inflammatory condition that causes pain or aching in the large muscle groups, especially around the shoulders and hips

polymyositis (pol"e-mi"o-si'tis) – chronic progressive inflammation of the muscles (myositis) with symmetrical weakness of the limb girdles, neck, and pharynx; it can occur in either children or adults

pruritus (proo-ri'təs) – an unpleasant itchiness of the skin

psoriatic arthritis (so ree a' tic) – abbreviated PA, this is arthritis in which the synovial membranes become inflamed

pseudogout (soo'do-gout") – inflammation caused by overproduction of calcium pyrophosphate crystals; sometimes referred to as calcium pyrophosphate disease (CPPD)

R

RA – <u>r</u>heumatoid <u>a</u>rthritis; a chronic systemic disease primarily of the joints, cause is unknown

Raynaud phenomena (ra-no') – intermittent bilateral ischemia (lack of blood) of the fingers, toes, and sometimes the ears and nose with severe pain; usually brought on by cold and relieved by heat

rheumatology (roo"mə-tol'ə-je) – a subspecialty of internal medicine consisting of the non-surgical evaluation and treatment of the rheumatic diseases and conditions involving the musculoskeletal system and the study of the immune system

RLS – <u>r</u>estless <u>l</u>eg <u>s</u>yndrome

RSI – <u>r</u>epetitive <u>s</u>train <u>i</u>njury

S

scleroderma (sklēr"o-dur'mə) – chronic hardening and thickening of the skin, a finding in various diseases; there are two primary forms: localized scleroderma and systemic scleroderma

seronegative (sēr"o-neg'ə-tiv) – serologically negative, showing negative results on serologic examination: a lack of antibody

seropositive (sēr"o-poz'ĭ-tiv) – serologically positive, showing positive results on serologic examination: a high level of antibody

SI – <u>s</u>acro<u>i</u>liac (joint)

Sjögren syndrome (shur'gren) – an autoimmune disease consisting of a symptom complex of unknown etiology occurring usually in middle-aged to elderly women. It is associated with rheumatoid arthritis and/or systemic lupus erythematosus, scleroderma, or polymyositis; also called sicca syndrome

SLE – <u>s</u>ystemic <u>l</u>upus <u>e</u>rythematosus

spondylitis (spon"də-li'tis) – inflammation of the vertebrae; called also rachitis

spondylitis rhizomelica (rī-zō-mel'-ih-kuh) – form of rheumatoid arthritis that affects the spine

spondyloarthropathy (spon"də-lo-ahr-throp'ə-the) – disease of the joints of the spine

stomatitis (sto"mə-ti'tis) – inflammation of the oral mucosa

styloid process (sti'loid) – resembling a pillar; there are several styloid processes in the human skeleton

T

TMJ – <u>t</u>empero<u>m</u>andibular <u>j</u>oints; joints in the mandible or jaw

trigger-point tenderness (tri-gər point) – there are trigger points throughout the body—found in the neck, knees, back, hips, chest, and even elbows—that when pressed are painful; out of the 18 trigger points, 11 of them must be painful to get a diagnosis of fibromyalgia; of equal importance, the pain must have been present for three months or more

trochanter (tro-kan'tər) – either of the two processes below the neck of the femur (long bone of the leg): the greater trochanter and the lesser trochanter

U

UCTS – <u>u</u>ndifferentiated <u>c</u>onnective <u>t</u>issue <u>s</u>yndrome

Transcription Tips

When transcribing arthritis/rheumatology dictation, it is helpful to be familiar with the terminology and abbreviations included in this chapter. In addition, familiarity with lab tests ordered by a rheumatologist (see below) will be beneficial. A review of orthopedics terminology in chapter 10 should prove valuable, as well, prior to transcribing dictation in arthritis/rheumatology. Physicians who specialize in arthritis/rheumatology, orthopedics, and podiatry often refer patients to each other, working together on the patients' clinical and surgical problems. While both orthopedists and podiatrists practice clinically and surgically, those in arthritis/rheumatology are strictly clinical. Perusing the information contained on the web sites listed below will also yield helpful information.

Laboratory and Diagnostic Testing

Some laboratory tests ordered by a rheumatologist might include the following.

- **antinuclear (ANA) antibodies** – blood test to identify antigen-antibody reactions. ANA antibodies are present in a number of autoimmune diseases.

- **complete blood count (CBC)** – blood tests done as part of a complete physical; those that include the platelet count results show a picture of the patient's hematologic system.

- **C-reactive protein (CRP)** – test on the serum; positive results can indicate rheumatoid arthritis, degenerative changes, acute inflammatory changes, and widespread metastasis.

- **erythrocyte sedimentation rate (ESR) [or Westergren sedimentation rate]** – nonspecific blood test that indicates inflammation anywhere in the body; also called a sed rate.

- **HLA-B27** – lab test ordered primarily to confirm a suspected diagnosis of autoimmune disorder, e.g., ankylosing spondylitis, reactive arthritis, or juvenile rheumatoid arthritis. This test is not definitive but can be used as evidence to support or rule out a diagnosis.

- **rheumatoid factor (RF)** – immunoglobulin is present in the serum of 50% to 95% of adults with rheumatoid arthritis.

- **uric acid blood test** – uric acid is shown to be increased in gout, arthritis, multiple myeloma, and rheumatism.

Anatomic Illustrations

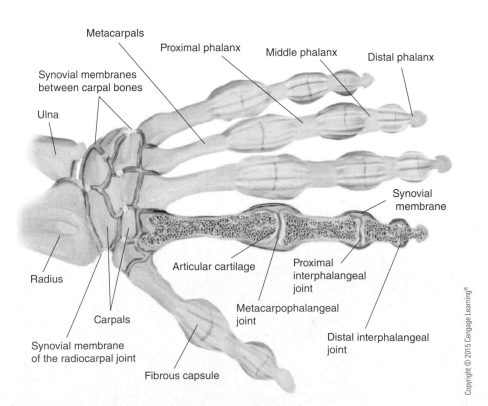

FIGURE 11-1   Anatomy of the wrist and hand

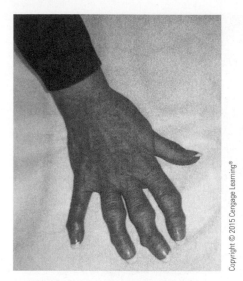

FIGURE 11-2   **Bouchard nodes and Heberden nodes**

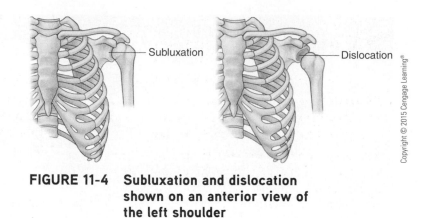

FIGURE 11-4   **Subluxation and dislocation shown on an anterior view of the left shoulder**

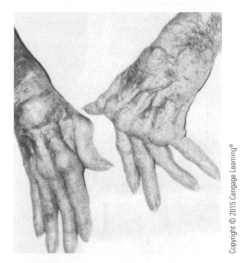

FIGURE 11-3   **Ulnar deviation**

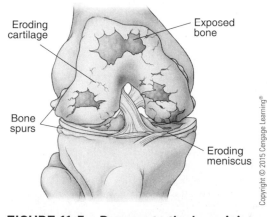

FIGURE 11-5   **Damage to the knee joint caused by osteoarthritis**

Supportive Web Sites

http://www.webmd.com/rheumatoid-arthritis/guide/most-common-arthritis-types	Contains information about rheumatoid arthritis with associated links.
http://www.vimovo.com/types-of-arthritis.aspx	Presents information on the three different types of arthritis.
http://www.vimovo.com/osteoarthritis-treatment.aspx	Contains information about treatment for arthritis.
http://www.vimovo.com/nsaid-therapy.aspx	Information here explains how NSAIDs work with arthritis pain.

http://arthritis.webmd.com/ankylosing-spondylitis-directory	Presents information about ankylosing spondylitis.
http://www.ncbi.nlm.nih.gov/pubmedhealth/PMH0002223/	Contains more general information on arthritis.
http://arthritis.about.com/od/arthritislearnthebasics/a/acronyms.htm	Presents information on acronyms associated with arthritis.
http://www.rheumatoidarthritis.com/ra/understanding-ra/signs-and-symptoms.htm	This site contains video and specific information about rheumatoid arthritis.

Index of Arthritis/Rheumatology Reports

Exercise#	Patient Name	Type of Report/Procedure
TE#1	Sarah Elizabeth Yoder	SOAP Note: Rheumatoid arthritis
TE#2	Robert Tyler Ford	SOAP Note: Ankylosing spondylitis
TE#3	Michael Jon Roberts	SOAP Note: Juvenile-onset rheumatoid arthritis
TE#4	Tara Lynn Abraham	SOAP Note: Osteoarthritis and fibromyalgia
TE#5	Cassandra M. Benito	SOAP Note: Systemic lupus
TE#6	Tess Burkholder	SOAP Note: Rheumatoid arthritis and a fatty liver
TE#7	Jessica L Kral	SOAP Note: Fibromyalgia and osteopenia
TE#8	Alice Nichols	HPIP Note: Postmenopausal osteoporosis
TE#9	Eric Alonzo	HPIP Note: Psoriatic arthritis
TE#10	David Emilson	Arthritis Clinic: Letter regarding medication

CHAPTER 12
PODIATRY

Introduction

Podiatry is devoted to the study, diagnosis, and treatment of disorders of the foot, ankle, and lower leg. The term *podiatry* denotes a Doctor of Podiatric Medicine (DPM), a specialist who is qualified by education and training to diagnose and treat conditions affecting the foot, ankle, and related structures of the leg.

Podiatrists can become Board Certified by passing The American Board of Podiatric Surgery examinations or The American Board of Podiatric Medicine examinations. Both Boards are located in California and have web sites where one can read more detailed information about the process of certification.

While the majority of podiatric physicians are in solo practice, there has been a movement toward larger group practices as well as the use of podiatrists in multi-specialty groups, including orthopedic groups and within the United States Department of Veterans Affairs, providing care to veterans of military service.

Different states allow DPMs a widely varying scope of practice. Many podiatrists perform office surgery, but most have surgical privileges for procedures of the foot in outpatient surgical facilities and hospitals. Some podiatrists have advanced training for reconstructive rear foot and ankle surgery. Some states allow surgery of the leg by podiatrists.

Some podiatrists complete additional fellowship training in reconstruction of the foot and ankle from the effects of diabetes or physical trauma. Other surgeons practice minimally invasive percutaneous surgery for correction of hammer toes and bunions. Podiatrists utilize medical, orthopedic, biomechanical, and surgical principles to maintain and correct foot deformities.

A podiatrist's office must contain all the tools, instruments, and supplies to help both his clinical and surgical patients with their activities of daily living, including products and shoes for diabetics, products for casting and splinting, and for edema, infection control, and wound care. They would also need an autoclave to keep surgical equipment sterile, x-ray equipment, and special chairs in which patients undergo their outpatient surgical procedures. Podiatry patients are admitted for inpatient surgery when the outpatient setting is inappropriate.

Critical Thinking Exercise

?

You have transcribed a preop H&P in which the podiatrist has dictated that this type 1 diabetic pediatric patient is to be given 5 units/kg/day Humulin R prior to hammertoe surgery. This seemed strange to you, and after checking your drug reference book, it is clear that this dose of Humulin R is incorrect. This is of concern to you—what are your options?

Podiatry Abbreviations

The abbreviations, acronyms, and terms in the following abbreviations and terminology sections are often dictated in this specialty. We offer abbreviated definitions here.

Please see an unabridged medical dictionary or the suggested web sites in this chapter for more information on each term.

call.rcd	callus reduced		**MPJ**	metatarsophalangeal joint
call.rdn	callus reduction		**NT&F**	nails trimmed and filed
enuc	enucleated		**O/C**	onychocryptosis
ESWT	extracorporeal shock wave therapy		**O/G**	onychogryphosis
HD	heloma durum, hard corn		**O/P**	onychophosis
HM	heloma molle, soft corn		**O/X**	onychauxis
Hmille	heloma miliaire, seed corn		**PIP**	proximal interphalangeal
HNV	heloma neurovasculare, neurovascular corn		**PNA**	partial nail avulsion
HV	heloma vasculare, vascular corn		**RSD**	reflex sympathetic dystrophy
IPJ	interphalangeal joint		**TNA**	total nail avulsion
mHBT	mild hyperbaric oxygen therapy		**VP**	verruca pedis

Anatomic Illustrations

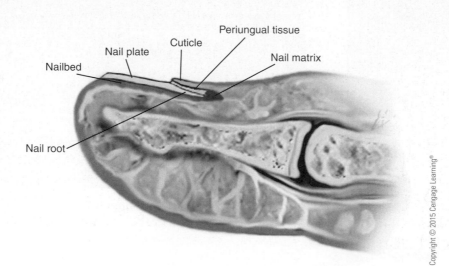

FIGURE 12-1   **Structures of the fingernails and toenails**

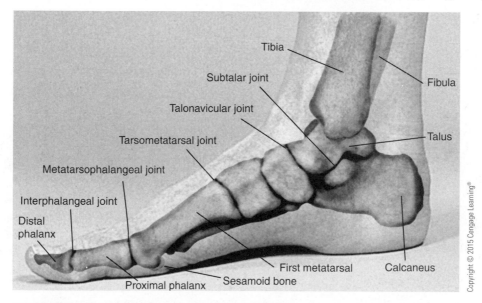

FIGURE 12-2   **Anatomy of the ankle and foot**

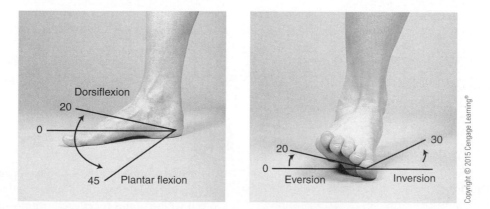

FIGURE 12-3   **Range of motion of the ankle and foot**

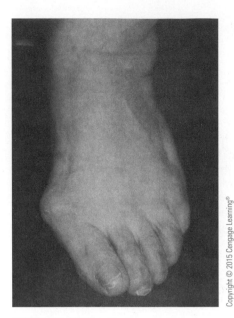

FIGURE 12-4   Hallux valgus

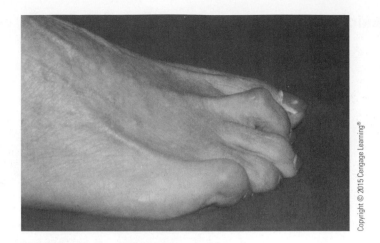

FIGURE 12-5   Hammertoe with corn

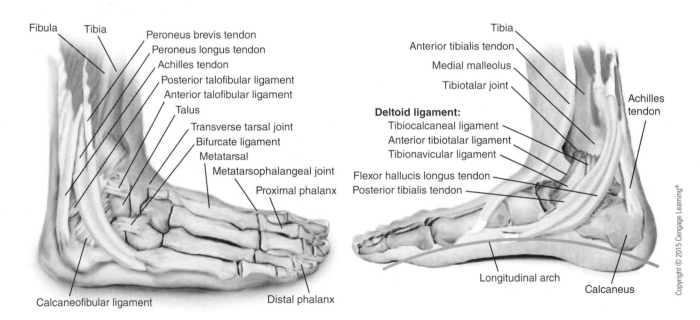

Fibula Tibia
Peroneus brevis tendon
Peroneus longus tendon
Achilles tendon
Posterior talofibular ligament
Anterior talofibular ligament
Talus
Transverse tarsal joint
Bifurcate ligament
Metatarsal
Metatarsophalangeal joint
Proximal phalanx

Calcaneofibular ligament
Distal phalanx

Tibia
Anterior tibialis tendon
Medial malleolus
Tibiotalar joint
Deltoid ligament:
Tibiocalcaneal ligament
Anterior tibiotalar ligament
Tibionavicular ligament
Flexor hallucis longus tendon
Posterior tibialis tendon

Achilles tendon

Longitudinal arch
Calcaneus

FIGURE 12-6   Ligaments of the ankle

Podiatry Terminology

A

Achilles tendon (ə-'kil-ēz) – a powerful tendon at the back of the heel that attaches the triceps surae muscle to the tuberosity of the calcaneus

apical (ā-pi-kəl) – on the apex, tip, or end of the toe

B

bone spurs (bōn spurz) – bone spurs are bony projections that develop along the edges of bones, often where bones meet each other—in the joints; also called osteophytes

bunion (bən-yən) – abnormal prominence of the inner aspect of the first metatarsal head, accompanied by bursal formation and resulting from a lateral or valgus displacement of the great toe; also known as hallux valgus

corn (kōrn) – a hard or soft hyperkeratosis of the sole of the human foot secondary to friction and pressure; a hard corn is usually over a toe joint, a soft corn is formed by pressure between two toes

callus (kal-əs) – noun; a composite mass of tissue that forms at a fracture site to establish continuity between the bone ends (syn. callosity)

callous (kal-əs) – adj.; relating to a callus; for example, a callous growth

dorsal (dȯr-səl) – adj.; pertaining to the back or any dorsum (syn. posterior)

dorsum – noun; the back of the body, the posterior surface

extracorporeal shock wave therapy (ESWT) (ek-strə kȯr-'pōr-ē-əl) – a therapy for the treatment of athletes with injuries to the elbow, knee, or ankle; actually, this therapy can be used throughout the whole body

fungus nails (fən-gəs) – thickened, deformed, rough nails due to a fungal infection; also known as *onychomycosis*

gout (gau̇t) – a complex form of arthritis that is characterized by sudden, severe attacks of pain, redness, and tenderness in joints, often the joint at the base of the big toe

Haglund deformity/disease (hahg" lund) – an abnormal prominence of the posterior superior lateral aspect of the os calcis; the back of the heel at the area of the insertion of the Achilles tendon

hallux varus (hal-əks var-əs) – angulation of the great toe toward the midline of the body, away from the other toes

hammertoe (ham-ər-'tō) – a deformity of the second, third, or fourth toes where the toe is bent at the middle joint (PIP), so that it resembles a hammer

heel spur (hēl spur) – a bony overgrowth on the bottom of the heel bone that is usually caused by an inflamed ligament (plantar fascia) on the bottom of the foot that attaches to the heel bone

heloma (he-lo'mə) – a corn; heloma durum is a hard corn; heloma molle is a soft corn

ingrown nail – a condition where the nail is cutting into the flesh

intractable plantar keratosis (in-'trak-tə-bəl plant-ər ker-ə-'tō-səs) – a severe form of callus that is discrete and focused on the plantar aspect of the forefoot

mild hyperbaric oxygen therapy (mHBT) (hi"pər-bar'ik) – a procedure whereby a person is exposed to increased atmospheric pressure inside an inflatable chamber; this allows more oxygen to reach the cells of the body, which contributes to healing

neuroma (nŏo-ro'mə) – a tumor growing from a nerve or made up largely of nerve cells and nerve fibers; an irritated, swollen nerve in the ball of the foot

onychatrophia (on"ĭ-kə-tro'fe-ə) – atrophy of a nail or nails

onychauxis (on"ĭ-kawk'sis) – marked overgrowth of the fingernails or toenails; also called *hyperonychia*

onychectomy (on"ĭ-kek'tə-me) – excision of a nail or nail bed; in animals, declawing

onychia (ō-'nik-ē-ə) – inflammation of the matrix of the nail; also known as *onychitis*

onychocryptosis (on"ĭ-ko-krip-to'sis) – ingrown nail

onychocyte (on'ĭ-ko-sīt") – one of the tightly packed keratinized cells arranged in layers to make up the nail plate

onychogenic (on"ĭ-ko-jen'ik) – producing or forming nail substance

onychograph (o-nik'o-graf") – an instrument for observing and recording the capillary blood pressure as shown by the circulation under the nail

onycholysis (on"ĭ-kol'ĭ-sis) – loosening of the nails, beginning at the free border, progressing proximally, and usually incomplete

onychomadesis (on"ĭ-ko-mə-de'sis) – complete shedding of the nails, usually associated with systemic disease

onychomalacia (on"ĭ-ko-mə-la'shə) – softening of a nail or nails

onychomycosis (on"ĭ-ko-mi-ko'sis) – very common fungal infection of the nails causing thickening, roughness, and splitting

onychopathology (on"ĭ-ko-pə-thol'ə-je) – the study of diseases of the nails

onychopathy (on"ĭ-kop'ə-the) – disease or deformity of the nails; also called *onychosis*

onychophosis (on"ĭ-ko-fo'sis) – a callus in a nail grove, such as one occurring with an ingrown toenail

onychoschizia (on"ĭ-ko-skiz'e-ə) – splitting of the nail plate, sometimes into layers, usually in a transverse (horizontal) direction at the free edge

onychotomy (on"ĭ-kot'ə-me) – surgical incision into a nail

paronychia (par"o-nik'e-ə) – suppurative inflammation of the nail fold surrounding the nail plate; may be due to bacteria or fungi

plantar – relating to the sole of the foot

plantar fasciitis (plant-ər fas"e-i'tis) – a common cause of heel pain; it involves pain and inflammation of a thick band of tissue, called the plantar fascia, that runs across the bottom (sole) of the foot and connects the heel bone to the toes

reflex sympathetic dystrophy (sim"pə-thet'ik dis'trə-fe) – a severe and debilitating condition that occurs when the nerves in the leg "go haywire"

shin splint – the tearing away of the anterior tibial muscle from the bone

stress fracture – a fracture caused by repetitive stress

subungual heloma durum (sub un" gwal he-lo'mə) – a hard corn beneath the fingernail or the toenail

synovial sarcoma (sĭ-no've-əl sahr-ko'mə) – a malignant soft tissue tumor; often misdiagnosed as plantar fasciitis

talipes (tal'-ih-pēz) – a congenital deformity of the foot, which is twisted out of shape or position

tarsal tunnel syndrome (tar' săl tŭn'ĕl) – occurs when the posterior tibial nerve becomes inflamed due to excessive pronation, arthritic problems, trauma, or even obesity; usually affects the inside aspect of the ankle

tenosynovitis (ten"o-sin"o-vi'tis) – inflammation of a tendon sheath

ulcers (ŭl'sĕrz) – lesions through the skin or mucous membrane resulting from loss of tissue, usually with inflammation; patients with diabetes have to watch their feet carefully for ulcers because of a lack of circulation

xerosis (zi-'rō-səs) – pathologic dryness of the skin or mucous membranes

Transcription Tips

In podiatry dictation, familiarity with terminology relative to the foot and ankle is essential. A review of transcription tips found in chapter 10 (orthopedics) should prove valuable in learning details about the practice of podiatry. Knowledge of the abbreviations and terms listed in podiatry as well as in orthopedics will aid in transcribing cases included in podiatry. Physicians who specialize in both podiatry and orthopedics often refer patients to each other, working together on the patient's specific foot and ankle problems. Orthopedists and podiatrists both practice clinically and surgically. Information included in the Supportive Web Sites section is also helpful to the healthcare documentation specialist learning podiatry.

Equipment/Supplies Found in a Podiatrist's Office

A podiatrist's office must contain all the tools, instruments, and supplies necessary for clinical and surgical patients. Vendors provide catalogs from which any of these can be ordered. They include but are not limited to the following:

Adhesive products	Surgical blades with handles in all sizes
Casting products	Sterile cleaners/disinfectants
Creams/ointments/powders	Diagnostic instruments and equipment
Gauze/cotton/bandages	Injectables/needles/syringes/sutures in all sizes
Orthopedic appliances/padding	Protective apparel—shoes and inserts
Sterilization equipment	X-ray equipment

Supportive Web Sites

http://www.webmd.com/	Search for "podiatry" and click on links of interest.
http://www.footlaw.com/glossary.html	Contains podiatry terminology.
http://foothealth.about.com/od/glossary/Glossary.htm	Contains definitions of common foot and ankle medical terms.
http://www.skatelog.com/feet/glossary.htm	Contains list of podiatry and foot-related terminology.

Index of Podiatry Reports

Exercise#	Patient Name	Type of Report/Procedure
TE#1	Rick Rodriguez	SOAP Note, onychogryphosis of toenails; hyperkeratosis of feet
TE#2	Minnie Fortunado	Followup Visit (FUV), neuritis of right foot
TE#3	Norberto Melizzo	Surgery, cheilectomy and unionectomy
TE#4	Norberto Melizzo	Postoperative Visit (letter)
TE#5	Barry Walsh	FUV, Achilles tendinitis and heel pain
TE#6	Josefina Gonzales	FUV, painful punctuate keratones
TE#7	Rowena M. Kinsey	Surgery, excision of foreign body, left foot
TE#8	Charles Newman	FUV, infected ingrown nail – letter
TE#9	Penny Buttel	FUV, painful right great toe – letter
TE#10	Bill Buhmann	FUV, tophaceous gout – letter
TE#11	Kathy Lozano	FUV, painful right heel
TE#12	Patsy Price	Bunionectomy, excision of ganglion, left foot

CHAPTER 13
PEDIATRICS/NEONATOLOGY

Introduction

Pediatrics is a specialized field of medicine that is concerned with disturbances of any system or function that might affect the health or orderly growth and development of the child. The pediatrician's commitment, extending beyond purely physical matters, is to secure for all children the opportunity to achieve their full native potential. In their role as understanding guardians of children's physical, mental, and emotional progress from conception to maturity, pediatricians are in the forefront of social concern for children and their families. Generally, pediatrics requires three years of residency training.

Neonatology is a subspecialized field of pediatrics that focuses on the human newborn. A *neonatologist* is an intensive-care physician who takes care of sick or premature infants. The neonatologist's knowledge of newborn physiology can assist in the management of congenital anomalies; surgical conditions of the neonate; failure to thrive; nutritional problems; genetic, neurologic, and biochemical diseases; and a host of conditions involving delayed maturity. Thus, neonatology is sharply limited in the age range it covers but broad in its study of the interaction of normal physiology and disease processes. Training for neonatology requires three years of fellowship after successful completion of a pediatric residency.

The classifications of humans with which pediatricians and neonatologists do their work include *neonates* or *newborns, infants, children,* and *adolescents, youth,* or *teenagers.* A *neonate* (newborn) is a child from birth to one month of age. An *infant* is a child from one month to 24 months of age, and a *child* is a boy or girl from 2 to 13 years of age. Boys and girls ages 13 through 17 years are known as *adolescents, youths,* or *teenagers.*

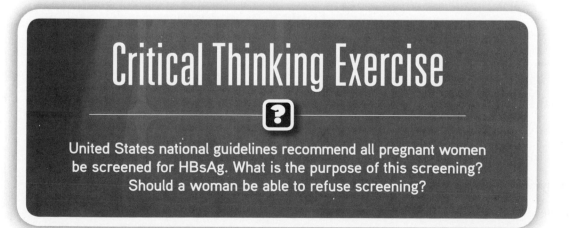

Critical Thinking Exercise

?

United States national guidelines recommend all pregnant women be screened for HBsAg. What is the purpose of this screening? Should a woman be able to refuse screening?

Pediatrics/Neonatology Abbreviations

The abbreviations, acronyms, and terms in the following abbreviations and terminology sections are often dictated in this specialty. We offer abbreviated definitions here.

Please see an unabridged medical dictionary or the suggested web sites in this chapter for more information on each term.

A&B	apnea and bradycardia
ABG	arterial blood gases
ACV	assist control ventilation or vent
ACAPI	anterior cerebral artery pulsatility index
ACHD	acyanotic congenital heart disease
AGA	appropriate for gestational age
alb	albumin
ALTE	acute life-threatening event
amp	ampicillin
ANC	absolute neutrophil count
AROM	artificial rupture of membranes
BAER	brain stem audioevoked response
BC	blood culture
bili	bilirubin
BMV	bag and mask ventilation
BPD	bronchopulmonary dysplasia
BS	blood sugar, bowel sounds, or breath sounds
BW	birth weight
CAH	congenital adrenal hyperplasia
CBG	capillary blood gas
CCHD	cyanotic congenital heart disease
CDH	congenital diaphragmatic hernia
CHD	congenital heart disease
CLD	chronic lung disease

CMV	cytomegalovirus
coag	coagulase
CP	cerebral palsy
CPAP	continuous positive airway pressure
CPIP	chronic pulmonary insufficiency of prematurity
Cr	creatinine
CRP	C-reactive protein
CSF	cerebrospinal fluid
DA	dopamine
DBM	donor breast milk
DOB	date of birth
DIC	disseminated intravascular coagulation
DM	diabetes mellitus
DNA	deoxyribonucleic acid
DOL	day of life
EBM	expressed breast milk
ECHO	echocardiogram
ECMO	extracorporeal membrane oxygenation
ENF	Enfamil
ET	expiratory time
ETT	endotracheal tube
FAS	fetal alcohol syndrome
Fe	iron
FEN	fluid/electrolytes/nutrition

FiO$_2$	fraction of inspired oxygen
FOC	frontal occipital circumference
GER	gastroesophageal reflux
glu	glucose, glutamate, glutamine
H flu	Haemophilus influenza
HBsAg	hepatitis B surface antigen
HBV	hepatitis B vaccine
HC	head circumference
Hct	hematocrit
HCTZ	hydrochlorothiazide
HFNC	high flow nasal cannula
Hgb	hemoglobin
H/H or H&H	hemoglobin and hematocrit
HIE	hypoxic-ischemic encephalopathy
HMD	hyaline membrane disease
HSV	herpes simplex virus
HUS	head ultrasound
ICH	intracranial hemorrhage
IDM	infant of diabetic mother
I-to-E	inspiratory-to-expiratory ratio
Ig	immunoglobulin
IMV	intermittent mandatory ventilation
IT	inspiratory time
I/T	immature total neutrophil ratio
ITP	idiopathic thrombocytopenic purpura
IUGR	intrauterine growth retardation
IVH	intraventricular hemorrhage
LBW	low birth weight
LGA	large for gestational age
LP	lumbar puncture

L-to-S	lecithin-to-sphingomyelin ratio (test of fetal lung maturity)
M	murmur
MAP	mean arterial pressure or mean airway pressure
MAS	meconium aspiration syndrome
MCA	multiple congenital anomalies
mec	meconium
MgSO$_4$	magnesium sulfate
MOM	mother's own milk
MSF	meconium-stained fluid
N cat	Neisseria catarrhalis
N gon	Neisseria gonorrhoeae
N men	Neisseria meningitidis
NB	newborn
NC	nasal cannula
NCPAP	nasal continuous positive airway pressure
NEC	necrotizing enterocolitis
neo	neonatal
NG	nasogastric
NICU	neonatal intensive care unit
NIV	noninvasive
NSVD	normal spontaneous vaginal delivery
N&V	nausea and vomiting
O&B	Ortolani and Barlow
OCT	oxytocin challenge test
OG	oral gastric or orogastric (feeding)
OI	oxygenation index
OM	otitis media
PaCO$_2$	arterial carbon dioxide tension
PaO$_2$	arterial oxygen tension

PBLC	preterm (premature) birth live child	**SIDS**	sudden infant death syndrome
PCN	penicillin	**SIM**	Similac
PDA	patent ductus arteriosus	**SIMV**	synchronized intermittent mechanical ventilation
PEEP	positive end-expiratory pressure	**SROM**	spontaneous rupture of membrane
PFC	persistent fetal circulation	**SSC**	Similac special care formula (followed by number = calorie count)
PFTs	pulmonary function tests		
PHH	posthemorrhagic hydrocephalus	**strep**	streptococcus
PIE	pulmonary interstitial emphysema	T_3	triiodothyronine
PIH	pregnancy-induced hypertension	T_4	levothyroxine
PIP	post (or peak) inspiratory pressure	**TAPVR**	total anomalous pulmonary venous return
PKU	phenylketonuria		
plts	platelets	**TBLC**	term birth live child
PPHN	persistent pulmonary hypertension of the newborn	**TOB**	time of birth
		TOF	tetralogy of Fallot
PPV	positive-pressure ventilation	**TOGV**	transposition of the great vessels
PPROM	preterm premature rupture of membranes	**toxo**	toxoplasmosis
PROM	prolonged or premature rupture of membranes	**TPN**	total parenteral nutrition
		TRIG	triglycerides
PS	pulmonary stenosis	**TSH**	thyroid-stimulating hormone
PUBS	percutaneous umbilical blood sampling	**TTN**	transient tachypnea of the newborn
PVL	periventricular leukomalasia	**TV**	tidal volume
RDS	respiratory distress syndrome	**UAC**	umbilical artery catheter
REM	rapid eye movement	**UC**	urine culture
ROM	rupture of membranes	**U/S**	ultrasound
ROP	retinopathy of prematurity	**UVC**	umbilical venous catheter
RRR	regular rate and rhythm	**VBG**	venous blood gas
S aureus	Staphylococcus aureus	**VCUG**	voiding cystourethrogram
S epi	Staphylococcus epidermidis	**VIT**	vitamin
SaO_2	arterial oxygen saturation	**VLBW**	very low birth weight
SEH	subependymal hemorrhage	**VSD**	ventricular septal defect
SGA	small for gestational age	**VSS**	vital signs stable

Anatomic Illustrations

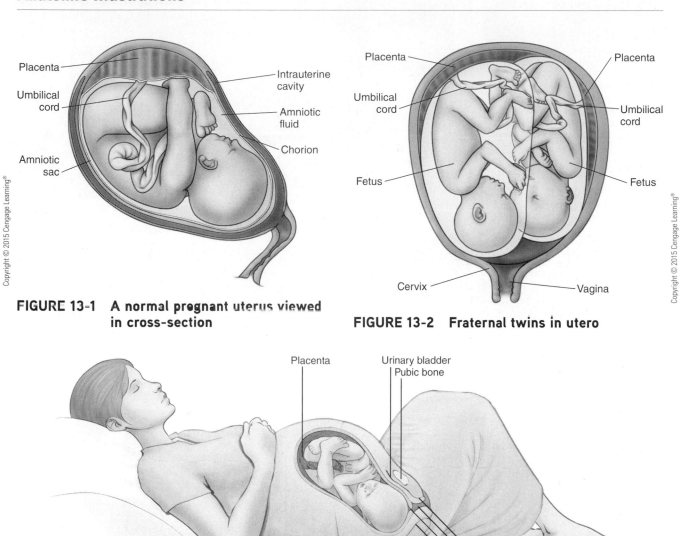

FIGURE 13-1   A normal pregnant uterus viewed in cross-section

FIGURE 13-2   Fraternal twins in utero

(A)

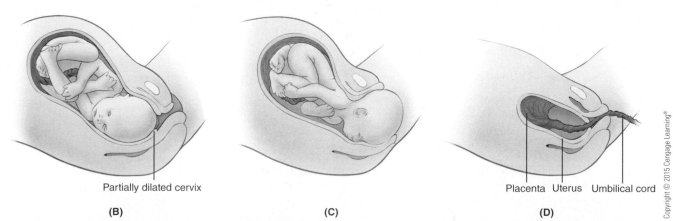

(B)　　　　(C)　　　　(D)

FIGURE 13-3   The stages of labor. (A) Position of the fetus before labor. (B) First stage of labor, cervical dilatation. (C) Second stage of labor, fetal delivery. (D) Third stage of labor, delivery of the afterbirth (placenta and fetal membranes).

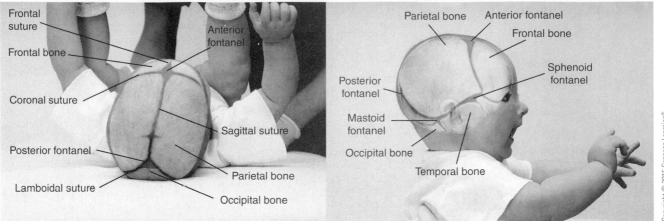

(A) Superior View   (B) Lateral View

FIGURE 13-4   Infant head structures

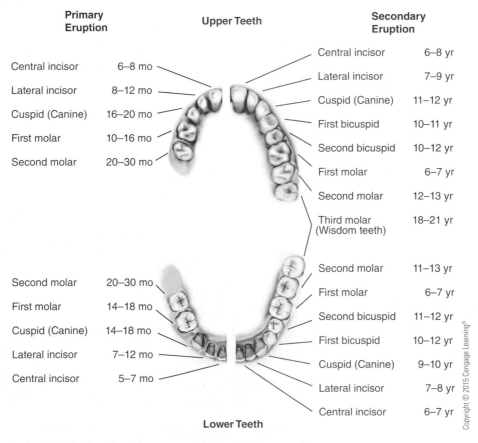

FIGURE 13-5   Deciduous and permanent teeth

Pediatrics/Neonatology Terminology

A

amniocentesis (am"-nē-ō -sen-tē'-sis) – transabdominal puncture of the amniotic sac using a needle and syringe in order to remove amniotic fluid

amnioscopy (am"-nē-ahss'-kuh-pē) – direct visual observation of the fetus, color of and amount of amniotic fluid by use of a specially designed endoscope inserted into the amniotic cavity via the abdominal wall

anencephaly (an"-en-sef'-uh-lē) – congenital absence of the cranial vault, with cerebral hemispheres completely missing or reduced to small masses attached to the base of the skull

apnea (ap'ne-ə) – the cessation of breathing

Apgar score (ap'-gar skōr) – a system of scoring the physical condition of infants at one and five minutes after birth; the heart rate, respiration, muscle tone, response to stimuli, and skin color are each rated 0 to 2; a total score of 8 to 10 indicates the best possible condition

arteriovenous malformation (AVM) (ahr-tēr"e-o-ve'nəs) – abnormal connection between the arteries and veins

ascites (ə-si'tēz) – a collection of fluid in the abdomen, usually due to poor cardiac function

asphyxia (as-fik'-sē-uh) – condition resulting from an insufficient intake of oxygen

atresia (ah-trē'-zē-uh) – congenital absence or closure of a normal body opening or tubular structure

B

bagging – the process of filling the lungs with air or oxygen by squeezing a bag connected to an endotracheal tube or attached to a mask fitted over the face; breathes for the baby when his own breaths are insufficient

bililights (bil"ĭ-litz) – distinctive lights used in the treatment of jaundice

bilirubin (bil"ĭ-roo'bin) – a breakdown product of red blood cells that is processed and excreted by the liver

bradycardia (brad"e-kahr'de-ə) – abnormally slow heart rate

C

caput succedaneum (kap'-it suk"-sē-dā'-nē-um) – swelling occurring in and under the fetal scalp during labor

cephalhematoma (sef"-ul-hē"-muh-tō'-muh) – a tumor or swelling filled with blood beneath the pericranium

chemstrip – a test in which a drop of blood is placed on a strip of special paper to determine the quantity of sugar in the blood (Chemstrip can be a brand name, as in Chemstrip BG test and Chemstrip dipstick; it depends on the test that is being done.)

chorioamnionitis (kō"-rē-ō-am"-nē-ō-nī'-tis) – inflammation of the fetal membranes by bacterial infection

circumcision (sur"kəm-sizh'ən) – a surgical procedure done to remove the foreskin of the penis; done only on request and normally before the baby is discharged after birth

cleft lip or palate (kleft lip or pal'ăt) – birth defect characterized by a split through the lip, the roof of the mouth, or the soft tissue in the back of the mouth resulting from failure of these structures to close normally during early fetal development

congenital (kən-jen'ĭ-təl) – existing at the time of birth

continuous positive airway pressure (CPAP) – a form of ventilator assistance that helps to keep the baby's lungs properly expanded; does not breathe for the baby but allows her to breathe into a "wind"; often dictated "C PAP"

craniotabes (krā"-nē-ō-tā'-bēz) – in infancy, abnormal softening of the skull bones

cyanosis (si"ə-no'sis) – blue color of the skin occurring when there is insufficient oxygen in the blood

Down syndrome – a variable combination of birth defects that include mental retardation and characteristic facial features

Eisenmenger syndrome (i'sɔn-meng"ər) – any situation in which increased pressure/flow in the lung vessels has resulted in cyanosis

endotracheal tube (ET tube) (en"do-tra'ke-əl) – a plastic tube that goes from the nose or mouth past the vocal cords and into the upper trachea (windpipe)

exchange transfusion (eks-chānj' trans-fyū'zhūn) – a treatment that removes the baby's blood in small quantities and replaces it with donor blood; used most frequently to lower the level of bilirubin in the baby's blood

extubation (eks"too-ba'shən) – the process of removing a tube that has been placed through the nose or mouth into the trachea

fontanelle (alt. sp. fontanel) (fahn"-tuh-nehl') – an unossified space or soft spot lying between the cranial bones of the skull of a fetus

foramen ovale (for-ā'-men ō'-vahl-ē) – in the fetal heart, the oval opening in the septum secundum; the persistent part of the septum primum acts as a valve for this interatrial communication during fetal life; postnatally it becomes fused to the septum secundum to close it

gastroschisis (gas-trahs'-kih-sis) – a congenital fissure that remains open in the wall of the abdomen

gavage feedings (gə-vahzh') – feedings carried by a small plastic tubing placed through the nose or mouth and down into the stomach when the

baby is too weak or too premature to suck and swallow

heel stick – a prick of the heel with a sterile instrument to obtain small blood samples for testing

hyaline membrane disease (hī'-uh-lin) – a disorder affecting newborn infants (particularly premature) characterized by the development of a hyaline-like membrane lining the terminal respiratory passages

hydrocephalus (hi"dro-sef'ə-ləs) – an abnormal accumulation of cerebrospinal fluid in the ventricles of the brain

hyperbilirubinemia (hī"per-bil"-ih-roo"-bih-nē'-mē-uh) – an excessive amount of bilirubin in the blood

hyperinsulinemia (hī"-per-in"-soo-lih-nē'-mē-uh) – an excessive amount of insulin in the blood

hypomagnesemia (hī"-pō-mag"-neh-sē'-mē-uh) – decreased magnesium in the blood; results in increased neuromuscular irritability

hypotonia (hī"-pō-tō'-nē-uh) – the condition of diminished tone of the skeletal muscles

hypoxia (hī-pok'-sē-uh) – deficiency of oxygen

I-to-E ratio – inspiratory to expiratory ratio; the ratio of the length of the forced breath provided by a ventilator to the length of the time between two breaths (dictated "I to E ratio")

inspiratory time (IT) (in-' spī-rə-, to' r-ē) – the length of a forced breath provided to the baby by a ventilator

intraventricular hemorrhage (IVH) (in"trə-ventrik'u-lər hem'ə-rəj) – a collection of blood in and around the ventricles (hollow portions) of the brain

intubation (in"too-ba'shən) – the procedure to place an endotracheal tube in the baby's trachea

intussusception (in"-tuh-suh-sep'-shun) – the slipping or receiving of one part of the intestine into another just below it

jaundice (jawn'dis) – yellow coloration of the skin and eyes caused by increased amounts of bilirubin in the blood

K

Klinefelter syndrome (klīn'-fel-ter) – a genetic disorder affecting males caused by an extra X chromosome; some have no symptoms but others have sparse body hair, enlarged breasts, wide hips, and small testicles

L

lactobezoar (lak"-tō-bē'-zōr) – a solid mass of milk products in the stomach or intestines of an infant

M

meconium (mē-kō'-nē-um) – first feces of a newborn infant; they are thick, sticky, and dark green to black in color

meconium aspiration (mē-kō'-nē-um as'pi-rā'shŭn) – the inhalation of meconium into the lungs; causes breathing problems after the baby is born

mucopolysaccharidosis (myoo"-kō-pahl"-ē-sak"-uh-rī-dō'-sis) – a genetic disorder caused by the lack of an enzyme essential for breaking down sugar molecules and used in building connective tissues in the body

myelomeningocele (mī"-eh-lō-meh-ning'-gō-sēl) – spina bifida with a portion of cord and membranes protruding

myringotomy (mih"-ring-got'-uh-mē) – surgery for otitis media in which the surgeon makes a small incision in the eardrum

N

nasal cannula (kan'u-lə) – clear plastic tubing that passes under the nose to provide supplemental oxygen

neonatal necrotizing enterocolitis (nē"-ō-nā'-tul nek'-rō-tī"-zing en"-ter-ō-kō-lī'-tis) – an infection of the wall of the intestines that may spread to the blood; premature babies are particularly vulnerable to this severe disease

neonatal septicemia (sep"-tih-sē'-mē-uh) – bacterial infection documented by a positive blood culture in the first four weeks of life

neonates (ne'o-nātz) – newborn infants

O

Ohtahara syndrome (ō-tah-hah'-rah) – a neurological disorder characterized by seizures, usually within the first three months of life

omphalocele (om'-fah-lō-sēl") – a congenital hernia of the navel

ostium primum (os'-tē-um prē-mum) – an opening in the lowest aspect of the septum primum of the embryonic heart, posteriorly, in the area of the atrioventricular valve

oxyhood (O$_2$ hood) – a clear plastic hood placed over the baby's head through which oxygen is delivered

P

parenteral nutrition (pə-ren'tər-əl) – protein and sometimes fats given intravenously along with sugars and salts when the baby cannot tolerate complete feedings by nipple or gavage; also known as total parenteral nutrition (TPN)

patent ductus arteriosus (PDA) (pā'-tent duk'-tus artēr"-ē-ō'-sus) – persistence of a communication between the main pulmonary artery and the aorta after birth

peak inspiratory pressure (PIP) (pēk in-spī'ră-tō'rē presh'ŭr) – the highest pressure delivered by the ventilator to the baby during a forced breath

PE tubes – polyethylene tubes utilized in tympanostomy (surgery for otitis media)

perinatology (pār"-ih-nā-tahl'-uh-jē) – study of the fetus and infant from 20 to 29 weeks of gestation to one to four weeks after birth

phototherapy (fō-tō-' ther-ə-pē) – treatment where the baby is placed under bright lights or on a special light blanket that helps bilirubin to be excreted into the intestine

phenylketonuria (PKU) (fenl-keto-n u're-a) – a rare disorder where one of the amino acids (a building block of protein) cannot be handled normally by the baby, leading to elevated levels in the blood; by law all babies are tested for PKU before leaving the nursery

pneumomediastinum (noo"mo-me"de-əs-ti'nəm) – leakage of air from the normal passageways of the lung into the space surrounding the heart inside the chest

pneumothorax (noo"-mō-thor'-aks) – presence of free air in the pleural cavity

polycythemia (pol"e-si-the'me-ə) – refers to excess red blood cells in the bloodstream that may be due to chronic cyanosis, among other things

positive end-expiratory pressure (PEEP) ('pä-zə-tiv 'end-ik-'spī'rä-tō'rē presh'ŭr) – the lowest pressure delivered by the ventilator to the baby between forced breaths

progeria (prō-jē'-rē-uh) – a form of infantilism that causes a child to age prematurely

renal agenesis (ā-jen'-eh-sis) – absence of one or both kidneys

respiratory distress syndrome (RDS) (res'pi-ră-tōr'ē di-'stres sin-drōm) – a common breathing problem for premature infants caused by insufficient surfactant in the baby's lungs; results in an excessive stiffness of the baby's lungs

retinopathy of prematurity (ROP) (ret"ĭ-nop'ə-the) – a problem of the retina (back part of the eye that "sees") occurring mostly in very premature infants; can threaten vision in one or both eyes; surgery is sometimes necessary to improve the chance for sight

septic workup – an assortment of laboratory tests performed on an infant who is suspected of having an infection

spina bifida (spī'-nuh bihf'-ih-duh) – a neural tube birth defect characterized by a malformation of vertebrae, involving malformation and protrusion of the spinal cord and spinal nerve roots

surfactant (sər-fak'tənt) – a material secreted by special cells within the alveoli (air sacs) of the lung that makes the lung flexible and helps to keep the lung from collapsing

tachypnea (tak"-ip-nē'-uh) – abnormal rapidity of respiration

tetralogy of Fallot (teh-trahl'-uh-jē fal-ō') – a combination of congenital cardiac defects characterized by pulmonary stenosis, interventricular septal defect, dextroposition of the aorta so that it overrides the interventricular septum and receives venous as well as arterial blood, and right ventricular hypertrophy

trisomy (trī'-sō-mē) – condition that occurs when an individual or a cell has an extra chromosome

truncus arteriosus (trun'-kus ar-tē"-rē -ō'-sus) – birth defect in which a large, single arterial vessel is present at the top of the heart, from which the aortic arch and the pulmonary and coronary arteries originate

tympanostomy (tim"-puh-nahs'-tuh-mē) – surgery for otitis media in which a tube is inserted into the eardrum to allow for continuous drainage of fluid from the middle ear

vernix caseosa (ver'-niks cās-ē-ō'-suh) – the white, clinging, greasy material found on the skin of newborn infants

vesicoureteral reflux disease (veh"-sih-kō-yoo-rē'-ter-ul) – condition in which urine stored in the bladder can "backwash" up the ureters to the kidney

Transcription Tips

Transcription in pediatrics/neonatology can be challenging. However, knowledge of related terminology, common NICU disorders, major congenital abnormalities, genetic disorders, reflexes of the newborn, respiratory problems of the neonate, and neonatal infections will make the task much easier. A neurological exam on a newborn or young infant may include terms such as the following:

blinking reflex due to loud noise	blinking reflex due to bright light
palmar grasp reflex	rooting reflex
trunk incurving	vertical suspension position
stepping response	tonic neck reflex
mass reflexes	Perez reflex

Some Common NICU Problems/Disorders

prematurity	meconium aspiration
respiratory distress syndrome (RDS)	jaundice
patent ductus arteriosus	intraventricular hemorrhage (IVH)
apnea	multiple births
infection	infants with congenital defects (defect present at birth)
necrotizing entercolitis (NEC)	infants born with congenital heart disease (heart defect present at birth)
retinopathy of prematurity (ROP)	
pneumothorax	infants needing a septic workup

Selected Major Congenital and Chromosomal Anomalies Identifiable in the Neonate

Body System/Tissue	Defect
central nervous system	hydrocephalus
	meningocele
	myelomeningocele
	spina bifida occulta
skeletal system	dislocation of hip
	talipes equinovarus (clubfoot)

Body System/Tissue	Defect
genitourinary	exstrophy of the bladder
	hypospadias
gastrointestinal tract	cleft lip and palate
	esophageal atresia with or without tracheoesophageal fistula
	imperforate anus
	intestinal stenosis or atresia
	omphalocele
abdominal wall	diaphragmatic eventration or paralysis
	diaphragmatic hernia
	heart disease
	Hirschsprung disease
	tracheoesophageal fistula

Potential Genetic Disorders

Aicardi syndrome (ĕ-kahr-de′) – rare disorder characterized by partial or complete absence of the structure that links the two hemispheres of the brain, infantile spasms, mental retardation, and an ocular abnormality of the retina of the eye

Angelman syndrome (ān′jəl-mən) – neurological disorder characterized by severe congenital mental retardation, unusual facial appearance, and muscular abnormalities

cleidocranial dysplasia (kli″do-kra′ne-əl) – genetic disorder of bone development

cloacal exstrophy (klo-a′kəl ek′stro-fe) – very rare and complicated birth defect involving eversion of the gastrointestinal tract

Coffin Lowry syndrome – rare genetic disorder characterized by craniofacial and skeletal abnormalities, mental retardation, short stature, and hypotonia

craniosynostosis (kra″ne-o-sin″os-to′sis) – a deformity of the infant skull that results when the skull sutures between various skull bones fuse prematurely

Crouzon syndrome (kroo-zon′) – one of a large group of birth defects in which there is abnormal fusion of the bones of the skull and face

equinovarus (ē-kwɪ n″-nō-vār′-us) – clubfoot; a common birth defect characterized by certain ankle and foot abnormalities, where the foot is twisted inward and downward

Fragile X syndrome – most common genetically inherited form of mental retardation

Friedreich ataxia (frēd′rīk) – inherited disease with sclerosis of the dorsal and lateral columns of the spinal cord that causes progressive damage to the nervous system

hereditary spherocytosis (sfēr″o-si-to′sis) – disorder of the red blood cell membrane characterized by spherocytosis, abnormal fragility of erythrocytes, jaundice, and splenomegaly

Hermansky-Pudlak syndrome (HPS) (hər-mahn′ske pood′lahk) – a genetic disorder characterized by a rare form of albinism that is associated with low visual acuity, bruising and prolonged bleeding, and lung fibrosis

holoprosencephaly (hōl″o-pros″ən-sef′ə-le) – disorder caused by failure of the forebrain of the embryo to divide to form bilateral cerebral hemispheres; results in a deficit in midline facial development

Hurler syndrome (hur'lər) – a rare genetic disease characterized by a missing enzyme essential for breaking down sugar molecules and used in building connective tissues in the body; a type of mucopolysaccharidosis (MPS)

hypospadias (hi"po-spa'de-əs) – relatively common birth defect in males; characterized by the urethra opening on the underside of the penis or on the perineum

Klippel-Feil syndrome (klĭ-pel' fīl') – rare disorder characterized by the congenital fusion of any two of the seven cervical vertebrae, resulting in shortness of the neck

Kostmann syndrome (kost'mahn) – inherited disorder of the bone marrow

leukodystrophy (leukodystrophies) (loo"ko-dis'trə-fe) – a group of genetic disorders characterized by imperfect development or maintenance of the myelin sheath covering nerve fibers in the brain

Menkes disease (meng'kəz) – genetic neurodegenerative disorder of copper metabolism

myotonia congenital (mi"o-to'ne-ə) – genetic neuromuscular disorder characterized by slow relaxation of the muscles

Refsum disease (syndrome) (ref'soom) – one of a group of genetic disorders called *leukodystrophies* that affect growth of the myelin sheath

Rothmund-Thomson syndrome (RS) (rot'moond tom'son) – hereditary disease characterized by progressive degeneration, scarring, and abnormal pigmentation of the skin together with stunting of growth, baldness, cataracts, depressed nasal bridge, and malformations of the teeth, nails, and bone

Sandhoff disease (zahnd'hof) – rare, genetic lipid-storage disorder that causes progressive deterioration of the central nervous system

Sturge-Weber syndrome (sturj' va'bər) – congenital disorder characterized by a vascular birthmark and neurological abnormalities

Tay-Sachs disease (ta' saks') – a fatal, inherited disease of the central nervous system; death occurs by age five

Treacher Collins syndrome (tre'chər kol'inz) – a genetic birth defect that may affect the size and shape of the ears, eyelids, cheek bones, and upper and lower jaws

Normal Reflexes of the Newborn

auditory blink reflex – infant's eyes quickly close if the examiner loudly claps his or her hands 3 cm above the infant's head

Babinski reflex – extension of the great toe and flaring of the outer toes when the sole of the foot is stimulated

crossed extensor reflex – when one leg is extended and the knee is held straight, while the sole of the foot is stimulated, the opposite leg will flex

Landau sign – when the baby is suspended horizontally, with the head depressed against the trunk and the neck flexed, the legs will flex and be drawn up to the trunk

Moro reflex – response to sudden loud noise; the body stiffens and the arms go up and out, then forward and toward each other

neck righting – when the head is turned to one side, the shoulder and trunk, followed by the pelvis, will turn to that side

optical blink reflex – when light is suddenly shined into the open eyes, the eyes will close quickly with a quick dorsal flexion of the head

palmar grasp – pressure on palm of hand will elicit grasp reflex

plantar grasp – pressure on sole of foot behind toes causes flexion of toes

positive-supporting reflex – when held in an erect position, baby will stiffen the lower extremities and support his or her weight

pupillary reflexes – ipsilateral constriction to light

rooting – when the corner of the mouth is touched and an object is moved toward the cheek, an infant will turn the head toward the object and open the mouth

tonic neck reflex – sudden jolt will cause head to turn to one side with the leg and arm on that side extended, while the extremities on the other side flex

Potential Respiratory Problems of the Neonate

chronic lung disease of the neonate

meconium aspiration syndrome

persistent pulmonary hypertension

pneumonias

- intrauterine (congenital) pneumonia

- neonatal pneumonia

pneumothorax and pneumomediastinum

pulmonary hypoplasia

pulmonary interstitial emphysema

retained lung fluid syndromes

Potential Infections of the Neonate

conjunctivitis

enteritis

meningitis

omphalitis

osteomyelitis

otitis media

peritonitis

septicemia

tetanus

tuberculosis

urinary tract infection

Nonbacterial (Viral) Infections

HIV/AIDS

herpes simplex

TORCH syndrome

T = toxoplasmosis,

O = other viruses and congenital syphilis,

R = rubella,

C = cytomegalovirus, and

H = herpes simplex

Supportive Web Sites

http://www.webmd.com/	Search for "pediatrics" or "neonatology" for links on these topics.
http://www.nlm.nih.gov/medlineplus/	Click on "health topics" then under "demographic groups," select "children and teenagers" for an extensive list of relevant topics; you can also search for "pediatrics" and "neonatology."
http://www.oncolink.com/	Provides an alphabetical list of cancer types, including "pediatric cancer."
http://www.tchin.org/	Click on "Resources," then "Resource Room," then on links of interest.
	Under "Dictionaries," click on "Glossary of Childhood Onset Heart Disease" for a list of words and definitions.

Index of Pediatrics/Neonatology Reports

Exercise#	Patient Name	Type of Report/Procedure
TE#1	Riley Houston	Neonatal H&P: Birth
TE#2	Riley Houston	Neonatal Discharge Summary
TE#3	Jacob Lively	Pediatric Sick Visit: Arthralgias
TE#4	John Cantu	Pediatric Well Visit: 2 year old
TE#5	Betina Bandel	Pediatric Urgent Care Visit: Acute sinusitis
TE#6	Mary Ellen Harley	Pediatric Orthopedics Consult: Scoliosis
TE#7	Lilly Hamilton	Pediatric Sick Visit: Acute URI
TE#8	Jonathan Cramer	Pediatric Memo: Counseling, meds
TE#9	Jonathan Cramer	Pediatric SOAP Note: Behavioral issues

CHAPTER 14
PLASTIC/RECONSTRUCTIVE SURGERY

Introduction

Simply stated, *plastic surgery* is the surgical method of repairing or reconstructing body structures that are defective or have been damaged by injury or disease. Some of these deformities may be present at birth; others are caused by burns, wounds, trauma, disease, or the aging process. This method of surgery is employed to restore both function and appearance.

The word *plastic* is defined simply as "giving form or shape to a substance." As might be thought by many, neither the word *plastic* nor the substance bearing this name have any relationship to commercially prepared synthetic plastic materials and products. It is true, however, that medical-grade plastic materials may be used in some areas of reconstructive and cosmetic surgery.

The essence of plastic surgery is *tissue transplantation* and repositioning. *Tissues,* which include nerves, skin, bone, cartilage, tendon, mucous membrane, and fat, can be moved from sites near the damaged area or from remote parts of the body. In the new location, such tissue can substitute for damaged, deformed, or lost tissue; it can protect exposed and functioning areas.

For optimum and lasting results, *grafts* are transferred from one part of the body to another part of the same individual. This would constitute an *autologous* donation. It is possible, though, for bone, cartilage, skin, and corneas to be transplanted from one person to another. Living related donors, designated donors, and even cadaveric donors are some terms used in the donor processes.

Reconstructive surgery is performed to repair extravisceral defects and malformations, both congenital and acquired, and to restore function, as well as to prevent further loss of function. Reconstructive procedures include Z-plasty to reposition a scar, skin cancer removal, and gynecomastia (male breast reduction).

Cosmetic surgery involves reconstruction of the cutaneous tissues around the neck and face as well as other parts of the body to restore function, correct defects, and remove the marks of time.

Recent years have seen many advances in plastic surgery. Improved techniques have enabled surgeons to repair cleft lips and palates so that the remaining scars are almost imperceptible. It is now common practice to transfer ultrathin sheets of good skin from one area to another by use of an instrument called the *dermatome.* New materials, such as the rubber-silicone compound *Silastic* and medical mesh grafts, are being used safely and successfully to round out facial contours and fill in depressions.

Critical Thinking Exercise

?

You have heard through the grapevine that your boss is scheduled for an abdominoplasty in the near future; you had one five years ago with major complications. She is apparently using the same physician you had. How can you discretely discuss with your boss the problems you encountered as a result of negligence on the part of the surgeon without jeopardizing your job? List how to approach your boss regarding this delicate, confidential situation.

Plastic surgeons are frequently called upon to treat patients who have been burned. Burns are classified as first, second, third, or fourth degree depending on the depth of the burn. In many cases, grafting of tissue is required to restore function and appearance to the affected area(s).

The practice of plastic and reconstructive surgery is not confined to the head and neck; it is successfully performed on all parts of the body, as needed. However, the plastic and reconstructive surgeon may work with otorhinolaryngology (ENT) surgeons on some head and neck procedures.

Plastic/Reconstructive Surgery Abbreviations

The abbreviations, acronyms, and terms in the following abbreviations and terminology sections are often dictated in this specialty. We offer abbreviated definitions here. Please see an unabridged medical dictionary or the suggested web sites in this chapter for more information on each term.

ATL	antitension line
BTX or BTX-A	botulinum toxin type A (Botox)
B-W	Braun-Wangensteen graft
CAD	cadaver donor
CL	cleft lip
CP	cleft palate
CRIF	closed reduction, internal fixation
DIP	distal interphalangeal
FTSG	full-thickness skin graft

ILP	intense light pulse
IP	interphalangeal
NHBP	non-heart-beating donor
PIP	proximal interphalangeal
RSTL	relaxed skin tension lines
STSG	split-thickness skin graft
TBSA	total body surface area
TMJ	temporomandibular joint
TRAM	transverse rectus abdominis myocutaneous procedure

Anatomic Illustrations

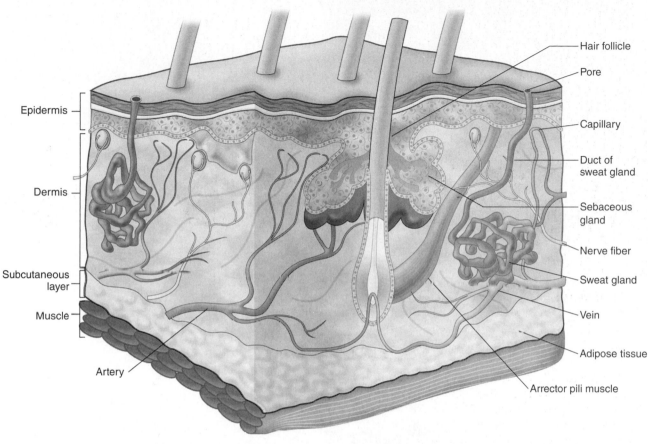

Epidermis

Dermis

Subcutaneous layer

Muscle

Artery

Hair follicle

Pore

Capillary

Duct of sweat gland

Sebaceous gland

Nerve fiber

Sweat gland

Vein

Adipose tissue

Arrector pili muscle

Copyright © 2015 Cengage Learning®

FIGURE 14-1   Structures of the skin; the sweat and sebaceous glands are associated structures of the skin

Plastic/Reconstructive Surgery Terminology

A

abdominoplasty (ab-dahm'-ih-nō-plas"-tē) – surgery to remove excess skin and tighten a protuberant abdomen; for example, one that can result from multiple pregnancies

allograft (syn. homograft) (al'-ō-graft, hō'-mō-graft) – graft from one individual to another in the same species

autograft (aw'-tō-graft) – graft from one place to another on the same individual

autologous (aw-tol'-uh-gus) – in transplantation, refers to transfer of an organ or other tissue from one location to another in the same person; regarding blood and blood components, refers to those donations the patient has previously made and receives at a later time, usually preoperatively

B

bariatric surgery (bar"e-at'rik) – a term that refers to several different types of weight-loss surgery: gastric bypass, gastric banding, lap banding, gastric sleeve, and duodenal switch

blepharochalasis (blef"-uh-rō-kal'-uh-sis) – relaxation of the skin of the eyelid due to atrophy of the intercellular tissue

blepharoplasty (blef'-uh-rō-plas"-tē) – surgery on the eyelids to correct blepharochalasis

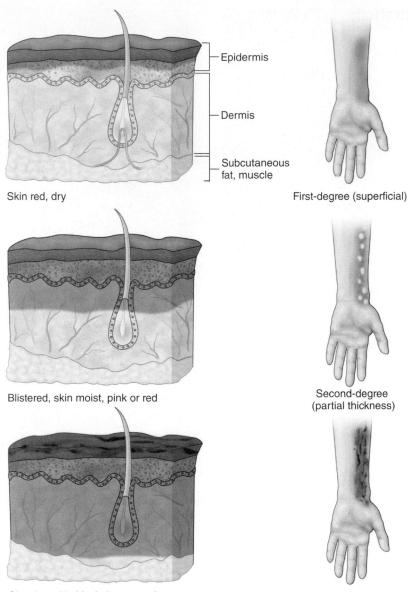

Skin red, dry

Epidermis

Dermis

Subcutaneous fat, muscle

First-degree (superficial)

Blistered, skin moist, pink or red

Second-degree (partial thickness)

Charring, skin black, brown, red

Third-degree (full thickness)

FIGURE 14-2 The degree of a burn is determined by the layers of skin involved

blepharoptosis (blef"-uh-rōp-tō'-sis) – drooping of upper eyelid(s) due to paralysis

brachioplasty (brā'-kē-ō-plas"-tē) – surgery to correct "batwing arms"; surgery to tighten or remove hanging skin of the inner arms

canthus (kan'-thus) – the angle at either end of the fissure between the eyelids; the points at which the upper and lower eyelids meet

cellulite (sel'u-līt) – subcutaneous fat deposits that cause a dimpled condition of the skin, such as on the thigh or buttock

cheilectomy (kī-lek'-tuh-mē) – excision of a lip

cheiloplasty (kī'-lō-plas"-tē) – surgical repair of a defect of the lip

chemical peel – also known as "chemexfoliation" or "derma-peeling"; a technique to improve the appearance of the skin whereby a chemical solution is applied to the skin that causes it to "blister," eventually peel off, leaving smoother and less wrinkled skin

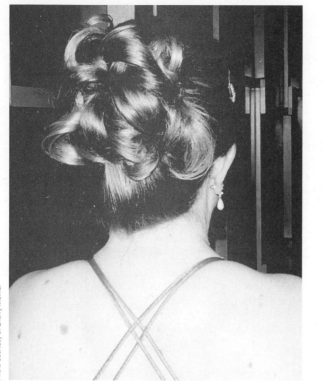

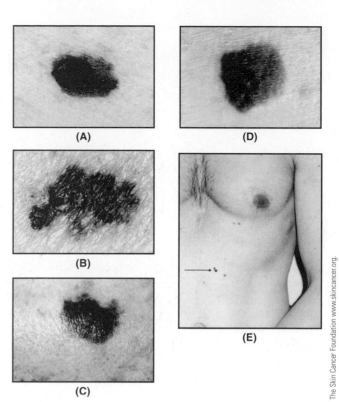

FIGURE 14-3 Left: Melanoma visible on the left shoulder blade. Right: The A-B-C-D-E signs of melanoma are (A) symmetry, (B) border irregularity, (C) color variation, and (D) diameter larger than a pencil eraser, (E) evolving, or changing in size, shape, or shade of color.

cicatrix (sik'-uh-triks, sik-ā'-triks) – the normal, nonraised scar left by a healed wound

cleft lip or palate (kleft lip or pal'ăt) – birth defect characterized by a split through the lip, the roof of the mouth, or the soft tissue in the back of the mouth resulting from failure of these structures to close normally during early fetal development; often, plastic surgery and otorhinolaryngology will work together on these surgical procedures

craniofacial reconstruction (krā"-nē-ō-fā'-shul) – surgery for head and facial deformities; often, plastic surgery and neurosurgery work together on these surgical procedures

D

dermabrasion (der"-muh-brā-zhun) – surgical removal of the frozen epidermis and as much of the dermis as necessary by mechanical means

dermatome (dur'mə-tōm) – instrument for incising the skin or for cutting thin slices for transplantation of skin

E

endovenous laser (en"do-ve'nəs) – an alternative for varicose vein treatment where a small laser fiber is placed inside the vein; pressure is then placed on the vein, and the laser delivers pulses of laser light, which cause the vein to collapse

electrodermatome (e-lek"tro-dur'mə-tōm) – an electrical dermatome for cutting off layers of skin from large areas in a short time; used in skin grafting, shaving scars, and the like

eschar (es'-kar) – a thick, coagulated crust or slough that develops following thermal burn, chemical burn, or physical cauterization of the skin; a scab

escharotomy (es-kar-ot'-uh-mē) – surgical incision into a burn eschar to lessen constriction

escutcheon (es-kuh'-chun) – the pattern of distribution of the pubic hair

exsanguinate (eks-sang'-gwih-nāt) – to deprive of blood; bloodless

fat grafting – a technique whereby fat cells are extracted from one area of the body and injected into another area where needed, such as in surgical buttock augmentation

facioplasty (fā'-shē-ō-plas"-tē) – reparative or reconstructive surgery of the face

genioplasty (jē'-nē-ō-plas"-tē) – a type of cosmetic surgery that is used to improve the appearance of a person's chin; also called "mentoplasty"

gynecomastia (gi"nə- jin"ə-ko-mas'te-ə) – excessive growth of the male mammary glands

hypermastia (hī"-per-mas'-tē-uh) – hypertrophy of the mammary gland

hypomastia (hī-pō-mas'-tē-uh) – abnormal smallness of the mammary glands

inframammary incisions (in"-fruh-mā'-uh-rē) – incisions made below the mammary gland

keloid (kē'-loyd) – a mass of raised, hyperplastic, fibrous connective scar tissue

keloplasty (kē'-lō-plas"-tē) – surgical removal of a scar or keloid

labiaplasty (la'be-ə-plas"te) – surgical procedure to reduce elongated labia (the external folds of skin surrounding the vaginal opening); also known as labioplasty or labial reduction surgery (sing. labium)

laser therapy (lā-zər ' ther-ə-pē) – with intense light pulse (ILP), it destroys tiny spider veins and small varicose veins with heat that causes scar tissue to form; this eventually closes off the vein, working more slowly than sclerotherapy

laserbrasion surgery (lā'-zur-brā'-zhun) – procedure that uses light beams to vaporize the top layers of the skin to minimize the appearance of wrinkles, scars, or birthmarks

lipectomy (lip-ek'-tuh-mē) – the excision of a mass of subcutaneous adipose tissue, as from the abdominal wall

liposuction (lī-pō"-suk'-shun) – surgical reduction of excess fatty deposits

mammaplasty (syn. mammoplasty) (mā'-uh-plas"-tē, mā'-ō-plas"-tē) – plastic reconstruction of the breast, as may be done to either augment or reduce its size

mammaplasty reduction – surgery to reduce breast size

mastopexy (mass'-tō-pek-sē) – mammaplasty performed to correct a pendulous breast

mentoplasty (men"-tō-plas'-tē) – surgery done on the chin to either augment or reduce; this results in a better definition of the face; also called "genioplasty"

microdermabrasion (mī"-krō-der'-muh-brā'-zhun) – a mini-peeling of the skin surface with minimal risk of dyspigmentation or scarring; also known as "power peel"

myocutaneous (mī"-ō-kyoo-tā'-nē-us) – denoting a parcel comprising a muscle and its investments, its vascular supply, the overlying skin, and intervening tissues

O

orthognathic surgery (or"-thahg-nā'-thik) – procedure performed in cooperation with a patient's dentist, orthodontist, or oromaxillofacial surgeon to correct problems with the "bite" or jaw alignment

otoplasty (ō'-tō-plas"-tē) – surgical correction of ear deformities and defects

palatoplasty (pal'-uh-tō-plas"-tē) – plastic reconstruction of the palate, including cleft palate correction

palatorrhaphy (pal"-uh-tōr-uh-fē) – suture of a cleft palate

palpebra (pl. palpebrae) (pal'-pē-bruh, pal'-pē'-brē) – (noun) eyelid(s)

palpebral (pal'-pē-bruhl) – (adj.) pertaining to an eyelid or the eyelids

Panas operation (pan-ahz') – attachment of the upper eyelid to the occipitofrontalis muscle for correction of ptosis

pharyngoplasty (fah-ring'-gō-plas"-tē) – plastic surgery operation on the pharynx

ptosis (pl. ptoses) (tō-sis, tō-sees) – a sinking down or prolapse of an organ or a part

punch biopsy – a cylindrical instrument used to obtain a plug of tissue for pathologic examination and diagnosis

radiofrequency ablation (ra"de-o-fre'kwən-se ab-la'shən) – a nonsurgical option for treatment of varicose veins where a small catheter delivers radiofrequency energy (instead of laser energy) directly into the vein wall, causing it to heat up and collapse

retinoids (ret'ĭ-noidz) – derivatives of vitamin A that minimize the appearance of wrinkles, bolster the thickness and elasticity of the skin, slow the breakdown of collagen, and lighten brown spots caused by sun exposure

rhinocheiloplasty (rī"-nō-kī'-lō-plas"-tē) – plastic surgery of the nose and lip

rhinoplasty (rī'-nō-plas"-tē) – plastic surgery of the nose, whether reconstructive, restorative, or cosmetic

rhinotomy (rī-not'-uh-mē) – incision into the nose

rhytidectomy (rit"ĭ-dek'tə-me) – also known as a "face lift"; a surgical procedure that removes excess skin and fat and tightens the skin of the face

rhytidoplasty (rit'-ih-dō-plas"-tē) – plastic surgery for the elimination of wrinkles from the skin

rhytidosis (rit"-ih-dō'-sis) – a wrinkling of the cornea

sclerotherapy (sklēr"o-ther'ə-pe) – a procedure for the treatment of spider and varicose veins whereby the physician injects a solution directly into the abnormal vein; the blood vessel is destroyed, becomes fibrotic, and eventually disappears

septorhinoplasty (syn. septoplasty) (sep"-tō-rī'-nō-plas"-tē, sep"-tō-plas"-tē) – a form of rhinoplasty performed to reconstruct the nasal passage or to relieve obstructions inside the nose to correct breathing problems

spider veins (spī-dər' vānz) – small, twisted blood vessels that are visible through the skin

suction lipectomy (lĭ-pek'tə-me) – body-contouring technique to aspirate fat by vacuuming from the buttocks, flanks, abdomen, thighs, upper arms, knees, ankles, or chin

tantalum (tan'-tuh-lum) – a noncorrosive and malleable metal that has been used for plates or disks to replace cranial defects, for wire sutures, and for making prosthetic appliances

tarsorrhaphy (tahr-sōr'-uh-fē) – the operation of suturing together a portion of or the entire upper and lower eyelids for the purpose of shortening or closing entirely the palpebral fissure

temporomandibular joint (tē"-pō-rō-man-dib'-yoolur) – the joint that connects the lower jaw to the mandible

vaginoplasty (vaj'ĭ-no-plas"te) – a plastic surgery procedure also called "colpoplasty" or "vaginal rejuvenation" whereby vaginal muscles that have been stretched due to childbirth are tightened

varicose veins (var'ĭ-kōs) – large blood vessels that are swollen and twisted; can develop anywhere in the body but are usually found on the legs and ankles

vermilion border (vur-mil'-yun) – the red boundary of the lips that represents the highly vascular

epithelial covering between the outer skin and moist oral mucosa of the mouth

xenograft (syn. heterograft) (zē'-nō-graft het' ər-o-graft") – graft transferred from an animal of one species to one of another species

xiphisternum (zif"-ih-ster'-num) – the xiphoid process

Transcription Tips

To be successful in completing plastic and reconstructive surgery dictation, become familiar with the accessory organs of the skin, in addition to the various layers of the skin, as in dermatology. Recognizing terminology used in cosmetic surgery is also helpful.

The following information provides data on types of grafts and more specialized plastic and reconstructive surgery procedures.

Types of Grafts

Most plastic surgery requires moving tissue from one part of the body to another. The moved tissue, or *graft*, is referred to as an *autograft*; skin, bone, cartilage, fat, fascia, muscle, or nerves may be taken.

Tissue transplanted from another person is called a *homograft (allograft)*. The tissue can be obtained from living persons or taken from bodies soon after death.

Heterografts (xenografts) consist of tissue from another species. Plastic surgery may be performed by means of free grafting—cutting tissue from one part of the body and moving it directly to another part.

Split-thickness grafts consist of the epidermis and varying thicknesses of the dermis. *Thin split-thickness grafts* have only a very thin layer of the dermis. *Intermediate* and *thick split-thickness grafts* have a thicker layer of dermis attached to the epidermis.

Full-thickness grafts are used primarily to cover small areas where matching skin color and texture are important, such as on the face.

Skin flaps are used when a large and deep defect is to be covered. "Sliding," "rotating," or "tubed" are a few of the terms used to identify various types of grafts that are never completely removed from the body at any one time, thereby maintaining a direct vascular supply.

Specialized Plastic/Reconstructive Surgery Procedures

cleft palate repair – surgery to repair a congenital fissure in the roof of the mouth

ear reconstruction for microtia – microtia exists when there is a congenital absence of part or all of the external ear

hypospadias repair – hypospadias is a congenital anomaly where the urethra ends on the top surface of the penis or in the perineum

repair of acute burns – skin grafting is utilized to repair tissue that has been severely burned

repair of syndactyly – syndactyly exists when the digits of the hand or feet are webbed

tattooing – useful in plastic surgery for changing the color of grafted skin so that it more closely resembles the surrounding skin

Supportive Web Sites

http://www.the-cosmetic-surgery-directory. com/procedures.html

Provides a list of cosmetic procedures available.

http://www.nlm.nih.gov/medlineplus/

Search for "plastic surgery" for links with detailed information.

http://www.plasticsurgery.org/

Click on "cosmetic" to see different types of cosmetic procedures; click on "reconstructive" to see types of reconstructive procedures.

Index of Plastic/Reconstructive Surgery Reports

Exercise#	Patient Name	Type of Report/Procedure
TE#1	Jamie Lynn Childers	Consultation: Breast cancer
TE#2	Jamie Lynn Childers	Office Visit: Recheck
TE#3	Jamie Lynn Childers	Office Visit: Recheck
TE#4	Jamie Lynn Childers	Preop Visit: Breast reconstruction
TE#5	Jamie Lynn Childers	Postoperative Visit
TE#6	Jamie Lynn Childers	Office Visit: Discuss implants
TE#7	Jamie Lynn Childers	Preop Visit: Replacement of implants
TE#8	Jamie Lynn Childers	Operative Report: Breast reconstruction
TE#9	Jamie Lynn Childers	Urgent Care Visit: Infection
TE#10	Jamie Lynn Childers	Office Visit: Recheck
TE#11	Jamie Lynn Childers	Office Visit: Discuss tattoos
TE#12	Lawrence V. Stewart	Bilateral upper lid blepharoplasty
TE#13	Anderson Lee	Punch biopsy procedure, chin

CHAPTER 15
PATHOLOGY

Introduction

Pathology is the branch of medicine dealing with the study of disease. It is divided into anatomic and clinical pathology. Clinical pathology deals with testing done in vitro (in glass or a test tube). Anatomic pathology deals with testing done in vivo (in the living body). Tissue specimens submitted from surgery are examined grossly and microscopically by a pathologist.

The *pathologist* is a physician who seeks to determine the cause of disease as well as the changes the disease causes in cells, tissues, organs, and the body as a whole. Additionally, the pathologist studies the form the disease may take, together with the complications that may follow. If the disease leads to death, an *autopsy* may be performed by the pathologist, providing additional clues to the process and termination of the disease.

Pathologists receive tissue for examination through the removal of specimens during surgical procedures. A *biopsy,* a small piece of tissue removed for pathological examination, is widely used for detection of malignant cells. Pathologic examinations, both *gross* and *microscopic,* at the time of surgery or autopsy provide the ultimate answer in assessing tissue and organ damage to the body. These examinations establish the cause or contributing cause of disease and death. The cytology lab is where cells from fluid specimens and Pap smears are processed. The histology lab is where tissue cells are processed.

Anatomic and Clinical Lab

The pathologist is in charge of the following subsections of the hospital laboratory. Each member of the group of pathologists contracted by the hospital would be Board Certified in Anatomic and Clinical Pathology.

Anatomic Lab:	Autopsy Room or Morgue
	Histology Lab
	Cytology Lab
Clinical Lab:	Blood Bank with Donor Room
	Hematology and Urinalysis Labs
	Chemistry and Special Chemistry Labs
	Microbiology Lab
	Serology Lab

Critical Thinking Exercise

?

As a healthcare documentation specialist working in a hospital pathology department, you notice that an acquaintance has been received into the morgue after surgery, and an autopsy is pending. The autopsy is being done without permission from the next of kin. Can an autopsy be done without permission? Explain why or why not.

 Pathology Abbreviations

The abbreviations, acronyms, and terms in the following abbreviations and terminology sections are often dictated in this specialty. We offer abbreviated definitions here. Please see an unabridged medical dictionary and/or the suggested web sites in this chapter for more information on each term.

ABG	arterial blood gas	**CPK**	creatine phosphokinase
ACTH	adrenocorticotropic hormone	**DJD**	degenerative joint disease
AFB	acid-fast bacilli	**DNA**	deoxyribonucleic acid
A/G	albumin-to-globulin ratio	**E coli**	Escherichia coli
AHT	antihyaluronidase titer	**ERA**	evoked response audiometry
AIDS	acquired immunodeficiency syndrome	**ET**	essential thrombocythemia, eustachian tube, exchange transfusion
ANF	antinuclear fluorescent antibodies	**FAN**	fluorescent antinuclear antibodies
ALT	alanine aminotransferase		
AST	aspartate aminotransferase	**FBS**	fasting blood sugar
BM	bone marrow, bone metastases, bowel movement, brain metastases	**FISH**	fluorescent in situ hybridization
		FS	frozen section
BMP	basic metabolic profile or panel	**FSH**	follicle-stimulating hormone
Bx	biopsy	**FTA**	fluorescent treponemal antibody
CMP	comprehensive metabolic profile or panel	**GGTP**	gamma-glutamyl transpeptidase

GTM	glucose tolerance meal
GTT	glucose tolerance test
HAA	hepatitis-associated antigen
HBD	hydroxybutyrate dehydrogenase
hCG	human chorionic gonadotropin
Hct	hematocrit
H&E	hematoxylin & eosin (stain)
Hgb, Hb	hemoglobin
HIAA	hydroxyindoleacetic acid
HNP	herniated nucleus pulposus
HPF	high-power field
IgG	immunoglobulin G
LAP	leucine aminopeptidase or leukocyte alkaline phosphatase
LDH	lactic dehydrogenase
LFT	liver function test
LP	lipid panel, lipoprotein, lumbar puncture
MCH	mean corpuscular hemoglobin
MCL	mantle cell lymphoma
MCHC	mean corpuscular hemoglobin concentration
MCV	mean corpuscular volume
mmHg	millimeters of mercury
MRSA	methicillin-resistant Staphylococcus aureus

MRSE	methicillin-resistant Staphylococcus epidermidis
OCP	ova, cysts, parasites
Pap	Papanicolaou stain, Pap smear
pH	hydrogen ion concentration, pH of arterial blood—always lowercase p
PKU	phenylketonuria
PPD	purified protein derivative (of tuberculin)
PPLO	pleuropneumonia-like organism
PRA	plasma renin activity
QNS	quantity not sufficient
Rh	Rhesus factor in blood
RIA	radioimmunoassay
RPE	retinal pigment epithelium
RPR	rapid plasma regain (test for syphilis)
SIDS	sudden infant death syndrome
SP GR	specific gravity
SSKI	saturated solution of potassium iodide
STS	serologic test for syphilis
TNTC	too numerous to count
TSH	thyroid-stimulating hormone
UCG	urinary chorionic gonadotropins
USG	urine specific gravity
VRE	vancomycin-resistant enterococcus
WBRT	whole-brain radiation therapy

Anatomic Illustrations

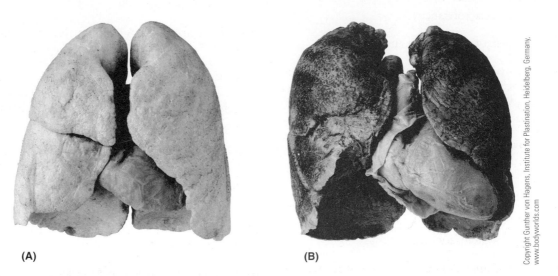

(A) (B)

FIGURE 15-1 **Photographs of actual lung and heart specimens: (A) healthy lungs of a nonsmoker; (B) damaged lungs of a smoker**

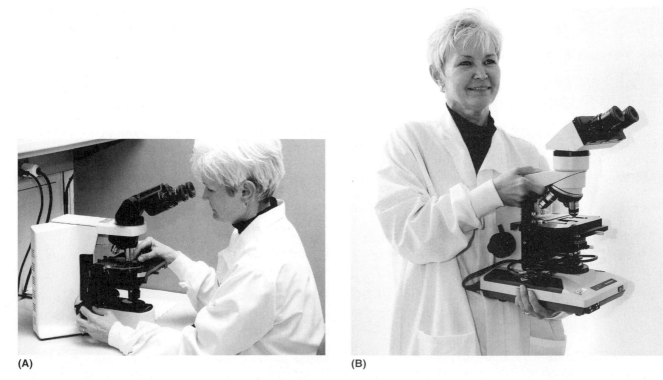

(A) (B)

FIGURE 15-2 **Use and care of the microscope: (A) observe slide and objectives when changing from high-power to oil-version objective; (B) correct way to transport a microscope**

Pathology Terminology

A

abscess – a localized collection of pus within tissues, organs, or confined spaces formed by the disintegration of tissue

adenoma (ad"ə-no'mə) – a benign epithelial tumor in which the cells form recognizable glandular structures or in which the cells are clearly derived from glandular epithelium

adenomyosis (ad"-ē-nō-mī-ō'-sis) – a benign condition characterized by ingrowth of the endometrium into the uterine musculature

agenesis (a-jen'ə-sis) – absence, failure of formation, or imperfect development of an organ

aleukemic (ā"-loo-kē'-mik) – marked by aleukemia, the absence or deficiency of leukocytes (white blood cells) in the blood

aleukocytic (ā-loo"-kō-sit'-ik) – showing no leukocytes

amelanotic (ā"-mel-uh-not'-ik) – containing no melanin; unpigmented

amitotic (ā"-mī-tot'-ik) – of the nature of amitosis; not occurring by mitosis

amorphous (uh-mor'-fuss) – without definite shape or form

angioma (an jē-ō'-muh) – a swelling or tumor resulting from proliferation with or without dilation of the blood vessels or lymphatics

apocrine (ap'-o-krīn, ap'-uh-krin) – denoting that type of glandular secretion in which the free end or apical portion of the secreting cell is cast off along with the secretory products that have accumulated therein

Armanni-Ebstein changes (ar-mah'-nē-eb-stīn) – epithelial tubule containing deposits of glycogen; occurs in diabetes mellitus

arrhenoblastoma (ah-re"-nō-blas-to'-muh) – a neoplasm of the ovary, arising from the ovarian stroma

Askanazy cells (as-kuh-nah'-zē) – follicular cells of the thyroid that show increased eosinophilia and nuclear enlargement, e.g., in Hashimoto disease (syn. Hürthle cells)

astrup (ass'-trup) – an instrument designed to determine the pH, partial carbon dioxide, and bicarbonates of the blood

atresia (ə-tre'zhə) – congenital absence or closure of a normal body orifice or tubular organ

Auer bodies (ow'-er) – elongated bacteria-like inclusions found in the cytoplasm of myeloblasts, myelocytes, monoblasts, and granular histiocytes; thought to be nucleoprotein material

autolysis (aw-tahl'-ih-sis) – the spontaneous disintegration of tissues or cells by the action of their own autogenous enzymes, such as occurs after death and in some pathological conditions

azure eosin (azh'-yoor ē'-ō-sin) – a stain for chromaffin

azurophilic (azh"-yoor-ō-fil'-ik) – staining well with blue aniline dyes

B

Bacteroides (bak"-ter-oy'-dēz) – a genus of non-sporulating obligate anaerobic filamentous bacteria occurring as normal flora in the mouth and large bowel; often found in necrotic tissues, probably as secondary invaders

Bartonella (bar"-tō-nel'-luh) – a genus of bacteria; these organisms multiply in fixed tissue cells

Bielschowsky stain (bē"-el-show'-skē) – a silver stain for demonstrating axons and neurofibrils

biopsy (bi'op-se) – (verb) process of removing tissue from patients for microscopic examination and diagnosis; (noun) a specimen obtained via biopsy procedure—many subcategories of biopsy exist

blood group – the ABO blood group consists of four major blood types: A, B, AB, and O.

Boeck sarcoid (bek sar'-koyd) – a nonmalignant, granulomatous disease with an unknown cause that affects mainly the lungs, skin, and bone

bone marrow aspiration (mer-ō as-pə-'rā-shən) – test for aplastic anemia, leukemia, certain cancers, and polycythemia; performed by aspirating (removing) bone marrow via a lumbar puncture

botryoid (bot're-oid) – resembling a bunch of grapes

Bouin solution (bwahn') – a fixation solution for tissue that is especially good for skin and other tissue in which cellular detail is important

calcospherite (kal"-kō-sfar'-īt) – one of the small globular bodies formed during the process of calcification

Call-Exner bodies (kahl"-eks'-ner) – the accumulations of densely staining material that appear among granulosa cells in maturing ovarian follicles and that may be intracellular precursors of follicular fluid

cancer – general term frequently used to indicate any of various types of neoplasms, most of which invade surrounding tissues; may spread to other sites, are likely to recur after attempted removal, and are likely to result in death unless treated adequately

carbolfuchsin stain (kar"-bahl-fook'-sin) – a stain for acid-fast bacteria

carcinoma (kar' sin o" muh) – any of various types of malignant neoplasm derived from epithelial cells, chiefly glandular or squamous cells; the most commonly occurring type of cancer

caseous (ka'se-əs) – having a consistency like that of cottage cheese

catarrh (kə-tahr') – inflammation of mucous membranes, especially in the air passages of the head and throat, with a free discharge of mucus

celloidin (seh-loy'-din) – a solution of pyroxylin in ether and alcohol, used for embedding histologic specimens

celloidin section (seh-loy'-din) – a microscopically thin section cut by a microtome from a specimen of tissue that has been embedded in celloidin

chondromyxofibroma (kon"-drō-mik"-sō-fi-brō'-muh) – a benign connective tissue tumor containing cartilage cells, fibrocytes, and a degenerated granular material (myxoid tissue)

chordoma (kor-dō'-muh) – a malignant tumor arising from the embryonic remains of the notochord

coccidiosis (kok"-sid-ē-ō'-sis) – infection by coccidian

condyloma (kon"-dih-lō'-muh) – a wart-like excrescence at the anus or vulva or on the glans penis

condyloma acuminatum (kon"-dih-lō'-muh ah-kyoo"-mih-nah'-tum) – a contagious projecting warty growth on the external genitalia or at the anus due to sexual contact with infection by human papillomavirus (syn. venereal wart, genital wart)

Coombs test (kooms) – a test using various antisera, usually employed to detect the presence of proteins on the surface of red cells

corpus (pl. corpora) (kor'-pus kor'-pō-ruh) – any body or mass; the main part of an organ as distinguished from the head or tail

corpora amylacea (kor'-pō-ruh am"-ī-lā'-shē-uh) – small ovoid or rounded bodies resembling grains of starch found in nervous tissue, in the prostate, and in pulmonary alveoli

corrugated ('korə, geɪ təd) – having a ripple-like distortion

cotyledon (kot"-ih-lē'-don) – any one of the subdivisions of the uterine surface, a placental unit

cyst – an abnormal sac filled with gas, fluid, or semi-solid material that is lined by a membrane

cystosarcoma phyllodes (sis"-tō-sar-kō'-muh fil'-uhdēz) – a low-grade malignant tumor of the human breast resembling a giant fibroadenoma and often containing cleft-like cystic spaces

cytology (sī-tol" ō-jē) – the study of the anatomy, physiology, pathology, and chemistry of the cell (syn. cellular biology)

deciduoma (dē-sid"-yoo-ō'-muh) – an intrauterine mass containing decidual cells

Demodex folliculorum (dem'-ō-deks fahl-ik"-yoo-lō'rum) – a species of mite found in hair follicles and in secretions of the sebaceous glands, especially of the face and nose

Diff-Quik™ (dihf'-kwik) – a product used to obtain histochemical stains or smears

diphtheritic membrane (dif"the-rit'ik) – a thin coating on the surface of an epithelial-lined organ that is composed of necrotic cellular debris, inflammatory cells, and fibrin

Diplococcus pneumoniae (dip"-lō-kok'-us noo-mō'-nē-uh) – a species of bacteria that is a common cause of lobar pneumonia

Döhle inclusion bodies (dō '-lē in-kloo'-zhun) – small coccus-shaped bodies occurring in the poly-nuclear leukocytes of the blood in several diseases, especially scarlet fever

dysgenesis (dis-jen'ə-sis) – defective embryonic development

dysplasia (dis-pla'zhə) – abnormal tissue development

dysontogenesis (dis"-ahn-tō-jen'-eh-sis) – defective embryonic development

ecchymosis (ek"ĭ-mo'sis) – a purplish patch caused by extravasation of blood into the tissues differing from petechiae only in size

Ehrlich™ (ār'-lik) – brand name for a test/staining method—Erlich test, acid hematoxylin stain, diazo reaction, triacid stain, triple stain, etc.

Ehrlichia (ār-lik'-ē-uh) – gram-negative bacteria; transmitted by ticks

enchondroma (en"-kahn-drō'-muh) – a benign growth of cartilage arising in the metaphysis of a bone

eosin (e'o-sin) – staining solution commonly used in histology; often combined with hematoxylin and dictated "H&E" for hematoxylin and eosin (**NB**: Do not transcribe "HNE" for H&E)

eroded (ē-rōd'd) – having a shallow or superficial ulceration

erythropoiesis (ē-rith"-rō-poy-ē'-sis) – the production of erythrocytes (red blood cells)

Escherichia coli (E coli) (esh"-er-ih'-kē-uh kohl'-ī) – a species of organisms constituting the greater part of the intestinal flora of humans and other animals; often dictated E coli

etiology (e"te-ol'ə-je) – the causative agent in a lesion

F

ferrugination (fuh-roo'-jih-nā-shun) – mineralization (with iron) of the blood vessels of the brain

fetus papyraceous (fē'-tus pap"-ih-rā'-shus) – extreme compression of a dead fetus by its living twin

fibrin (fi'brin) – a filamentous protein formed from the precursor fibrinogen by the enzyme thrombin; it forms the essential portion of a blood clot

Fibrindex™ test (fi'-brin-deks) – a test to determine the adequacy of fibrinogen of the blood

flocculent (flok'u-lənt) – containing downy or flaky masses

friable (fri'ə-bəl) – easily pulverized or crumbled

G

gemistocytic (jem-is"-tō-sih'-tik) – composed of large round cells (gemistocytes)

Giemsa™ stain (gem'-sah) – a solution used for staining protozoan parasites, such as trypanosomes; also Giemsa method

gitter cell (git'-er) – a honeycombed cell packed with a number of lipoid granules

glioma (gli-o'mə) – a broad category of brain and spinal cord tumors that come from glial cells, the main brain cells that can develop into cancer

glomangioma (glō-man"-jē-ō'-muh) – a benign, often painful tumor derived from a neuromyoarterial glomus, usually occurring on the distal portions of the fingers and toes, in the skin, or in deeper structures

Gomori™ methenamine silver stain (guh-mōr'-ē meth"-en-am'-ēn) – stain used specifically for fungus; there are several other Gomori staining methods/procedures

granuloma (gran"u-lo'mə) – a focal collection of activated macrophages

gross (grōs) – large enough to be visible to the naked eye; macroscopic

grumous (groo'məs) – clotted or lumpy

gynandroblastoma (jī-nan"-drō-blas-tō'-muh) – a rare ovarian tumor containing histological features of both arrhenoblastoma and granulosa cell tumor

Hamman-Rich syndrome (ham'-un rich) – a disease characterized by widespread fibrosis of the lung parenchyma

Hassall corpuscles (hass'-ul kor'-puh-suhlz) – small concentrically striated bodies in the thymus

hemangiopericytoma (hē-man"-jē-ō-pār"-ē-sih-tō'muh) – a tumor composed of spindle cells with a rich vascular network, which apparently arises from pericytes

hematoma (he"mə-to'mə) – a localized collection of blood, usually clotted, in an organ, space, or tissue, usually due to a break in the wall of a blood vessel

hematoxylin stain (hēm"-ah-tok'-sih-lin) – an intense blue stain used in the preparation of microscopic tissue specimens; stains the nucleus of the cell (see eosin above)

hemosiderin (hē"-mō-sid'-er-in) – an insoluble form of storage iron in which the micelles of ferric hydroxide are so arranged as to be visible microscopically, both with and without the use of specific staining methods

histology (his-tol" o-jē) – the science concerned with the minute structure of cells, tissues, and organs in relation to their function (syn. microscopic anatomy)

Hürthle cells (her'-tul) – follicular cells of the thyroid that show increased eosinophilia and nuclear enlargement, e.g., in Hashimoto disease (syn. Askanazy cells)

hyperemia (hi"pər-e'me-ə) – presence of an increased amount of blood in a part or an organ

hypereosinophilia (hī"-per-ē"-ō-sin-ō-fil'-ē-uh) – excessive eosinophilia, the formation and accumulation of an abnormally large number of eosinophils in the blood

hypertrophy (hi-pur'trə-fe) – the enlargement or overgrowth of an organ or part due to an increase in size of its constituent cells

hypogammaglobulinemia (hī"-pō-gam"-uh-glob"-yoolin-ē'-mē-uh) – an immunological deficiency state generally characterized by an abnormally low level of all classes of gamma globulin in the blood

hypoplasia (hi"po-pla'zhə) – incomplete or underdevelopment of a tissue or organ usually due to a decrease in the number of cells

iatrogenic (ī"-at-rō-jen'-ik) – resulting from the activity of physicians

indurated (in'du-rāt"əd) – abnormally hard

infarct (in'fahrkt) – a localized area of ischemic necrosis produced by the occlusion of the blood vessels—either arterial supply or venous drainage

in vitro (in vē'trō) – in glass or in a test tube

in vivo (in vē'vō) – in the living body

Jakob-Creutzfeldt disease (yak'-ob-kroytz'-felt) – a progressive dementia involving gray matter and basal ganglia

Kaposi sarcoma (kap'-uh-sē) – a multifocal, metastasizing, malignant reticulosis with features resembling those of angiosarcoma, mainly involving the skin, manifest as reddish blue or brownish soft nodules and tumors; the signature lesion of patients with full-blown AIDS

karyolysis (kār"-ē-ol'-ih-sis) – destruction of the nucleus of a cell by swelling and loss of affinity of its chromatin for basic dyes

keratoacanthoma (kār"-uh-tō-ak"-an-thō'-muh) – a rapidly growing papular lesion, with a crater filled with a keratin plug, which reaches maximum size and then resolves spontaneously within four to six months of onset

Kerckring folds (kerk'-ring) – circular folds of mucous membranes that form elevations in the inner wall of the small intestine

Krukenberg tumor (kroo'-ken-berg) – a metastatic carcinoma of the ovary, usually bilateral and secondary to a mucinous carcinoma of the stomach containing signet ring cells filled with mucus

Kupffer cells (koop'-fer) – large star-shaped or pyramidal cells with a large oval nucleus and a small prominent nucleolus

L

Lambl excrescence (lam'-bul eks-kress'-ens) – small papillary projections on the cardiac valves seen postmortem on many adult hearts

Langhan cells (lahng'-hahn) – polyhedral (many-sided) epithelial cells constituting cytotrophoblasts

lesion (le'zhən) – an alteration or abnormality in a tissue or cell; a pathological change

Letterer-Siwe disease (let'-er-er-sī'-wē) – a serious disease characterized by a proliferation of reticulo-endothelial cells in many organs, especially lymph nodes, spleen, and bone

leucine aminopeptidase (loo'-sin am-ē"-nō-pep'-tihdāz) – an enzyme found in the pancreas

Leydig cells (lī'-digz) – the interstitial cells of the testes that furnish the internal secretion of the testicle

lines of Zahn (zahn) – the white lines that are present in thrombosed blood clots and consist of coagulated blood serum that has separated from cellular components

lutein (loo'-tē-in) – a yellow pigment (lipochrome) from the corpus luteum, from fat cells, and from the yolk of eggs

Lutembacher syndrome (loo'-tem-bak"-er) – atrial septal defect with mitral stenosis

lymphangiectasia (lim-fan"je-ək-ta'zhə) – dilation of the intestinal lymphatic vessels that may be congenital or acquired

M

macrogametocyte (mak"-rō-gah-mē'-tō-sīt) – the infected red blood cell containing the female form of the malarial parasite which, when transferred from a human to a mosquito, becomes a macrogamete

malpighian corpuscles (mal-pig'-ē-un kor'-puh"-sulz) – ovoid collections of lymphocytes that are present around the small penicilliary blood vessels in the spleen

malposition (mal"pə-zish'ən) – faulty or abnormal position of a part of the body

May-Grunwald stain (mā-groon'-wawld) – an alcoholic neutral mixture of methylene blue and eosin

Mayer mucicarmine stain (mā'-er myoo"-sih-kar'-mīn) – a tissue stain for the substance mucin

megakaryocyte (meg"-uh-kār'-ē-ō-sīt) – the giant cell of bone marrow

mesenchymoma (meh"-zeng-kī-mō'-muh) – a mixed mesenchymal tumor composed of two or more cellular elements not commonly associated, not counting fibrous tissue as one of the elements

mesothelium (mez"o- me"zo-the'le-əm) – the layer of flat cells that line the body cavity of the embryo; in the adult it forms the simple squamous epithelium that covers all true serous membranes (peritoneum, pericardium, pleura)

molluscum contagiosum (mō-lus'-kum kon-tā'-jē-ō-sum) – a mildly contagious viral disease characterized by lesions in the skin or trunk, face, and genital areas

morphologic diagnosis (mȯr-'fä-lə-jēk) – the interpretation of abnormalities in terms of severity, time, lesion, and anatomic site, i.e., severe, chronic glomerulonephritis

mosaicism (mō-zā'-ih-sih-zum) – the presence of cells that have different chromosomal constitution

mucicarmine stain (myoo"-sih-kar'-mīn) – a reddish stain designed to show selectively the presence of mucinous material

myelin (mi'ə-lin) – the lipid substance forming a sheath around the axons of certain nerve fibers; serves as an electrical insulator

myelophthisis (mī"-eh-lof'-thih-sis) – reduction of the cell-forming functions of the bone marrow

N

necropsy (nek'-rop-sē) – examination of a body after death; autopsy

neoplasm (nē"-ō-plazm) – abnormal tissue that grows by cellular proliferation more rapidly than normal and continues to grow; usually forms a distinct mass of tissue that may be either benign or malignant (syn. new growth, tumor)

O

osseocartilaginous (oss"-ē-ō-kar"-tih-laj'-ih-nus) – pertaining to or composed of bone and cartilage

osteoid (os'te-oid) – resembling bone

P

pacchionian bodies (pak"-ē-ō'-nē-un) – smooth, granular structures found in the meninges of the brain

pacinian corpuscles (puh-sin'-ē-un kor'-puh'-sulz) – small, but enlarged, nerve endings concerned with the perception of pressure

palisade (pal"i-sād) – in pathology, a row of elongated nuclei parallel to each other

Paneth cells (pah'-nat) – narrow, pyramidal, or columnar epithelial cells with a round or an oval nucleus close to the base of the cell

panniculus (pə-nik'u-ləs) – a thin layer of membrane

Papanicolaou stain (Pap smear) (pap"-uh-nik"-ō-lā'-oo) – smear of vaginal or cervical cells obtained for cytological study

papillary (pap'ĭ-lar"e) – having small nipple-shaped projections

papule (pap'ūl) – a small circumscribed, superficial, solid elevation of the skin

parenchyma (pə-reng'k ĭ-mə) – the essential or functional elements of an organ

patent (pa'tənt) – open, exposed, or unobstructed

pedunculated (pə-dung'ku-lāted) – elevated, as on a stem (peduncle)

Pel-Ebstein fever (pehl-eb'-stīn) – a fever in which the temperature rises by steps over several days and then goes down in steps the same way; common in Hodgkin disease

petechia (pl. petechiae) (pə-te'ke-ə, pə-te'ke-e) – a pinpoint, nonraised, purplish-red spot caused by intradermal or subcutaneous hemorrhage

phagocytized (fag'-ō-sit"-īzd) – said of particles engulfed by an active call (a phagocyte), especially a histiocyte

phthisis (tī'-sis) – a wasting away of the body or a part of the body; tuberculosis, especially of the lungs

pilomatricoma (pi"lo-ma"tr ĭ-ko'mə) – calcifying epithelioma of Malherbe

plicae palmatae (plī'-sē pahl'-mah-tuh) – the grooves in the cervical canal

poikilocyte (poy'-kī-lō-sīt") – a red blood cell showing abnormal variation in shape

polyp (pol'ip) – an abnormal growth protruding from a mucous membrane

proteinaceous (prō"-tē-in-ā'-shus) – compounds to or of the nature of a protein

Proteus vulgaris (prō'-tē-us vul-gār'-is) – species of a bacteria containing gram-negative rods and occurring primarily in fecal matter and putrefying materials; some species of Proteus can cause diarrhea, urinary tract infections, and gastroenteritis

pseudohypha (syoo"-dō-hī'-fuh) – a chain of easily disrupted fungal cells that is intermediate between a chain of budding cells and a true hypha, marked by constrictions rather than septa at the junctions

Pseudomonas aeruginosa (syoo"-dō-mō'-nus ār-oo-jihnō'-suh) – a bacterial species found in soil, water, and commonly in clinical specimens, e.g., wound infections, burn lesions, urinary tract infections; the causative agent of blue pus

punch biopsy – removing a small cylindrical specimen for biopsy by means of a special instrument that pierces the organ or skin directly, making a small incision

puncture – to make a hole with a small pointed object, such as a needle; as in lumbar puncture or spinal tap; see bone marrow aspiration

Purkinje cells (pur-kin'-jē) – the layer of large neuron cell bodies in the middle layer of the cerebellar cortex

purpura (pur'pu-rə) – any of a group of conditions characterized by ecchymoses or other small hemorrhages in the skin, mucous membranes, or serosal surfaces

pus (pŭs) – a liquid inflammation product made up of leukocytes, a thin fluid, and cellular debris

pyknosis (pik-nō'-sis) – condensation and increased basophilic staining of a cell nucleus

Queyrat erythroplasia (kā-rah' ē-rith"-rō-plā'-zē-uh) – squamous cell carcinoma in situ that manifests as a circumscribed, velvety, erythematous papular lesion on the glans penis, coronal sulcus, or prepuce, leading to scaling and superficial ulceration

Recklinghausen disease (rek'-ling-how"-zen) – a disease characterized by multiple neurocutaneous fibromas

reniform (ren' ĭ -form) – shaped like a kidney

rete pegs (rē'-tē) – the downward, sawtooth-like projections of the epidermis into the dermis; also rete ridges

Rokitansky-Aschoff crypts (rō"-kih-tan'-skē-ash'-ahff kriptz) – small folds of the gallbladder mucosa that extend into the muscular wall

Rokitansky disease, tumor (rō"-kih-tan'-skē) – acute yellow tumor atrophy of the liver

saprophytic actinomycosis (sap"-rō-fit'-ik ak"-tih-nō-mī-kō'-sis) – nonpathogenic form of actinomycosis

Schimmelbusch disease (shim'-el-boosh") – a form of productive mastitis marked by the production of many small cysts

scrofuloderma (skrof"-yoo-lō-der'-muh) – suppurating abscesses and fistulous passages opening on the skin, secondary to tuberculosis of lymph nodes, most commonly those of the neck and sometimes of bones and joints

serrated (ser'āt-ed) – having a saw-like edge

sessile (ses'il) – having a broad base of attachment; not pedunculated, as with a stalk

siderogenous (sid"-er-oj'-eh-nus) – producing or forming iron

squamocolumnar (skwah"-mō-kō-lum'-nahr) – pertaining to the junction between a stratified

squamous epithelial surface and one lined by columnar epithelium

suppurative (sup'u-ra"tiv) – containing pus

sympathicoblastoma (sim-path"-ih-kō-blas-tō'-muh) – a malignant tumor containing sympathicoblasts

syncytium (sin-sish'-ē-um) – a multinucleate mass of protoplasm produced by the merging of cells

syringocystadenoma (sih-ring"-gō-sis"-tad-ē-nō'-muh) – adenoma of the sweat glands

telangiectasia (tel-an"-jē-ek-tas'-ia) – (noun) a vascular lesion formed by dilatation of a group of small blood vessels and is the basis for a variety of angiomas

telangiectatic (tel-an"-jē-ek-tat'-ik) – (adj.) pertaining to or characterized by telangiectasia

thyroglobulin (thī-rō-glob'-yoo-lin) – an iodine-containing protein secreted by the thyroid gland and stored in its colloid substance

tissue processor (tish'yū prō'ses-sŏr) – an instrument in which selected tissue sections are successively passed through different solutions by a timed mechanism in preparation for sectioning, staining, and mounting on microscopic slides

trabeculae carneae (trah-bek'-yoo-lē kar'-nē-ā) – rounded, ridge-like elevations on the interior walls of the ventricles of the heart

ulcerated (ul'sər-ā ted) – to form an ulcer; damaged so that the surface tissue is lost or necrotic

umbilicated (əm-bil' ĭ -kāt" əd) – marked by depressed spots resembling the umbilicus

van Gieson stain (van-gē'-suhn) – a stain for connective tissue, consisting of acid fuchsin and an aqueous solution of trinitrophenol

Vater-Pacini corpuscles (fah'-ter-puh-sē'-nē kor'-puh'-sulz) – sensory nerve structures deep in the hands and feet and around joints serving a proprioceptive function

Verhoeff elastic stain (ver'-hef) – a stain for demonstrating elastic tissue

vernix caseosa (ver'-niks cās-ē-ō'-suh) – the white, clinging, greasy material found on the skin of newborn infants

Verocay bodies (vuhr'-ō-kā) – small groups of fibrils surrounded by rows of palisaded nuclei; seen in nerve tumors

verruca (və-roo'kə) – (noun) a wart

verrucous (və-roo'kəs) – (adj.) rough; wart-like

Virchow-Robin spaces (ver'-kō-rō-bēn') – the spaces around the blood vessels where they enter the brain

viscous (vis'kəs) – thick, coagulated; sticky or gummy

Zenker fixation (zeng'-ker) – a method of hardening tissue in preparation for sectioning (microscopic slide preparation)

Ziehl-Neelsen method, stain (zēl-nel'-sen) – a staining procedure for demonstrating acid-fast microorganisms

Transcription Tips

Transcribing pathology and cytology dictation is one of the most interesting tasks for healthcare documentation specialists. The vocabulary is complex, as it includes both anatomic and clinical laboratory terminology. Recently published (within five years) pathology/cytology reference books, including a good abbreviation book, will make the task easier.

Pathology reports detail the pathological or disease-related findings from the analysis of tissue (histology) and fluids (cytology). Samples of tissue may be taken via biopsy, surgery, special procedures, e.g., a bone marrow biopsy or a lumbar puncture, or at autopsy. Specimens come to the pathologist in sterile form from a doctor's office, a clinic, the hospital surgery department, or the morgue.

Autopsies are done on patients who die in the hospital unless the family refuses. It is possible for a limited autopsy to be done. However, if the cause of death is in question for any reason, it becomes a medical examiner's case, a legal case. The family has no jurisdiction, and the body is removed from the hospital to the medical examiner's office. In some cases, the medical examiner might perform the autopsy in the hospital morgue. (See Model Report #10).

Note on Model Reports 4A and 4B: Model 4A illustrates a "gross only" report, which means that no tissue was sent for microscopic analysis. The gross description is done with the naked eye, and then the report is transcribed and signed out. Model 4B illustrates specimens described grossly, then sent to histology to be prepared for microscopic examination. The microscopic description/diagnosis is done after the tissue has been prepared, mounted on a glass slide, examined under a microscope, and diagnosed. This takes overnight, so the report is dictated, transcribed, and signed out the next working day.

Cytology reports done on bodily fluids and smears obtained from patients include Pap smears. The cytology reports can be signed out on lab slips rather than being transcribed by the HDS. There are times, however, that a typed report is necessary.

Familiarity with the components of the anatomic and clinical lab, together with the tests performed in both, will assist the HDS in the transcription of pathology and cytology reports. Knowledge of bacteria, viruses, fungi, and microorganisms is also helpful. See the information presented in Chapter 3: Infectious Diseases.

Lab Tests Done in Vitro Include the Following:

ABO Rh blood typing with Rh factor
Basic metabolic profile (BMP)
Blood urea nitrogen (BUN)
Blood ethanol
Complete blood count (CBC)
  includes hemoglobin, hematocrit, white blood cell
    count, red blood cell count, platelet count, red
    blood cell indices
Comprehensive metabolic profile (CMP)
Creatinine
Drug screen—6 panel or 10 panel
Electrolytes (lytes)
  includes sodium, potassium, chloride, bicarbonate
Healthy Heart panel
Hepatitis panel, acute
Hepatitis panel, comprehensive
International Normalized Ratio (INR)
Lipid panel
  includes cholesterol, HDL, LDL, triglycerides

Liver function tests or panel
  includes bilirubin, alkaline phosphatase,
    AST, ALT, LDH
Partial thromboplastin time (PTT)
Prenatal profile, comprehensive
Prenatal profile, routine
Prostate specific antigen (PSA)
Prothrombin time (PT or pro time)
Renal panel or hepatic panel
  includes albumin, total bilirubin, alkaline
    phosphatase, AST, ALT, total protein
Sedimentation rate (sed rate) or erythrocyte
  sedimentation rate (ESR)
Serum pregnancy test
Thyroid function tests (TFTs)
Urinalysis (UA) or microscopic urinalysis
  includes glucose, protein, specific gravity, pH,
    WBC, RBC, presence of bacteria
Urine pregnancy test

Lumbar Puncture (LP) is Done in Vivo

When spinal fluid needs to be examined microscopically, an LP is the procedure. The fluid is obtained via lumbar puncture, otherwise known as a spinal tap. While the patient lies on his or her side with the back slightly rounded and knees flexed toward the abdomen, a puncture is made into the subarachnoid space of the lumbar region at L3-4.

Spinal fluid is obtained for either diagnostic or therapeutic purposes. This fluid can be sent to the laboratory where it is examined for color, pressure, protein level, chloride, glucose, lymphocytes, etc. It may be cultured for the presence of bacteria, parasites, or a virus.

Supportive Web Sites

https://www.med.illinois.edu/m2/pathology/ PathAtlasf/titlepage.html#vol2contents
This site provides an extensive list of terms related to pathology.

http://medmark.org/path/
Click on "pathology" and other links of interest.

http://www.nlm.nih.gov/medlineplus
Search for pathology, organisms, viruses, etc.

ology Reports

	Patient Name	Type of Report/Procedure
	Barbara C. Anello	Stomach biopsies
	Evan Merida	Urinary bladder biopsies
TE#3	Evan Merida	Urinary bladder/prostate biopsies
TE#4	Nancy Lee Richards	Punch biopsy of the skin
TE#5	Patrick Shannon	Hemorrhoids
TE#6	Ramona W. Whitted	Cytology Report
TE#7	Ramona W. Whitted	Abdominal pelvic mass
TE#8	Cathy Jo Myles	Biopsy abdominal mass
TE#9	Samuel Fairbrother	Aortic insufficiency, endocarditis
TE#10	Stella D. Norris	Bone marrow aspiration and biopsy

CHAPTER 16
RADIOLOGY/DIAGNOSTIC IMAGING

Introduction

The medical discipline of *radiology* originated with the discovery of an unknown ray by German physicist Wilhelm Conrad Roentgen in 1895. He named this unknown ray an x-ray. The specialty of radiology (also called *roentgenology*) employs electromagnetic radiation and ultrasonics for the diagnosis and treatment of injury and disease.

Diagnostic imaging is the medical evaluation of body tissues and functions by means of still or moving radiologic images. Physicians employed in the field of diagnostic imaging are *radiologists, nuclear physicians,* and *radiation oncologists*. Radiologists specialize in the practice of diagnostic, therapeutic, or interventional radiology. Nuclear physicians are radiologists who administer nuclear medicine procedures used in diagnosis. Radiation oncologists are skilled in treating disease using radiation, primarily in the management of malignancies.

Diagnostic techniques employed by personnel in diagnostic imaging are computerized axial tomography scans (CT or CAT scans), contrast studies, fluoroscopy, interventional radiology, tomography, ultrasound (US), and magnetic imaging or magnetic resonance imaging (MRI).

Interventional radiology is the nonsurgical treatment of disease using radiologic imaging to guide catheters, balloons, filters, and other tiny instruments through the body's blood vessels and other organs. Fallopian tube catheterization, balloon angioplasty, chemoembolization, and thrombolysis are examples of interventional radiologic procedures.

Nuclear medicine is the branch of radiology that uses small amounts of radioactive substances to image the body and diagnose disease. The amount of radiation used in diagnosis is quite small and poses little hazard to the patient or to any medical employee. Treatment (thyroid ablation) requires larger doses and thus special precautions are required. Nuclear medicine personnel consider both the physiology and anatomy of the body in establishing diagnosis and treatment.

Nuclear imaging techniques give physicians a way to look inside the body using computers, detectors, and radioactive substances. These techniques include cardiovascular imaging, bone scanning, positron emission tomography (PET), and single photon emission computer tomography (SPECT). Medical conditions such as tumors, aneurysms, irregular or inadequate blood flow to tissues, blood cell disorders, and inadequate functioning of organs, such as thyroid and pulmonary function deficiencies, can be detected using nuclear imaging techniques.

Various body systems are tested through the administration of intravenous medications (IV) found in the nuclear medicine department. Almost any of the body systems can be evaluated by intravenous, or noninvasive, method through the use of one or more different drugs tagged with *technetium,* a *radionuclide*. Because radionuclides emit gamma rays that can be detected and recorded in many ways, thus providing statistical information or images, they are commonly used in many phases of medicine.

Critical Thinking Exercise

?

Healthcare documentation specialists who work remotely for national companies have to use critical thinking to know what time it is in each time zone.

(a) How does one figure this out? What exceptions might there be?

(b) Where in the United States and its territories is Daylight Saving Time not used?

Of the techniques mentioned, contrast studies, CT scans, fluoroscopy, and tomography use x-rays. Ultrasonography uses ultrasound waves, and magnetic resonance imaging (MRI) utilizes magnetic and radio waves.

After the diagnostic study is completed, the report is interpreted and dictated by a radiologist. The healthcare documentation specialist (HDS) transcribes it, and it is signed by the radiologist; the definitive report is the radiologist's responsibility.

Radiology/Diagnostic Imaging Abbreviations

The abbreviations, acronyms, and terms in the following abbreviations and terminology sections are often dictated in this specialty. We offer abbreviated definitions here. Please see an unabridged medical dictionary or the suggested web sites in this chapter for more information on each term.

angio	angiography		**Ci**	curie (a measure of radioactivity)
ASIS	anterior-superior iliac spine		**CPB**	competitive protein binding
AV	arteriovenous		**C-spine film**	cervical spine film
Ba	barium		**CXR**	chest x-ray
BI-RADS™	breast imaging reporting and data system		**decub**	decubitus position (lying down)
BPD	biparietal diameter		**DI**	diagnostic imaging
CT or CAT	computerized tomography, computerized axial tomography		**DISH**	diffuse idiopathic skeletal hyperostosis
CC	costochondral or cardiac catheterization		**DOBI**	dynamic optical breast imaging system
cGy	centigray (a rad that is one-hundredth of a gray)		**DSA**	digital subtraction angiography
			EGD	esophagogastroduodenoscopy

ERCP	endoscopic retrograde cholangio-pancreatography		**MPL**	maximum permissible level or limit
ESD	esophagus, stomach, and duodenum		**MPR**	multiplanar reconstruction
GM	Geiger-Muller (counter)		**MRI**	magnetic resonance imaging
Gy	gray (unit of radiation equal to 100 rads)		**MUGA**	multiple-gated acquisition scan (radioactive test to show heart function)
HEG	high energy gamma		**N**	neutron
HI-RADS™	head injury imaging reporting and data system		**PAP**	pulmonary artery pressure
HVL	half-value layer or hippocampal volume loss		**PBI**	protein-bound iodine
ICA	internal carotid artery		**PET**	positron emission tomography
ICS	intercostal space		**PICC**	peripherally inserted central catheter
IHSA	iodinated human serum albumin		**PTA**	percutaneous transluminal angioplasty
IV	intravenous		**PTC**	percutaneous transhepatic cholangiography
IVP	intravenous pyelogram		**PTEA**	pulmonary thromboendarterec-tomy
keV/kev	kilo (thousand) electron volts		**R**	Roentgen (unit of exposure)
kHz	kilohertz		**rad**	radiation-absorbed dose or roentgen-administered dose
KUB	kidneys, ureters, bladder		**RAIU**	radioactive iodine uptake (test)
LAO	left anterior oblique		**RAO**	right anterior oblique
LD	lethal dose		**RAQ**	right anterior quadrant
LI-RADS™	liver imaging reporting and data system		**REG**	radiation exposure guide
LS	lumbosacral		**RIA**	radioimmunoassay
LS films	lumbosacral spine films		**RISA**	radioiodinated serum albumin
mCi	millicurie (measure of radiation)		**SPECT**	single-photon emission computer tomography
MFB	metallic foreign body		**TBI**	total body irradiation
MHz	megahertz		**Tc**	technetium
MIP	maximum intensity projection		**Tc99m or ⁹⁹ᵐTc**	radioactive technetium used in brain, skull, thyroid, liver, spleen, bone, and lung scans
MLD	median lethal dose			
MLO	mesiolinguo-occlusal			
MPC	maximum permissible concentration		**TD**	total dose
MPD	maximum permissible dose			

TIPS	transjugular intrahepatic portosystemic shunt	US, U/S	ultrasound
TSD	target-skin distance	V/Q	ventilation-perfusion lung scan
UGI	upper gastrointestinal series	XOP	x-ray out of plaster
		XRT	radiation therapy

Anatomic Illustrations

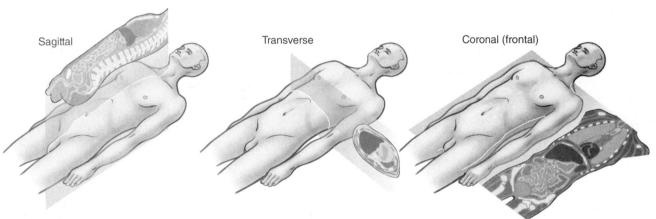

Sagittal   Transverse   Coronal (frontal)

FIGURE 16-1 Computed tomography (CT scan) provides cross-sectional views of different body planes

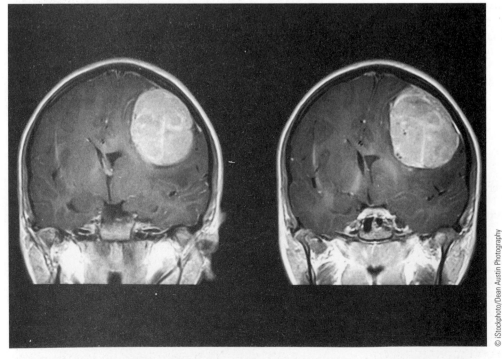

FIGURE 16-2 An MRI of the brain with a tumor visible in the upper right

Radiology/Diagnostic Imaging Terminology

A

air bronchogram (brong'-kō-gram) – radiographic appearance of an air-filled bronchus surrounded by fluid-filled airspaces

angiocardiography (an"-jē-ō-kar'-dē-og'-ruh-fē) – examination of the chambers of the heart and pulmonary circulation after injection of radiopaque material

angiogram (an'-jē-ō-gram") – an x-ray of blood vessels filled with a contrast medium

aortogram (ā-or'-tuh-gram") – an x-ray of the aorta after injection of contrast fluid

appendicolith (uh-pen"-dih-kō'-lith") – a calcified concretion in the appendix visible on an abdominal radiograph

arteriogram (ar-tē'-rē-uh-gram") – an x-ray of an artery

arthropneumoradiograph (ar"-thrō-noo"-mō-rā'-dē-uh-graf") – radiographic examination of a joint after it has been injected with air

attenuation (ah-ten"-yoo-ā'-shun) – the process by which a beam of radiation is reduced in energy when passed through tissue or other material

B

BI-RADS™ (bī'-radz) – breast imaging reporting and data system; mammographic findings dictated by using BI-RADS categories numbered 0 to 6; BI-RADS category 0: Additional imaging evaluation or comparison to prior mammograms is needed; BI-RADS category 6: Known biopsy-proven malignancy, appropriate action should be taken

C

Cardiolite™ (kar'-dē-ō-līt") – an imaging agent

cephalometric radiograph (cephalogram) (sef"-uh-lō-meh'-trik sef'-uh-lō-gram") – a radiographic view of the jaws and skull permitting measurement

cesium 137 (sē'-zē-um) – radionuclide used for internal radiation therapy of cancer

choledochogram (kō-led'-ō-kō-gram") – an x-ray of the common bile duct

cineangiography (sin"-ē-an"-jē-og'-ruh-fē) – the photographic recording of fluoroscopic images of the blood vessels by motion picture techniques

cineradiography (sin"-e-ra"-dē-og'-run-fē) – x-ray motion pictures

cisternography (sis"-ter-nog'-ruh-fē) – the roentgenographic study of the basal cisterns of the brain after the subarachnoid introduction of an opaque or other contrast medium or a radiopharmaceutical

collimator (kahl'-ih-mā"-tur) – a diaphragm or system of diaphragms made of an absorbing material, designed to identify the dimensions and direction of a beam of radiation

colpostat (kahl'-pō-stat) – an appliance for retaining sources of radiation, such as iridium, in the vagina

Combidex™ (kahm'-bih-deks) – multifunctional imaging agent

computed tomography (CT) (tō-mog'-ruh-fē) – a diagnostic x-ray procedure where a cross-section coronal, sagittal image of a specific body segment is generated; many subclasses of CT scans exist

curie (Ci) (kyoo'-rē) – a unit for measurement of radioactivity

cyclotron (sī'-klo-tron) – an accelerator that produces high-speed ions (e.g., protons and deuterons) under the influence of an alternating magnetic field for bombardment and disruption of atomic nuclei

cystogram (sis'-tuh-gram) – an x-ray of the urinary bladder

cystourethrogram (sis"-tō-yoo-rē'-thruh-gram) – an x-ray of the urinary bladder and ureters

D

diathermy (dī'-uh-ther"-mē) – heating of the body tissues due to their resistance to the passage of high-frequency electromagnetic radiation

Digirad 2020tc Imager™ (dih'-jih-rad ih'-muh-jer) – a digital gamma camera used in nuclear medicine

diskography (dis-kog'-ruh-fē) – radiographic demonstration of an intervertebral disk by injection of contrast media into the nucleus pulposus

dosimeter (dō-sim'-eh-ter) – an instrument for measuring the dose of radiation

echogenic (ek-ō-gē'-nik) – containing internal interfaces that reflect high-frequency sound waves

encephalogram (en-sef'-uh-lō-gram") – an x-ray made after the injection of contrast material, usually air, into the cerebrospinal fluid in order to outline the spinal cord and brain

Explorer ST™ – fixed curve diagnostic catheters

Explorer 360°™ – rotational diagnostic catheter

Explorer X 70™ – intraoral radiography system

fluorescence (floo"-ur-es'-ens) – the characteristic of certain substances to emit light when exposed to certain types of light radiation

fluoroscopy (floo"-ur-os'-kuh-pē) – use of a fluoroscope for medical diagnosis or for testing various materials by roentgen rays

GE Senographe 2000D™ (sen'-uh-graf) – fully digital system for mammography manufactured by General Electric—a company that produces many radiographic devices

Gore 1.5T Torso Array™ – MRI surface coil for imaging chest, abdominal, and pelvic areas

hilar shadow (hī'-lur) – radiographic hilum of the lung; a composite radiographic shadow of the central

pulmonary arteries and veins with associated bronchial walls and lymph nodes within the right or left lung

Hypaque™ (hi-pāk') – imaging agent; there are several Hypaque imaging agents, including Hypaque swallow

hyperechoic area/region (hī"-per-ē-kō'-ik) – denoting an area or region in an ultrasound image in which the echoes are stronger than normal or than surrounding structures

hysterogram (hiss'-ter-uh-gram) – an x-ray of the uterus

hysterosalpingography (hiss"-ter-ō-sal"-ping-gahg'-ruh-fē) – x-ray study of the uterus and uterine tubes after injection of a contrast medium

interstitial therapy (in"-ter-stih'-shul) – the procedure in which radioisotopes are surgically inserted into a tumor, usually in the form of seeds or needles.

intracavitary therapy (in"-truh-kāv'-ih-tair"-ē) – the process in which radioisotopes are placed within a body cavity adjacent to a tumor

iridium (Ir 192) (ih-rid'-ē-um) – a radioisotope used for selected cases of cancer

irradiation (ih-rā"-dē-ā'-shun) – exposure to the action of electromagnetic radiation, e.g., heat, light, x-rays

isotope (ī'-suh-tōp) – one of a series of chemical elements that have nearly identical chemical properties but differ in their atomic weights and electric charge; many are radioactive

laminagram (lam'-ih-nuh-gram) – an x-ray of a selected layer of the body made by body-section roentgenography

laminagraphy (lam"-ih-nag'-ruh-fē) – the taking of x-rays at varying levels of tissue

LINAC linear accelerator – a device imparting high velocity and energy to atomic and subatomic particles; an important device for radiosurgery

lymphangiography (lihm-fan"-jē-og'-ruh-fē) – x-ray study of the lymphatic system after the injection of a contrast medium

megavoltage (meg"-uh-vōl'-tij) – high-energy radiation generated by a machine; used in curative and palliative x-ray therapy for cancer

meglumine (meg'-loo-mēn) – a chemical used in the preparation of certain radiopaque media

microcurie (mī"-krō-kyoo'-rē) – unit for measuring the activity of a radionuclide in a tracer dose

millicurie (mCi) (mil"-ih-kyoo'-rē) – unit for measuring the activity of a radionuclide in a therapeutic dose

myelogram (mī'-eh-lō-gram) – an x-ray of the spinal cord

myelography (mī"-eh-log'-ruh-fē) – x-ray study of the spinal cord after injection of a radiopaque substance into the subarachnoid space

myelopathic (mī"-eh-lō-path'-ik) – relating to myelopathy (disease of the spinal cord)

Myoscint™ (mī'-ō-cent) – an imaging agent

Myoview™ (mī'-ō-vyoo) – an imaging drug in scintigraphy

NeoSpect™ (nē'-ō-spekt") – diagnostic imaging agent

nephrogram (nef'-ruh-gram) – an x-ray of the kidney

nephrotomography (nef"-rō-tuh-mog'-ruh-fē) – body-section roentgenography as applied to the kidney

neurosonography (nyoo"-rō-suh-nog'-ruh-fē) – a diagnostic technique in which pulses of ultrasonic waves are projected through the head from both sides, and echoes from the midline structures of the brain are recorded as graphic tracings

nonopaque (non"-ō-pāk') – not opaque to the roentgen ray; translucent

nuclide (noo'-klīd) – a general term denoting all nuclear species of chemical elements, both stable and unstable, used synonymously with isotope

opaque (ō-pak') – neither transparent nor translucent; blocking the passage of radiant energy

orifice (or'-ih-fiss) – the entrance or outlet of any body cavity

oxycephalic (ok"-sē-seh-fal'-ik) – pertaining to or characterized by a condition in which the top of the head is peaked or pointed

Pantopaque™ (pan-tō-pāk') – contrast medium or radiopaque dye used in x-ray studies

photoscan (fōt'-ō-skan) – a representation of the concentration of a radioisotope outlining an organ in the body

picogram (pī'-kō-gram) – a unit of weight of the metric system; also called a micromicrogram or one-trillionth of a gram

pneumothorax (noo-mō-thor'-aks) – an accumulation of air or gas in the pleural space; may occur spontaneously, as a result of trauma or a pathological process, or be introduced deliberately

portogram (por'-tuh-gram) – an x-ray of the portal vein

pyelogram (pī'-el-uh-gram") – an x-ray in which the pelvis of the kidney is shown filled with contrast material, which may be injected directly into the urinary system through a catheter or into a vein to reach the kidneys through the blood

pyeloureterography (pyelography) (pī"-el-ō-yoo-rē"-ter-og'-ruh-fē, pī"-el-og'-ruh-fē) – radiologic study of the kidney and renal collecting system, usually performed with the aid of a contrast agent

radiodense (rā'-dē-ō-dens") – the property of a substance that does not allow for the passage of x-rays

radioimmunoassay (RIA) (rā"-dē-ō-ih"-myoo-nō-as'-ā) – an in vitro procedure whereby radioactive chemicals and antibodies are combined to detect minute quantities of hormones, enzymes, or other substances in the blood

radioisotope (rā"-dē-ō-ī'-suh-tōp) – an isotope of a chemical element made radioactive by bombardment with neutrons; term has become obsolete – radionuclide is the current term

radiolucent (rā-dē-ō-loo'-sent) – allows the passage of most x-rays; radiolucent structures appear black on x-ray film

radionuclide (rā"-dē-ō-noo'-klīd) – a nuclide that displays the property of radioactivity

radiopaque (rā"-dē-ō-pāk') – not permitting radiant energy, such as x-rays, to pass

radiopharmaceutical (rā"-dē-ō-fahr"-muh-syoo'-tih-kul) – a radioactive chemical or pharmaceutical preparation labeled with a radionuclide in tracer or therapeutic concentration used as a diagnostic or therapeutic agent

Reno-M-DIP™ – a radiopaque contrast agent

roentgen (rent'-gen) – the international unit of x- or γ-radiation (gamma radiation)

roentgenography (rent"-gen-og'-ruh-fē) – picture of an organ or a region by means of roentgen rays

roentgenology (rent"-gen-ol'-uh-jē) – the study of x-rays; radiology

scintigram (sin'-tih-gram) – a two-dimensional representation (map) of the gamma rays emitted by a radioisotope, revealing its varying concentration in a specific tissue of the body, such as the brain, kidney, or thyroid gland

scintillation scan (sin-tih-lā'-shun) – image made by a scintillation counter to determine the size of a tumor, goiter, or other involvement and to locate aberrant, metastatic lesions

scintiscan (sin'-tih-skan) – the use of scintiphotography to create a map of scintillations produced when a radioactive substance is introduced into the body

scybalum (sib'-uh-lum) – a dry, hard mass of fecal matter in the intestine

selenium (seh-len'-ē-um) – a metallic element chemically similar to sulfur

sialogram (sī-al'-uh-gram) – radiographic visualization of the salivary glands and ducts after injection of radiopaque material

stereoroentgenography (star"-ē-ō-rent"-gen-og'-ruh-fē) – the making of an x-ray giving an impression of depth as well as width and height

strontium (Sr 90) (stron'-shē-um) – radionuclide used for lesions of the eye and removal of benign small tumors

supratentorial (soo"-pruh-ten-tō'-rē-ul) – above the tentorium of the cerebellum

tagging – the process of attaching a radionuclide to a chemical and following its course in the body

technetium (Tc 99m) (tek-nē'-shē-um) – a radionuclide used in brain, thyroid, parotid, and heart-blood pool scans

technetium-labeled sulfur colloid (tek-nē'-shē-um kahl'-oyd) – radionuclide used in liver, spleen, and bone marrow scans

Telepaque™ (tel'-eh-pāk) – contrast media, or radiopaque dye, used in x-ray studies

teleroentgenogram (tel"-eh-rent"-gen'-uh-gram) – the picture or film obtained by teleroentgenography

thallium 201 (²⁰¹TI) (thal'-ē-um) – one of many radionuclide imaging agents

tomography (tuh-mog'-ruh-fē) – a special technique to show detailed images of structures lying in a predetermined plane of tissue, while blurring or eliminating detail in images of structures in the other planes

transjugular intrahepatic portosystemic shunt (TIPS) (tranz-jug'-yoo-lur in"-truh-hē-pat'-ik por"-tō-sis"-teh'-mik) – an interventional radiology procedure to relieve portal hypertension

UltraSure DTU-one™, DTU-one UltraSure™ – imaging system for assessment of osteoporotic fracture risk

uptake (ŭp'tāk) – refers to the rate of absorption of a radionuclide into an organ or tissue

ureteropyelogram (yoo-rē"-ter-ō-pī'-eh-lō-gram") – an x-ray of the ureter and pelvis of the kidney

Valsalva maneuver (val-sal'-vuh) – any forced expiratory effort against a closed airway to increase intrathoracic pressure and impede venous return to the right atrium; used to study cardiovascular effects of raised peripheral venous pressure and decreased cardiac filling and cardiac output

ventilation/perfusion studies (ven"-tih-lā'-shun per-fyoo'-zhun) – studies in which a radiopharmaceutical is inhaled (ventilation) or injected (perfusion) and its passage through the respiratory tract is imaged

ventriculography (ven-trik"-yoo-log'-ruh-fē) – x-ray study of the head following removal of cerebrospinal fluid from the cerebral ventricles and its replacement by air or other contrast medium

xenon (^{133}**Xe**) (zē'-non) – radionuclide imaging agent and/or clearance technique

Xplore 1000™ (eks"-plor') – digital x-ray imaging

Xplore™ (eks"-plor') – filmless high-resolution digital radiography imaging system

yttrium (Y 90) (ih'-trē-um) – radionuclide used for ascites and effusions associated with malignant metastatic involvement; i.e., hepatomegaly, splenomegaly, chronic leukemia, and polycythemia

Transcription Tips

As a healthcare documentation specialist learning radiology/diagnostic imaging reports, basic concepts with which a student should be familiar include x-ray views (or positions of the patient), anatomical planes of the body, nuclear medicine tests, confusing terms, and typical formatting of x-ray reports.

X-ray Views or Positioning

AP view (anteroposterior) – patient positioned so that the front of the body is to the x-ray machine

PA view (posteroanterior) – patient upright with back to the x-ray machine and chest to film

lateral view – x-ray beam passes from one side of the body toward the other to reach the film

oblique view – body part to be imaged is positioned at an angle to x-ray tube

supine – patient lying face up with head turned to one side; x-rays pass through body from front to back

prone – patient lying face down with head turned to one side; x-rays pass from back to front of body

Anatomical Planes

sagittal (lateral) – a lengthwise vertical plane through the longitudinal axis of the trunk dividing the body into two portions

midsagittal or **median** – a vertical plane through the anterior-posterior midaxis that divides the body into right and left halves

frontal (coronal) – a plane dividing the body into front (anterior) and back (posterior) portions

transverse (cross-sectional) – a plane running across the body parallel to the ground that divides the body into upper and lower portions

Nuclear Medicine Tests

scans – scans of the blood and heart, bone, brain, liver and spleen, thyroid, and PET (positron emission tomography)

radioactive iodine uptake – reflects the rate of hormone synthesis by the thyroid gland

SPECT (single-photon emission computed tomography) – used to detect liver tumors, cardiac ischemia, and bone disease of the spine

Typical Formats for Radiology/Diagnostic Imaging Reports

The formatting of x-ray reports differs from one facility to another; therefore, the health documentation specialist should be flexible in this. In some facilities, x-ray documents are typed on plain paper (sometimes of a specific color to identify them as such); other facilities have a prepared form onto which the dictation is transcribed. Some prepared forms include a line at the bottom of the page for the signature of the radiologist. Others will use an electronic signature that includes the dictator's name plus the date and time the report was dictated. The sign-off block will be necessary under any circumstances, as this gives the date and sometimes the time the HDS completed the transcription. (See Model Report #6).

Currently many medical facilities provide equipment that allows the HDS to download patient information and demographics directly onto the report. The HDS selects account information, copying all relevant information automatically into the document. Then the HDS begins keying the dictation concerning the procedure immediately and enters no patient information manually.

If results of a particular procedure are found to be normal, most physicians have prerecorded a "normal" template. The physician gives the HDS instructions to retrieve a copy of a "normal 1" or a "normal 2," for example. When a "normal" is to be used, the HDS downloads the "normal" text, entering in only pertinent dictated changes. The use of "normal" templates helps to prevent errors and saves time for both the HDS and the physician.

Supportive Web Sites

http://www.webmd.com	Search on "diagnostic imaging," "nuclear medicine," or "interventional radiology"; click on other links as desired.
http://www.howstuffworks.com	Search on "nuclear medicine"; click on other links as desired.
http://www.nlm.nih.gov/medlineplus	Search on "diagnostic imaging," "nuclear medicine," or "interventional radiology"; click on other links as desired.
	See The American College of Radiology (ACR) website for details on BI-RADS, HI-RADS, and LI-RADS.

Index of Radiology/Diagnostic Imaging Reports

Exercise#	Patient Name	Type of Report/Procedure
TE#1	Duane Leroy Capps	Venous Doppler, left lower extremity
TE#2	Janet L. Clark	Bilateral diagnostic mammograms
TE#3	Belinda Jo Arollo	MRI, cervical spine
TE#4	Jo Ann Crum	Bone density hip and spine x-ray
TE#5	Marsha Crowell	Nuclear medicine total body scan
TE#6	Kevin R. Donovan	Bilateral venous mapping ultrasounds
TE#7	John Austin Rowen	MRI, left knee, without contrast
TE#8	Janet L. Clark	CT abdomen, contrast enhanced
TE#9	Victor F. Hirsch	Nuclear medicine bleeding scan
TE#10	Janet L. Clark	PET scan
TE#11	Susan Whatley	Renal ultrasound
TE#12	Samuel Fairbrother	MRI, head, with contrast
TE#13	Samuel Fairbrother	MRA, head, without contrast
TE#14	Jamie Pierce	Ultrasound, bilateral breasts
TE#15	Mary Lou Garcia	Fluoro-guided PICC line

CHAPTER 17
RESPIRATORY/PULMONARY MEDICINE

Introduction

Physicians specializing in *respiratory/pulmonary medicine* treat diseases of the *respiratory system*. This system embraces all the structures concerned with the exchange of carbon dioxide and oxygen between the blood and the atmosphere. Components of the respiratory system include the *lung tissue*, where this gaseous exchange takes place; and the *respiratory tract*, a system of tubes that carry air to and from the lungs.

The respiratory system is divided into upper and lower tracts. The *upper tract* consists of the *nose, mouth, nasopharynx, oropharynx, laryngopharynx,* and *larynx.* The *lower tract* is subdivided into the *conducting airways (trachea, primary bronchi, lobar,* and *segmental bronchi)* and the *acinus,* which is the area of gas exchange (respiratory *bronchioles, alveolar ducts,* and *alveoli).*

Air travels through the following pathway from the nose to capillaries of the lungs:

nose
↓
nasal cavities and paranasal sinuses
↓
pharynx
↓
larynx
↓
trachea
↓
bronchi
↓
bronchioles
↓
alveoli
↓
lung capillaries

The *lungs* and accessory structures—*pleura, thoracic cavity,* and *mediastinum*—form significant parts of the respiratory system. Straddling the heart, the cone-shaped lungs fill the thoracic cavity. The right lung is shorter and broader than the left. Above and behind the heart lies the *hilum,* the opening through which pass the lung's root structures—primary *bronchus, pulmonary* and *bronchial blood vessels, lymphatics,* and *nerves.*

The *pleurae* totally enclose the lungs and are composed of a *visceral* layer and a *parietal* layer. The *thoracic cavity* is the area within the chest wall; it is bounded below by the *diaphragm,*

Critical Thinking Exercise

[?]

The healthcare documentation specialist supervisor of a transcription firm is asked by her boss to falsify the monthly production numbers so he can make the operation look good to his Board of Directors. What should be done? Is this ethical? Should she make her boss happy? Risk being fired by refusing?

above by the *scalene muscles* and the fascia of the neck, and circumferentially by the *ribs, intercostal muscles, vertebrae, sternum,* and *ligaments.*

The *mediastinum* is the space between the lungs, which includes the heart; the thoracic aorta, pulmonary artery, and veins; the vena cavae and azygos veins; the thymus, lymph nodes, and vessels; the trachea, esophagus, and thoracic duct; and the vagus, cardiac, and phrenic nerves.

Physicians and surgeons concerned with the treatment of the respiratory system treat such conditions as *bronchitis, pneumonia, asthma, emphysema, cystic fibrosis, tuberculosis, asbestosis, pleurisy,* and *cancerous* conditions that occur throughout the respiratory tract.

A thoracotomy is a surgical cut that a thoracic or pulmonary surgeon makes to open the chest wall. Lung surgery is surgery to repair or remove lung tissue. Several common lung surgeries performed include:

- Biopsy of an unknown growth
- Lobectomy, to remove one or more lobes of a lung
- Lung transplant

- Pneumonectomy, to remove a lung
- Surgery to prevent the buildup or return of fluid to the chest (pleurodesis)
- Surgery to remove an infection or blood in the chest cavity (empyema)
- Surgery to remove small balloon-like tissues (blebs) that cause lung collapse (pneumothorax)
- Wedge resection, to remove part of a lobe in a lung

Respiratory/Pulmonary Medicine Abbreviations

The abbreviations, acronyms, and terms in the following abbreviations and terminology sections are often dictated in this specialty. We offer abbreviated definitions here. Please see an unabridged medical dictionary or the suggested web sites in this chapter for more information on each term.

ABG	arterial blood gas		**ASO**	antistreptolysin-O titer
AC	assist control (ventilation)		**BAL**	bronchoalveolar lavage
AFB	acid-fast bacillus		**BOOP**	bronchitis obliterans-organized pneumonia
ARD	acute respiratory disease		**bronch**	bronchoscopy
ARDS	adult (or acute) respiratory distress syndrome		**CF**	cystic fibrosis

COLD	chronic obstructive lung disease	**IRDS**	infant respiratory distress syndrome
COP	cryptogenic organizing pneumonia	**IRV**	inspiratory reserve volume
COPD	chronic obstructive pulmonary disease	**JVD**	jugular vein distention
CPPT	chest percussion and postnasal drainage	**KOH**	potassium hydroxide
CPT	chest physiotherapy	**LAM**	lymphangioleiomyomatosis
CPR	cardiopulmonary resuscitation	**LL**	left lung
CT	computer tomography (scan)	**LLL**	left lower lobe
CTA	clear to auscultation	**LUL**	left upper lobe
CVD	cerebrovascular disease	**MAC**	Mycobacterium avium complex
CXR	chest x-ray	**MAI**	Mycobacterium avium-intracellulare
DIP	desquamative interstitial pneumonitis	**MAIC**	Mycobacterium avium-intracellulare complex
DLCO	diffusing capacity for carbon monoxide	**MBC**	maximal breathing capacity
DPT	diphtheria, pertussis, tetanus	**MOTT**	mycobacteria other than tubercle
EBUS	endobronchial ultrasound	**MUGA**	multigated (radionuclide) angiogram
ERV	expiratory reserve volume	**MV**	minute volume
ET	endotracheal	**MVV**	maximum voluntary ventilation or maximum ventilatory volume
FEF	forced expiratory flow	**NTM**	nontuberculosis mycobacterium
FEV	forced expiratory volume	**PACO$_2$**	partial pressure (tension) of carbon dioxide, alveolar
FEV$_1$	FEV in 1 second	**PaCO$_2$ or PCO$_2$**	partial pressure (tension) of carbon dioxide, artery
FFB	flexible fiberoptic bronchoscopy		
FIF	forced inspiratory flow	**PaO$_2$**	arterial oxygen pressure (tension)
FNA	fine-needle aspirate or aspiration	**PO$_2$**	partial pressure (tension) of oxygen, artery
FVC	forced vital capacity		
HBOT	hyperbaric oxygen therapy	**PAH**	pulmonary arterial hypertension
HMD	hyaline membrane disease	**PC**	pressure control
HPS	Hantavirus pulmonary syndrome	**PCP**	Pneumocystis carinii pneumonia
HRCT	high-resolution CT scan	**PCV**	pressure-controlled ventilation
IC	inspiratory capacity	**PE**	pleural effusion, pulmonary embolus
IMV	intermittent mandatory ventilation	**PEEP**	positive end-expiratory pressure
IPF	idiopathic pulmonary fibrosis	**PEFR**	peak expiratory flow rate
IPPB	intermittent positive-pressure breathing	**PET**	position emission tomography

PFT	pulmonary function test
PND	paroxysmal nocturnal dyspnea, postnasal drip
PPD	purified protein derivative
PPH	primary pulmonary hypertension
PPY	packs per year
PSV	pressure support ventilation
PTE	pulmonary thromboembolus
R	respiration
RAD	reactive airways disease (bronchial asthma)
RD	respiratory disease
RDS	respiratory distress syndrome
RLL	right lower lobe

RUL	right upper lobe
RV	residual volume
SARS	severe acute respiratory syndrome
SOB	shortness of breath
TB	tuberculosis
TBNA	transbronchial needle aspiration
TTNAB	transthoracic needle aspiration biopsy
TLC	total lung capacity
TV	tidal volume
UIP	usual interstitial pneumonitis (pneumonia)
URI	upper respiratory infection
VC	vital capacity
V/Q scan	ventilation perfusion (lung) scan

Anatomic Illustrations

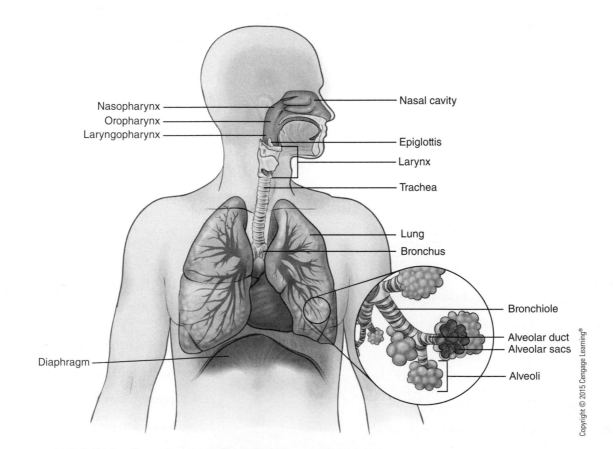

Copyright © 2015 Cengage Learning®

FIGURE 17-1   Structures of the respiratory system

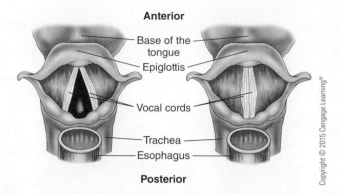

FIGURE 17-2 **View of the larynx and vocal cords from above. Shown on the left, the vocal cords are open during breathing. On the right, the vocal cords vibrate together during speech.**

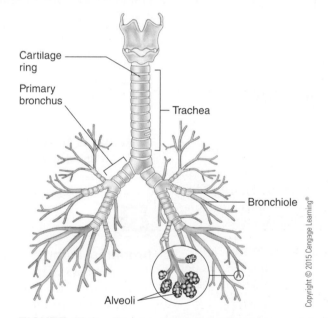

FIGURE 17-3 **The trachea, bronchial tree, and alveoli**

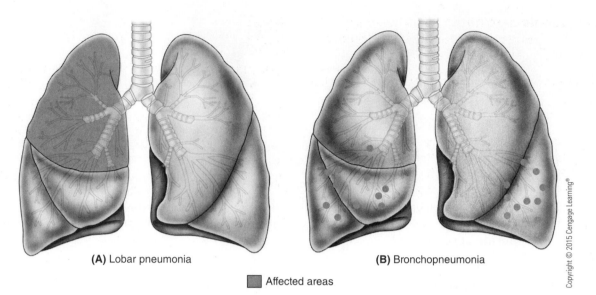

(A) Lobar pneumonia   **(B)** Bronchopneumonia

■ Affected areas

FIGURE 17-4 **Types of pneumonia are usually named for the area of the lung that is involved or for the causative agent. (A) Lobar pneumonia affects larger areas of the lungs. (B) Bronchopneumonia affects the bronchioles and surrounding alveoli.**

■ Respiratory/Pulmonary Medicine Terminology

##

acute interstitial pneumonitis (in"tər-stish'əl noo"mo-ni'tus) – a sudden, severe interstitial lung disease that often requires life support

acute respiratory distress syndrome (ARDS) – a type of severe, acute lung dysfunction affecting all or most of both lungs that occurs as a result of illness or injury

alveolus (pl. alveoli) (al-ve' o-lus, al-ve'o-li) – an air sac in the lung

anoxia (uh-nok'-see-uh) – absence or lack of oxygen from arterial blood or tissues

apical (ap'-ih-kul) – pertaining to the apex, the uppermost portion of the lung

asbestosis (as"-beh-sto'-sis) – an interstitial lung disease caused by inhalation of asbestos particles

asphyxia (as-fik'-see-uh) – absent or impaired exchange of oxygen and carbon dioxide on a ventilatory basis; suffocation

asthma (az'mə) – a chronic disease of the respiratory system that causes inflammation and narrowing in the bronchial tubes; difficulty breathing, wheezing, coughing, and tightness in the chest can result

atelectasis (at"-eh-lek'-tuh-sis) – loss of air space as a result of collapse of lung tissue

B

bronchial asthma (brong'-kee-ul) – a condition of the lungs characterized by narrowing of airways throughout the lungs; results in dyspnea and wheezing due to spasmodic contraction of the bronchi

bronchiectasis (brong"-kee-ek'-tuh-sis) – chronic dilatation of the bronchi as a result of inflammatory disease or obstruction; irreversible lung disease

bronchiole (brong'kee-ōl) – one of the finer subdivisions of the bronchi, all smaller than 1 mm in diameter

bronchiolitis (brong"kee-o-li'tis) – inflammation of the bronchioles, often associated with bronchopneumonia; several subcategories of bronchiolitis exist

bronchiolus (brong-ki"o-ləs) – one of the finer subdivisions of the bronchi (syn. bronchiole)

bronchitis (brong-ki'tus) – inflammation of the mucous membrane of the bronchial tubes

bronchogenic carcinoma (brong-kee-o-jen'-ik) – lung cancer; applied generally to any primary malignancy of the lung or bronchial tract

bronchoscopy (brong-kos'-kuh-pee) – examination of the interior of the tracheobronchial tree through a bronchoscope

bronchus (pl. bronchi) (brong'-kus, brong'-ki) – one of two subdivisions of the trachea (windpipe) serving to convey air to and from the lungs; right main bronchus, left main bronchus

Cheyne-Stokes respiration (chān' stōks') – a common and bizarre breathing pattern characterized by a period of apnea lasting 10 to 60 seconds followed by gradually increasing depth and frequency of respirations

chronic thromboembolic disease (thräm'-bō-em-bō'lik) – the condition resulting from a pulmonary embolism that is not reabsorbed by the body, resulting in multiple small blood vessels in the lungs becoming diseased

chronic bronchitis (brong-ki'tus) – inflammation of the mucous membranes of the bronchi characterized by cough, hypersecretion of mucus, expectoration of sputum, and associated with frequent bronchial infections; usually due to inhalation, over a prolonged period, of air contaminated by dust or noxious gasses

cilia (sil'e-ə) – thin hairs attached to the mucous membrane epithelium lining the respiratory tract

constrictive bronchiolitis (brong"ke-o-li'tus) – obstruction of bronchioles by scarring

cor pulmonale (kor pul"mo-na'le) – hypertrophy (enlargement) of the right ventricle resulting from disease of the lungs

cryptogenic organizing pneumonia (COP) (krip"to-jen'ik) – an interstitial lung disease that mimics pneumonia but without an infection present; also called bronchiolitis obliterans with organizing pneumonia (BOOP)

cystic fibrosis (sis'-tik fi-bro'sis) – a congenital disorder of exocrine glands affecting the sweat glands and pancreatic acini as well as the lungs, in which abnormally thick mucus plugs the bronchioles, causing a chronic inflammatory reaction and leading to collapse and consolidation of alveoli

desquamative interstitial pneumonitis (des-kwə-māt-iv in"tər-stish'əl noo"mo-ni'tus) **(DIP)** – diffuse proliferation of alveolar epithelial cells, which desquamate into the air sacs and become filled with macrophages; gradual onset of dyspnea and nonproductive cough occurs

diaphragm (di'ə-fram) – the muscle separating the chest and the abdomen

dyspnea (disp-nee"-uh) – difficulty or distress in breathing, shortness of breath

emphysema (em"fə-se'mə) – a condition of the lungs characterized by an increase in the size of air spaces with destructive changes in their walls and reduction in their number; there are many subcategories of emphysema

empyema (em"pi-e'mə) – a pocket of pus between visceral and parietal pleura

expectoration (ek-spek "tə-ra'shən) – the process of coughing up and spitting out sputum from the lungs

Hantavirus pulmonary syndrome (hahn"-tuh-vi"-rus) – a potentially deadly disease carried by rodents, especially the deer mouse

hemithorax (hem"e-thor'aks) – one side of the chest

hemoptysis (he-mop'tĭ-sis) – the spitting of blood derived from the lungs or bronchial tubes as a result of pulmonary or bronchial hemorrhage

histoplasmosis (his"to-plaz-mo'sis) – a disease caused by the fungus Histoplasma capsulatum that can cause acute or chronic lung disease

hypersensitivity pneumonitis (hi"pər-sen"sĭ-tiv'ĭ-te noo"mo-ni'tis) – an interstitial lung disease caused by constant inhalation of dust, mold, or other irritants

hypoxia (hi-pok"see-uh) – decrease below normal levels of oxygen in arterial blood or tissues without reaching anoxia

idiopathic pulmonary fibrosis (id"e-o-path'ik pool'mo-nar"ee fi-bro'sis) – an inflammatory lung disorder characterized by abnormal formation of fibrous tissue (fibrosis) between tiny air sacs (alveoli) or ducts in the lungs

interstitial lung disease (int-ər-' stish'-əl) – refers to many different lung conditions, all of which affect the interstitium, a lace-like network of tissue that spreads throughout both lungs

laryngostasis (lah"-ring-gos'-tuh-sis) – acute obstruction of upper airway in infants and children characterized by barking cough with difficult and noisy respiration; croup

Legionella pneumonia (le"jə-nel'ə) – an acute infectious disease with flu-like symptoms and a rapidly rising high fever, followed by severe pneumonia; Legionnaires disease

leukoplakia (loo"ko-pla'ke-ə) – a disease characterized by the development of white, thickened patches on the mucous membrane of the cheeks or tongue that cannot be rubbed off

lobectomy (lo-bek'tə-me) – excision of a lobe of the thyroid, liver, brain, or lung

lymphangioleiomyomatosis (lim-fan"je-o-li"o-mi"o-mə-to'sis) – a rare lung disease characterized by an unusual type of muscle cell that invades the tissue of the lungs

mediastinoscopy (me"de-as"tĭ-nos'kə-pe) – visual examination of the mediastinum via a surgical procedure

mediastinum (me"de-ə-sti'nəm) – the region between the lungs in the chest cavity

mesothelioma (me"zo-the"le-o'mə) – a malignant tumor arising in the pleura

mycoplasmal pneumonia (mi"ko-plaz'məl) – primary atypical pneumonia

naris (pl. nares) (na'ris, na'rēz) – nostril(s)

orthopnea (or"-thop'-nee-uh) – discomfort in breathing that is brought on by lying flat; sometimes dictated as one-pillow orthopnea, two-pillow orthopnea, or three-pillow orthopnea, depending upon how many pillows a patient needs to sleep comfortably

oximeter (ok-sim'ə-ter) – an instrument for determining the oxygen saturation of a sample of blood

oximetry (ok-sim'ə-tree) – procedure using a device (oximeter) to measure the oxygen saturation of a sample of blood

pleura (ploor'-uh) – the double-folded membrane enveloping the lungs and lining the walls of the pulmonary cavities

pleural effusion (ploor'-ul ə-fu'zhən) – escape of fluid into the pleural cavity

pleural rub – the grating sound produced by the motion of pleural surfaces rubbing each other

pleurisy (ploor'ĭ-se) – inflammation of the pleura, with exudation into its cavity and upon its surface; many subcategories of pleurisy exist

pleurodesis (ploŏ-rod'ə-sis) – surgical creation of a fibrous adhesion between the visceral and parietal layers of the pleura

pneumoconiosis (noo"mo-ko"ne-o'sis) – inflammation commonly related to fibrosis of the lungs due to irritation from inhalation of dust incident to an occupation

pneumonectomy (noo"mo-nek'tə-me) – the excision of lung tissue, particularly of the entire lung

pneumonia (noo-mo'-nĕă) – inflammation of the lungs with consolidation; many subcategories of pneumonia exist

pneumothorax (noo"-mo-thor'-aks) – air in the pleural cavity

psittacosis (sit"ə-ko'sis) – a disease caused by a strain of Chlamydia psittaci; may cause flu-like syndrome; in severe disease, symptoms of bronchopneumonia

pulmonary arterial hypertension (ar-tē'rē-ăl) – the condition of increased blood pressure in the arteries that carry blood from the heart to the lungs

pulmonary edema (e-dē'mă) – an abnormal buildup of fluid in the air sacs of the lungs, which leads to shortness of breath; usually caused by heart failure

pulmonary embolism (em'bə-liz-əm) – the condition that occurs when a blood clot breaks off from a deep vein (usually in the leg), travels into the right heart, and is forced into the lungs

pulmonary fibrosis (fi-bro'sis) – scarring of the lungs

pulmonary parenchyma (pah-reng'-kihmuh) – the key cells of the lung, those performing its main function; the air sacs and small bronchioles

pulmonary tuberculosis (too-ber"-kyoo-lo'-sis) – tuberculosis of the lungs

pulmonary vascular disease (vas'kyū-lăr) – disease affecting the blood vessels that lead to or from the lungs

pulmonary venous hypertension (vē'nŭs) – condition of increased blood pressure in the veins that carry blood from the lungs to the heart

respiratory papillomatosis (pap"ĭ-lo-mə-to'sis) – a rare viral disease characterized by multiple benign growths (papillomata) in the middle and lower respiratory tract

respiratory syncytial virus (RSV) (sin-' sish-(ē-) əl) – a viral infection causing minor respiratory infection with rhinitis and cough in adults; is capable of causing severe bronchitis and bronchopneumonia in young children

rhonchi (rong'-ki) – abnormal, rumbling sounds heard during expiration (sing., ronchus)

sarcoidosis (sar"-koy-do'-sis) – a systemic granulomatous disease of unknown cause, especially

involving the lungs with resulting interstitial fibrosis

severe acute respiratory syndrome (SARS) – a disorder caused by a type of coronavirus, a family of viruses that often cause mild to moderate upper respiratory illness, such as the common cold; also known as SARS-CoV

silicosis (sil"-ih-ko'-sis) – pneumoconiosis due to the inhalation of silica dust, with formation of generalized nodular fibrotic changes in both lungs

supraglottic (soo"-pruh-glot'-ik) – located above the glottis

thoracentesis (thor"-uh-sen'-tu-sis) – surgical puncture of the chest wall for drainage of fluid (syn. thoracocentesis)

thoracostomy (thor"-uh-kos'-tuh-mee) – surgical creation of an opening in the chest cavity for the purpose of drainage

thoracotomy (thor"-uh-kot'-uh-mee) – surgical incision into the chest wall

trachea (tra"ke-uh) – the air tube extending from the larynx into the thorax to the level of the fifth or sixth thoracic vertebra where it bifurcates into the right and left bronchi (syn. windpipes)

tracheobronchial tree (tra"ke-o-brong'ke-əl) – pertaining to the trachea and bronchi

tracheostomy (tra"ke-os'tə-me) – the creation of an opening into the trachea through the neck and insertion of a tube to create an airway

tuberculosis (too-bur"ku-lo'sis) – an infectious disease that attacks the lungs; it is caused by bacteria and is spread through the air

turbinate (tur'-bih-nat) – shaped like a top, such as a turbinate bone, especially in the nose

V

visceral pleura (viss'-er-ul ploor'-uh) – the inner fold of pleura lying closest to the lung tissue

Transcription Tips

Students will find it easier to transcribe dictation about respiratory/pulmonary medicine if they are familiar with the terms that describe the functions and structures that make respiration possible. A study of information presented in the chapter introduction, types of drugs commonly used, plus lab and diagnostic tests commonly used to delineate disease processes in respiratory/pulmonary medicine will make the task smoother.

Commonly Used Classes of Drugs

antihistamines

antitussives

corticosteroids

expectorants

antituberculosis agents

bronchodilators

decongestants

mucolytics

Common Laboratory and Diagnostic Testing

- acid-fast bacilli (AFB)
- antistreptolysin (ASO)
- bronchoscopy
- culture of mucous membranes (nasal passages, throat), sputum, etc.

- laryngoscopy
- nasopharyngography
- pulmonary function tests
- rhinoscopy

Common Lung Function Tests

- *Arterial blood gases* (ABGs) – determine the amount of oxygen and carbon dioxide in the bloodstream
- *Body plethysmography* – measures the total amount of air the lungs can hold (total lung volume)
- *Carbon monoxide diffusing capacity* – measures how well the lungs transfer a small amount of carbon monoxide gas into the blood

- *Gas dilution tests* – measure the amount of air that remains in the lungs after complete exhalation (residual volume)
- *Spirometry* – measures how quickly the lungs move air in and out

Common Measurable Lung Function Values

- Diffusing capacity for carbon monoxide (DLCO)
- Forced expiratory volume (FEV)
- Maximum voluntary ventilation (MVV)
- Peak expiratory flow rate (PEFR)

- Residual volume (RV)
- Tidal volume (TV)
- Total lung capacity (TLC)
- Vital capacity (VC)

Supportive Web Sites

http://chorus.rad.mcw.edu/	Click on "Respiratory System" for an extensive terminology list.
http://www.mayoclinic.com	Search for "respiratory" or "pulmonary" for many informative sites; click on "Health Information" to look up a particular condition or disease.
http://www.nhlbi.nih.gov	Under "Health Topics" click on "Lung Diseases" then on "Other Lung Diseases."
http://www.nlm.nih.gov	Search for "respiratory" and "pulmonary" and select links of interest; click on "Health Information" to search for different diseases and conditions.

Index of Respiratory/Pulmonary Medicine Reports

Exercise#	Patient Name	Type of Report/Procedure
TE#1	Paulo Angelotti	Chest Film: Check PICC line
TE#2	Jonathan Olivier	OP Report: Rhoracoscopic wedge resection, left upper lobectomy, mediastinal lymph node dissection
TE#3	Josiah Lynch	Pulmonary Function Study
TE#4	Pamela Pendergast	OP Report: Tracheostomy at bedside
TE#5	Diane M. Fisher	Pulmonary Consult (letter): Lung mass
TE#6	Martha Korman	Pulmonary Consult (letter): CT chest
TE#7	Alex Prieto	Pulmonary Function Study
TE#8	Gertrude Denmark	OP Report: Robotic surgery

CHAPTER 18
UROLOGY/NEPHROLOGY

Introduction

Urology is the study of the urinary tract in the male and female as well as the reproductive system in the male. *Nephrology* is the study of the kidneys, their anatomy, physiology, pathology, and disorders.

The urinary system is made up of two *kidneys,* which form and excrete urine, thereby removing various toxins from the body; two *ureters,* which carry urine from the kidneys down to the bladder; the urinary *bladder,* which serves as a collecting reservoir for urine; and the *urethra,* which transports the urine to the outside of the body. Other terms by which the urinary system may be identified include the genitourinary system, the excretory system, the renal-urologic system, and the urogenital system.

A *urologist* is a physician who practices both clinically and surgically. Some of the problems a urologist treats include surgical disorders of the kidneys, ureters, bladder, and the male reproductive system. In addition, the urologist treats such disorders as kidney stones, hematuria, cystitis, stress and urge incontinence, sexually transmitted diseases, and both prostate and impotence problems in men.

The scientific study of the kidney, its anatomy, physiology, pathology, and pathophysiology is done by a physician who specializes in nephrology, a *nephrologist,* who, like the urologist, also practices both clinically and surgically.

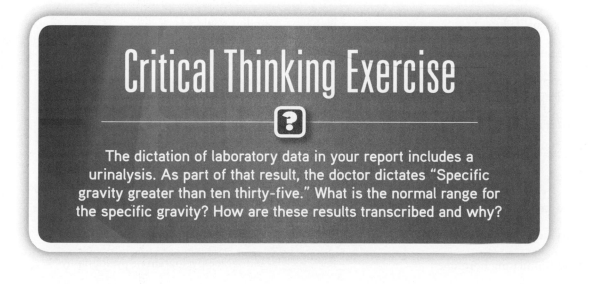

Critical Thinking Exercise

The dictation of laboratory data in your report includes a urinalysis. As part of that result, the doctor dictates "Specific gravity greater than ten thirty-five." What is the normal range for the specific gravity? How are these results transcribed and why?

Urology/Nephrology Abbreviations

The abbreviations, acronyms, and terms in the following abbreviations and terminology sections are often dictated in this specialty. We offer abbreviated definitions here. Please see an unabridged medical dictionary or the suggested web sites in this chapter for more information on each term.

ACTH	adrenocorticotropic hormone	**GBM**	glomerular basement membrane
ADH	antidiuretic hormone	**GFR**	glomerular filtration rate
A/G	albumin/globulin ratio	**G6PD**	glucose-6-phosphate dehydrogenase
AGN	acute glomerulonephritis	**HD**	hemodialysis
ANA	antinuclear antibody	**HPF**	high-power field
ARF	acute renal failure	**IC**	interstitial cystitis
ATN	acute tubular necrosis	**I&O**	intake and output or ins and outs
AV	arteriovenous	**IPD**	intermittent peritoneal dialysis
BNO	bladder neck obstruction	**IVP**	intravenous pyelogram
BPH	benign prostatic hypertrophy	**K**	potassium
BUN	blood urea nitrogen	**KUB**	kidneys, ureters, bladder
CAPD	continuous ambulatory peritoneal dialysis	**LDH**	lactic dehydrogenase (enzyme in blood and tissues)
CC	clean catch	**LH**	luteinizing hormone
CGN	chronic glomerulonephritis	**LPF**	low-power field
CMG	cystometrogram	**Na**	sodium
CRF	chronic renal failure	**NaCl**	sodium chloride
C&S	culture and sensitivity	**PD**	peritoneal dialysis
CURLL	cystoscopy, ureteral dilatation, laser lithotripsy	**pH**	hydrogen ion concentration (pH of arterial blood—always a lower case "p")
cysto	cystoscopic exam	**PKU**	phenylketonuria
ECF	extracellular fluid	**PSA**	prostate-specific antigen
ESRD	end-stage renal disease	**PSP**	phenolsulfonphthalein
ESWL	extracorporeal shock-wave lithotripsy	**PUL**	percutaneous ultrasonic lithotripsy
FEP	free erythrocyte protoporphyrin	**PVC**	postvoiding cystogram
FSH	follicle-stimulating hormone	**RP**	retrograde pyelogram or pyelography

SP GR	specific gravity
STD	sexually transmitted disease
TUE	transurethral extraction
TUNA	transurethral needle ablation
TUR	transurethral resection
TURB	transurethral resection, bladder
TURP	transurethral resection, prostate
UA	urinalysis

UPJ	ureteropelvic junction
UTI	urinary tract infection
UVJ	ureterovesical junction
VCUG	voiding cystourethrogram or vesicoureterogram
XC	excretory cystogram
XU	excretory urogram

Anatomic Illustrations

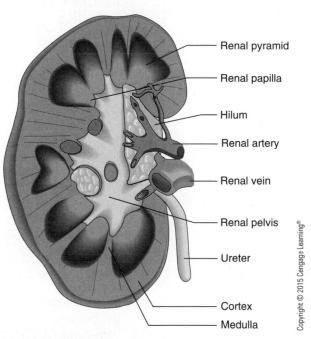

Renal pyramid

Renal papilla

Hilum

Renal artery

Renal vein

Renal pelvis

Ureter

Cortex

Medulla

Copyright © 2015 Cengage Learning®

FIGURE 18-1   The kidney

Urology/Nephrology Terminology

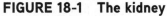

A

albuminuria (al"-byoo-mih-nyoo'-rē-uh) – presence of serum albumin in the urine

aminoaciduria (ah-mē"-nō-as"-ih-dyoo'-rē-uh) – an excess of amino acids in the urine

anorchism (an-or'-kizm) – congenital absence of the testis; this may occur unilaterally or bilaterally

antidiuretic (an"-tī-dī"-yoo-ret'-ik) – agent used to suppress the rate of urine formation

anuria (ah-nyoo'-rē-uh) – absence of excretion of urine from the body

aspermia (ā-sper'-mē-uh) – failure of formation or emission of semen

athrocytosis (ath"-rō-sī-tō'-sis) – absorption of macromolecules from the lumen of the renal tubules

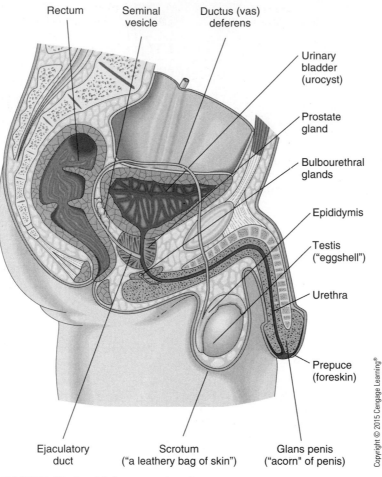

Rectum Seminal vesicle Ductus (vas) deferens

Urinary bladder (urocyst)

Prostate gland

Bulbourethral glands

Epididymis

Testis ("eggshell")

Urethra

Prepuce (foreskin)

Copyright © 2015 Cengage Learning®

Ejaculatory duct Scrotum ("a leathery bag of skin") Glans penis ("acorn" of penis)

FIGURE 18-2 Male reproductive organs

by renal tubular cells, by means of a process similar to phagocytosis (cells eating bacteria)

azoospermia (ā-zō"-ō-sper'-mē-uh) – the absence of living sperm

bacteriuria (bak-tēr"-ē-yoo'-rē-uh) – the presence of bacteria in the urine

balanitis (bal"-uh-nī'-tis) – inflammation of the glans penis

barbotage (bahr"bo-tahzh') – repeated injection and withdrawal of fluid

Bence Jones protein (behns jōnz) – proteins with unusual thermosolubility found in the urine of

patients with multiple myeloma—***NB***: this phrase takes no hyphen

brachytherapy (brak"-ē-thār'-uh-pē) – a procedure used to permanently implant tiny radioactive "seeds" into cancerous prostate glands; the seeds emit low-level radiation for several months

bulbourethral (bul"-bō-yoo-rē'-thrul) – pertaining to the bulb of the urethra

calculus (kal'-kyoo-lus) – an abnormal concretion occurring within the body; usually composed of mineral salts, but a stone analysis must be done to confirm the composition

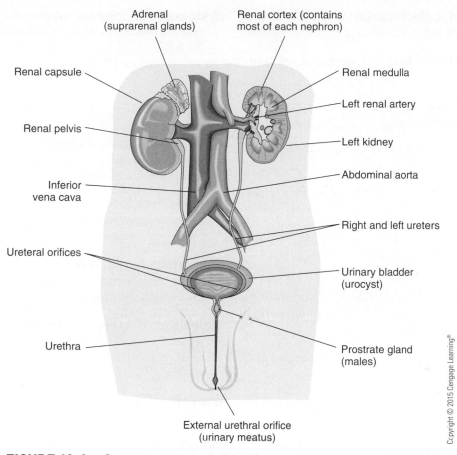

Adrenal (suprarenal glands)

Renal cortex (contains most of each nephron)

Renal capsule

Renal medulla

Renal pelvis

Left renal artery

Left kidney

Inferior vena cava

Abdominal aorta

Right and left ureters

Ureteral orifices

Urinary bladder (urocyst)

Urethra

Prostrate gland (males)

External urethral orifice (urinary meatus)

Copyright © 2015 Cengage Learning®

FIGURE 18-3   Gross anatomy of the urinary system

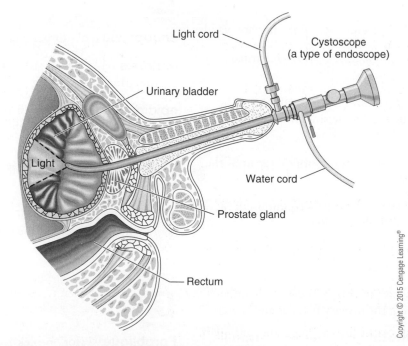

Light cord

Cystoscope (a type of endoscope)

Urinary bladder

Light

Water cord

Prostate gland

Rectum

Copyright © 2015 Cengage Learning®

FIGURE 18-4   Endoscopy of the urinary bladder

caliectasis (syn. calicectasis) (kal"-ē-ek'-tuh-sis, kal"-ih-sek'-tuh-sis) – dilatation of a calix of a kidney

calyx (syn. calix) (kā'-liks) – a cup-shaped organ or cavity

capsulectomy (kap"-suh-lek'-tuh-mē) – surgical excision of a capsule

capsulotomy (kap"-suh-lot'-uh-mē) – surgical incision into a capsule

chyluria (kī-loo'-rē-uh) – the presence of chyle in the urine, giving it a milky appearance

cloaca (klō-ā'-kuh) – the terminal end of the hindgut before division into the rectum, bladder, and genital primordia

cryptorchidism (krip-tōr'-kih-dizm) – a developmental defect characterized by failure of the testes to descend into the scrotum

crystalluria (kris-tuh-loo'-rē-uh) – the excretion of crystals in the urine, causing renal irritation

cystine (sis"-teen) – sometimes occurs as a deposit in the urine or forms a vesical calculus

cystinosis (Fanconi syndrome) (sis"-tih-nō'-sis, fankō'-nē) – a congenital hereditary disease in which the body accumulates cystine

cystinuria (sis"-tih-nyoo'-rē-uh) – the occurrence of cystine in the urine

cystitis (sis-tī'-tis) – inflammation of the urinary bladder

cystogram (sis'-tuh-gram) – x-ray of the urinary bladder

cystolithectomy (sis"-tō-lih-thek'-tuh-mē) – the removal of a calculus by incising into the urinary bladder

cystoplasty (sis'-tō-plas"-tē) – surgical repair of the urinary bladder

cystorrhagia (sis"-tō-rā'-jē-uh) – condition of blood bursting forth from the bladder

cystoscope (sis'-tō-skōp") – instrument used for examining the bladder

cystoureteritis (sis"-tō-yoo-rē"-ter-ī'-tis) – inflammation involving the urinary bladder and ureters

cystoureterolithotomy (sis"-tō-yoo-rē"-ter-ō-lih-thot'-uh-mē) – cystoscopy and ureterolithotomy for removal of calculus

cystourethroscopy (sis"-tō-yoo"-rē-thrah'-skuh-pē) – examination of the bladder and posterior urethra

dartos (syn. tunica dartos) (dar'-tōs, too'-nih-kuh) – a layer of smooth muscle fibers situated in the superficial fascia of the scrotum

Denonvilliers fascia (deh-nawn-vēl-yāz' fā'-shē-uh) – a membranous partition separating the rectum from the prostate and urinary bladder

descensus testis (dē-sen'-sus tes'-tis) – the descent of the testis from its fetal position in the abdominal cavity to the scrotum

dialysis (dī-al'-ih-sis) – a form of filtration to separate crystalloids from colloid substances in solution using a semipermeable membrane; a method of artificial kidney function

diuresis (dī"-yoo-rē'-sis) – increased secretion of urine

dysuria (dis-yoo'-rē-uh) – painful or difficult urination

endopelvic (en"-dō-pel'-vik) – within the pelvis

enuresis (en"-yoo-rē'-sis) – involuntary discharge of the urine; bed-wetting

epididymis (ep"-ih-did'-ih-mus) – a set of coiled tubes that lie alongside and connect the testes to the vas deferens

epididymitis (ep"-ih-did"-ih-mī'-tis) – inflammation of the epididymis

epispadias (ep"-ih-spā'-dē-us) – a congenital defect in which the urethra opens on the dorsum or underside of the penis

Foroblique™ (for"-ō-blēk') – an obliquely forward, visual telescopic system used in certain cystoscopes

funiculitis (fyoo-nik"-yoo-lī'-tis) – inflammation of the spermatic cord

glomerular (glō-mer'-yoo-lar) – pertaining to or of the nature of a glomerulus, especially a renal glomerulus

glomerulitis (glō-mer"-yoo-lī'-tis) – inflammation of the glomeruli of the kidney, with proliferative or necrotizing changes of the endothelial or epithelial cells or thickening of the basement membrane

glomerulonephritis (glō-mer"-yoo-lō-neh-frī'-tis) – a variety of nephritis characterized by inflammation of the capillary loops in the glomeruli of the kidney

glomerulosclerosis (glō-mer"-yoo-lō-skleh-rō'-sis) – fibrosis and scarring, which result in senescence of the renal glomeruli

glomerulus (pl. glomeruli) (glō-mer'-yoo-lus, glō-mer'-yoo-lie) – a tuft or cluster; often used alone to designate one of the glomeruli of the kidney

glycosuria (glī"-kō-syoo'-rē-uh) – the presence of an abnormal amount of glucose (sugar) in the urine; especially the excretion of an abnormally large amount of glucose in the urine

gonadectomy (gō"-nah-dek'-tuh-mē) – surgical removal of an ovary or a testis

gonococcal (gon"-ō-kok'-ul) – pertaining to gonococci, an individual microorganism of the species Neisseria gonorrhoeae, the organism causing gonorrhea

gonorrhea (gon"-ō-rē'-uh) – infection due to Neisseria gonorrhoeae, a sexually transmitted disease

hematuria (hēm"-ah-tyoo'-rē-uh) – blood in the urine

hemoglobinuria (hē"-mō-glō"-bih-nyoo'-rē-uh) – the presence of free hemoglobin in the urine

hemorrhagic (hem"-ō-raj'-ik) – pertaining to or characterized by hemorrhage; descriptive of any tissue into which bleeding has occurred

hermaphroditism (her-maf'-rō-dih-tizm") – a condition characterized by the presence of both male and female sex organs

Hesselbach triangle (hes'-ul-bok) – the area on the inferoanterior abdominal wall bounded by the rectus abdominis muscle, the inguinal ligament, and the inferior epigastric vessels

hydrocele (hī'-drō-sēl) – a collection of fluid in the membranes surrounding the testes

hypercalciuria (hī"-per-kal"-sē-yoo'-rē-uh) – an excess of calcium in the urine

hyperoxaluria (hī"-per-oks"-ah-loo'-rē-uh) – the excretion of an excessive amount of oxalate in the urine

hyperuricuria (hī"-per-yoo"-rih-kyoo'-rē-uh) – excess of uric acid in the urine

hypocitruria (hī"-pō-sih-troo'-rē-uh)—low levels of citric acid in the urine

hypospadias (hī"-pō-spa'-dē-us) – a developmental anomaly in the male in which the urethra opens on the dorsum (underside) of the penis or on the perineum

incontinence (in-kon'tĭ-nəns) – inability to hold or control urination or defecation

interstitial cystitis (in'tĕr-stish'ăl) – chronically irritable and painful inflammation of the bladder wall

intrarenal (in"-truh-rē'-nul) – within the kidney

kraurosis (kraw-rō'-sis) – a dry, shriveled condition of a part, especially of the vulva

leukocyturia (lyoo"-kō-sī-tyoo'-rē-uh) – the discharge of leukocytes in the urine

lipiduria (lip"-ih-dyoo'-rē-uh) – the presence of lipids in the urine

lithiasis (lih-thī'-uh-sis) – a condition characterized by the formation of calculi and concretions (stones)

litholapaxy (lih-thol'-uh-pak"-sē) – the crushing of a calculus in the bladder, followed at once by the washing out of the fragments

meatotomy (mē"-uh-tot'-uh-mē) – surgical incision into the urinary meatus to enlarge it

micturition (mik"-tyoo-rih'-shun) – the passage of urine; urination

myoglobinuria (mī"-ō-glō"-bih-nyoo'-rē-uh) – the presence of myoglobin in the urine

neobladder (ne"o-blad'ər) – an artificial reservoir for urine created as continent urinary diversion to re-place the bladder following cystectomy, constructed from a detubularized bowel segment or from a segment of the stomach, with implantation of the ureters and urethra

neocystostomy (nē"-ō-sis-tos'-tuh-mē) – recent cystostomy

nephrectomy (neh-frek'-tuh-mē) – surgical excision of a kidney

nephritis (neh-frī'-tis) – inflammation of a kidney

nephroblastoma (neh"-frō-blas-tō'-muh) – a malig-nant renal tumor of young children, often inherited, also called Wilms tumor

nephrocystitis (neh"-frō-sis-tī'-tis) – inflammation of the kidney and bladder

nephrolithotomy (neh"-frō-lih-thot'-uh-mē) – the removal of renal calculi by incising through the body of the kidney

nephropathy (neh-frahp'-uh-thē) disease of the kidneys

nephropexy (neh'-frō-pek"-sē) – the fixation or sus-pension of a floating kidney

nephrosclerosis (neh"-frō-skleh-rō'-sis) – hardening of the kidney; the condition of the kidney caused by renovascular disease

nephrosis (neh-frō'-sis) – any disease of the kidney

nephroureterectomy (neh"-frō-yoo"-rē-ter-ek'-tuh-mē) – surgical excision of a kidney and the whole, or a part of, the ureter

neuropathy (noŏ-rop'ə-the) – pathological disease of a kidney

nocturia (nok-tu're-ə) – urination during the night

oligospermia (ō"-lih-gō-sper'-mē-uh) – deficiency in the number of spermatozoa in the semen

oliguria (ō"-lih-gyoo'-rē-uh) – scanty, decreased amount of urine

orchialgia (or"-kē-al'-jē-uh) – pain in a testis

orchiopexy (or"-kē-ō-pek'-sē) – surgical fixation in the scrotum of an undescended testis

orchitis (or-kī'-tis) – inflammation of a testis

paraphymosis (pār"-uh-fi-mō'-sis) – condition in which the foreskin is stuck behind the head of the penis and cannot be pulled back down into a normal position

pelviolithotomy (pel"-vē-ō-lih-thot'-uh-mē) – surgical procedure in which a renal calculus is excised from the pelvis of the kidney

penoscrotal (pē'-nō-skrō'-tul) – relating to the penis and the scrotum

percutaneous ultrasonic lithotripsy (per"-kyoo-tā'-nē-us lith'-ō-trip"-sē) – the use of ultrasound to crush a kidney stone

peritoneal dialysis (pār"-ih-tō-nē'-ul) – use of a peritoneal catheter and dialysis to separate waste from the blood

periurethral (pār"-ē-yoo-rē'-thrul) – occurring around the urethra

Peyronie disease (pā-rō-nēz') – penile deformation characterized by a plaque or hard lump that develops on the upper or lower side of the penis in the layers containing erectile tissue

phallus (fal'-us) – the penis

pheochromocytoma (fē-ō-krō"-mō-sī-tō'-muh) – a tumor of chromaffin tissue, most commonly of the adrenal medulla; usually benign and often hereditary

phimosis (fĭ-mō'-sis) – tightness of the foreskin so that it cannot be drawn back over the glans

prevesical (prē-veh'-sih-kul) – situated in front of the bladder

priapism (prī'-uh-pihzm) – persistent abnormal erection of the penis, usually without sexual desire, and accompanied by pain and tenderness

prostate gland (pros'tāt) – structure surrounding the ejaculatory ducts that produces some of the components of sperm

proteinuria (prō"-tē-in-yoo'-rē-uh) – the presence of an excess of serum proteins in the urine

pyelectasis (pī"-eh-lek'-tuh-sis) – dilatation of the renal pelvis

pyelitis (pī"-eh-lī'-tis) – inflammation of the pelvis of the kidney

pyelocaliectasis (pī"-eh-lō-kal"-ē-ek'-tuh-sis) – dilatation of the kidney, its pelvis and calices

pyelonephritis (pī"-eh-lō-neh-frī'-tis) – inflammation of the kidney and its pelvis

pyonephrosis (pī"-ō-neh-frō'-sis) – suppurative destruction of the parenchyma of the kidney, with total or almost complete loss of renal function

R

renal colic (rē'năl kol'ik) – sharp, severe pain in the lower back over the kidney, radiating forward into the groin

renin (re'nin) – an enzyme produced by the kidney and elevated in some types of hypertension

residual urine (rē-zid'yū-ăl) – urine that is left in the bladder after urination

S

seminiferous tubules (seh"-mih-nif'-er-us too'-byoolz) – tiny coiled tubes in the testes that produce sperm

seminoma (seh"-mih-nō'-muh) – a malignant tumor of the testis thought to arise from primitive gonadal cells

smegma (smeg'-muh) – a foul-smelling, pasty accumulation of desquamated epidermal cells and sebum that has collected in moist areas of the genitalia

Sonolith Praktis™ (sōn'-ō-lihth prak'-tis) – a portable lithotripter used to treat stones in the kidney and ureters

specific gravity (spĕ-sif'ik grav'itē) – weight of a substance compared with an equal amount of water; a test done as part of the urinalysis

spermaturia (syn. seminuria) (sper"-muh-tyoo'-rē-uh, seh"-mih-nyoo'-rē-uh) – the presence of semen in the urine

stress incontinence – condition in which coughing, laughing, sneezing, or some other involuntary stress results in leaking of urine (see vesicourethropexy below)

synorchism (sin-or'-kizm) – fusion of the two testes into one mass that may be located in the scrotum or in the abdomen

T

Tenckhoff™ catheter (tenk'-hawf) – a catheter inserted into the peritoneum for peritoneal dialysis; also a silicone Tenckhoff catheter

testosterone (tess-tos'-ter-ōn) – the major male sex hormone

transvesical (trans-veh'-sih-kul) – through the urinary bladder

trigonitis (trig"-uh-nī'-tis) – inflammation or localized hyperemia of the trigone of the urinary bladder

urachus (u'rə-kəs) – the derivative of the allantoic stalk in the fetus that connects the urinary bladder with the umbilicus; it persists throughout life as a fibrous cord

urea (yoo-rē'-uh) – a white, crystalline substance found in the urine, blood, and lymph

ureter (yoo"-rē-ter) – one of the tubes that conducts the urine from the renal pelvis to the urinary bladder; *NB*: do not confuse this word with urethra; remember, there are two ureters and one urethra

ureterectasis (yoo-rē"-ter-ek'-tuh-sis) – distention of a ureter

ureteritis (yoo"-rē-ter-ī'-tis) – inflammation of a ureter

ureteroenteric (yoo-rē"-ter-ō-en-tār'-ik) – pertaining to or connecting the ureter and the intestine

ureterolithiasis (yoo-rē"-ter-ō-lih-thī'-uh-sis) – the formation of a calculus in the ureter

ureterolithotomy (yoo-rē"-ter-ō-lih-thot'-uh-mē) – the removal of a calculus from the ureter by incision

ureteropathy (u-re"tər-op'ə-the) – disease of the ureter

ureteropelvic (yoo-rē"-ter-ō-pel'-vik) – pertaining to or affecting the ureter and the renal pelvis

ureteroureterostomy (yoo-rē"-ter-ō-yoo-rē"-ter-os'-tuh-mē) – end-to-end anastomosis of the two portions of a transected ureter

urethra (yoo-rē"-thra) – the canal leading from the urinary bladder, discharging urine externally;

NB: do not confuse this word with ureter; remember, there is one urethra and two ureters

urethrovesical (yoo-rē"-thrō-veh'-sih-kul) – pertaining to or communicating with the urethra and the urinary bladder urge incontinence – condition in which the urge to urinate is strong and immediate; involuntary leaking of urine is common

uriniferous (yoo"-rih-nih'-fer-us) – transporting or conveying the urine

urostomy (yoo"-rahs'-tuh-mē) – surgical opening in the urinary bladder

urotoxia (yoo"-rō-tok'-sē-uh) – the toxicity of the urine; the toxic substance of the urine

varicocele (vār'-ih-kō-sēl") – varicose condition of the veins of the scrotum

vasectomy (vah-sek'-tuh-mē) – surgical removal of the ductus (vas) deferens, or of a portion of it; done in association with prostatectomy or to induce infertility

vesical (ves"-ee-kl) – relating to any bladder, but usually the urinary bladder; *NB*: do not confuse this word with *vesicle*, which means a small sac containing liquid or gas

vesicourethropexy (veh"-sih-kō-yoo-rē'-thrō-pek"-sē) – surgical fixation of the urinary bladder and urethra for correction of stress incontinence in a female

Transcription Tips

Students will find it easier to transcribe dictation in urology/nephrology if they are familiar with the names of the organs of the renal-urologic system, their locations, and their functions. Also study the confusing terms, the meanings of roots and combining forms, prefixes, and suffixes relevant to this system. Knowledge of the common laboratory testing and diagnostic procedures and disorders affecting the male reproductive system used in this specialty will also be beneficial.

Common Laboratory Testing and/or Diagnostic Procedures

blood urea nitrogen (BUN) – blood test to assess the amount of urea excreted by the kidneys

creatinine – blood test to determine amount of creatinine present

creatinine clearance – urine test to determine the glomerular filtration rate (GFR)

cystoscopy (cysto) – visual examination of the bladder and urethra using a lighted cystoscope

intravenous pyelography (IVP) – test conducted with the use of radiopaque substance injected intravenously to see the kidneys, ureters, and bladder

kidney, ureters, bladder (KUB) – x-ray of the abdomen to reveal the size and position of the kidneys, ureters, and bladder

magnetic resonance imaging (MRI) – procedure that uses magnetic waves to make images that are evaluated by a radiologist

radioisotope studies – pictures taken of kidneys following injection of a radioactive substance (isotope) into the bloodstream

renal biopsy – surgical removal of tissue from the kidney

retrograde pyelography – use of a contrast medium in radiology to see the kidneys, ureters, and bladder

ultrasonography of the kidneys – the use of high-frequency sound waves to view the kidneys

urine culture – test on urine (culture) to determine the presence of microorganisms

voiding cystourethrogram (VCUG) – x-ray of the bladder and urethra as patient expels urine, after the bladder has been filled with contrast material

Other Urology/Nephrology Procedures

dialysis – the separation of waste materials from the bloodstream when the kidneys no longer function properly; treatment includes both diffusion and ultra-filtration via any of the following methods:

- continuous ambulatory peritoneal dialysis (CAPD)
- continuous cycling peritoneal dialysis (CCPD)
- equilibrium dialysis
- intermittent peritoneal dialysis (IPD)
- hemodialysis dialysis (HD), also called kidney dialysis or renal dialysis
- lymph dialysis
- sustained low-efficiency dialysis (SLED)

lithotripsy – the crushing of a urinary calculus or gallstone within the body followed at once by the washing out of the fragments. Formerly done surgically, it can now be done by various noninvasive methods, including:

- ballistic lithotripsy
- electrohydraulic lithotripsy
- extracorporeal shock-wave lithotripsy (ESWL)
- laser lithotripsy
- percutaneous ultrasonic lithotripsy (PUL)

renal transplantation – procedure in which someone with renal failure receives a new kidney from either a living related donor, a living unrelated donor, or a cadaver donor—each of these is called an allograft or an allogeneic transplant. Syngraft is a graft between genetically identical individuals, also called isograft or an isogeneic transplant.

Disorders Affecting the Male Reproductive System (including penile disorders)

ambiguous genitalia	bifed penis
epididymitis	hydrocele
hypospadias	inguinal hernia
micropenis	phimosis
testicular cancer	testicular torsion
testicular trauma	undescended testicles

Supportive Web Sites

http://www.atnephrology.com	Click on links of interest.
http://www.cancer.gov	Click on "Cancer Information," then "Types of Cancer" ; also search for "urology" or "nephrology."
http://chorus.rad.mcw.edu/	Click on "Genito-Urinary System," then on other related links for an extensive terminology list.
http://www.my.webmd.com	Under "Medical Info," click on "Diseases and Conditions."
http://www.niddk.nih.gov	Click on "Health Information," then on "Kidney and Urologic Diseases."
http://www.nlm.nih.gov	Click on "Health Information," then "MEDLINEplus," then search for "urology."
http://www.thekidney.org/	Click on links of interest.

Index of Urology/Nephrology Reports

Exercise#	Patient Name	Type of Report/Procedure
TE#1	Evan Merida	Ambulatory Surgery: Cystoscopy, biopsy
TE#2	Evan Merida	Ambulatory Surgery: Cystoscopy, biopsy
TE#3	Evan Merida	Preoperative History and Physical Examination
TE#4	Evan Merida	Laparoscopic radical cystoprostatectomy with lymph node dissection
TE#5	Evan Merida	Urinary bladder reconstruction
TE#6	Evan Merida	Consultation, postoperative
TE#7	Randy Applewhite	Robotic-assisted laparoscopic radical retropubic prostatectomy
TE#8	Anna Kate Tippin	Preoperative H&P Evaluation
TE#9	Anna Kate Tippin	Ambulatory Surgery: Cystoscopy
TE#10	Anna Kate Tippin	Ambulatory Surgery: Retrograde pyelogram
TE#11	L. Victor Stuart Jr	SOAP Note: Microhematuria
TE#12	L. Victor Stuart Jr	CT, stone protocol

CHAPTER 19

CORRESPONDENCE AND PROOFREADING

Part A: Correspondence

Introduction

Part A presents three correctly formatted letters and two memos. Letter #1 illustrates a block style two-page letter; notice that "continued" is placed as the last line of page one and a correct heading is the first thing listed on page two of the letter. Letter #2 presents a letter formatted in modified block style. Letter #3 is formatted in the simplified letter style. Finally, two memoranda are shown that illustrate the use of military date and time.

Critical Thinking Exercise

?

While your doctor is dictating a patient's chart note, he includes insulting information about a nurse of his. He dictates about her inappropriate care of his patient and the disciplinary actions to be taken. What should be done? Transcribe as dictated in the patient's chart note? Leave it out? Transcribe it in a separate document?

Part A: Examples of Letters and Memos

Letter 1—Block Style Letter Format: All lines start at the left margin.

Merwin B. Moore Memorial Clinic
6249 Broad Street
Lebanon, TN 37106
Phone 615.555.2500

August 17, ----

James C. Thompson Memorial Clinic
ATTN: Savant Oswalt, MD, Hematology/Oncology
#1 Lincoln Circle
Paris, TN 37904

Patient Name: Martha Cordova   **DOB**: 07/10/----

Dear Dr. Oswalt:

Ms. Martha Cordova, 57 years old, returned to the office on August 18. As you may know, she was hospitalized for several weeks at Forrest General after returning from visiting family in California. She initially presented with pneumonitis. She has been hospitalized on a couple of occasions at Forrest General, and it was felt that this could be related to her Afinitor. She was readmitted to Forrest General and treated with antibiotics for a bacterial pneumonitis. I was consulted during that 3rd hospitalization. It was felt that she could be having a delayed Afinitor reaction, and we placed her on steroids as well. She was seen in consultation by pulmonary services and had a bronchoscopy done. Pathology was negative for lymphangitic spread of her tumor, as there was some suggestion of this on her CT scan. Cultures were negative as well.

While hospitalized, the patient also developed headaches. CT and MRI scans revealed the presence of brain metastases. She was therefore started on radiotherapy to her brain. Her condition initially declined, and hospice was considered with supportive care; however, her condition did improve somewhat, and she was discharged home.

Ms. Cordova has now been home a week, and despite some continued fatigue, she actually looks a fair amount better. On exam, her lungs are clear today. Her heart is regular, but she has trace edema in her lower extremities.

I had a long discussion with the patient and her family regarding other therapies. I think the Afinitor played a large role in her pulmonary problems, and these appear to have improved somewhat. She continues to be treated for her brain metastases with radiation therapy. I discussed other systemic treatments, and we are going to give her a trial of Nexavar. She understands that her condition is quite tenuous; however, this will at least give her an opportunity for further treatment. The patient understands and agrees with the above plan. We are referring Ms. Cordova and her family to Dr. Cynthia Gonzales for counseling.

(Continued)

Savant Oswalt, MD
Patient Name: Martha Cordova
August 17, ----
Page 2

Again, I appreciate the opportunity to participate in Ms. Cordova's care; I will be happy to follow her along with you as needed.

Sincerely,

Tonya Warren, MD
Hematology/Oncology

TW:xx

cc: Cynthia G. Gonzales, PhD, Psychology/Social Services

Letter 2—Modified Block Style Letter Format: Date and closing lines begin at center

Greater Nashville Gastroenterology Associates, P.A.
1200 Superior Street NW
Nashville, TN 37189
Phone 615.555.2600

August 17, ----

Merwin B. Moore Memorial Clinic
ATTN: Anderson Phipps, MD
Family Medicine/Geriatrics
6249 Broad Street
Lebanon, TN 37106

Patient Name: Clara Short   **DOB**: March 10, ----

Dear Dr. Phipps:

Thanks so much for allowing me to see Clara Short. As you know, this is a pleasant, 69-year-old black female who underwent cervical spine surgery at Forrest General Medical Center on January 18, ----. She has been recovering at Pebble Hill Skilled Care Facility.

Medications include saline and narcotics. Patient has a known history of gastroesophageal reflux and is on proton pump inhibitor therapy. She recently complained of morning regurgitation of fluid into her mouth while at Pebble Hill. This has been described as clear fluid with a yellowish tinge. There is no solid component to this. There has been no heartburn currently. She has had no dysphagia, no significant abdominal pain, no constipation, and no diarrhea.

On physical exam, vital signs are stable. Exam is limited to the GI system. Abdomen is soft and non-tender with positive bowel sounds.

Clara presents with some fluid regurgitation in the mornings, likely related to her history of gastro-esophageal reflux, also likely related to her use of narcotics and other medications. The patient will be advised to follow a strict anti-reflux regimen and to raise the head of her bed at night. Continue omeprazole and decrease her use of narcotics as much as possible.

The patient will begin Reglan at a level of 10 mg at bedtime. We will check later to make sure that she is comfortable with that dosage level. This can be increased if necessary. She will also have followup labs. Her clinical progress will be monitored, and she will be re-evaluated in two weeks. An upper endoscopy can be repeated if necessary.

Thanks for allowing me to participate in the care of this interesting patient. If I can be of any further assistance, please let me know.

Yours truly,

Doris Robertson, MD, Gastroenterology

DR:xx

c: Pebble Hill Skilled Care Facility

Letter 3—Simplified Letter Style: Salutation and complimentary close are omitted

The Nashville Diagnostic Clinic
12221 N. Cleary Expressway
Nashville, TN 37758
Phone 615.901.1111

August 17, ----

Merwin B. Moore Memorial Clinic
ATTN: Anderson Phipps, MD
        Family Medicine/Geriatrics
6249 Broad Street
Lebanon, TN 37106

Patient Name: Fanny Eubanks   **DOB**: 01/26/----

I had the pleasure of seeing Ms. Fanny Eubanks, a 67-year-old black female, in the office today in followup for her myelodysplastic syndrome. She is doing very well and has no complaints.

Physical examination today is unremarkable. We obtained a CBC, which revealed a white count of 7, hemoglobin of 14.4, hematocrit 45.3, and a platelet count of 546,000. Ms. Eubanks' counts remain stable. I have instructed her to continue her Hydrea. We will continue to follow her, and I will have her return to my office in four months for a followup visit.

It is a pleasure to participate in the care of this most pleasant patient, and I will continue to keep you informed.

Tonya Warren, MD, Hematology/Oncology
Dictated By: Greg Farrow, FNP

GF:xx

Memorandum 1– Military Style Date and Time

The Nashville Diagnostic Clinic
12221 N. Cleary Expressway
Nashville, TN 37758
Phone 615.901.1111

Memorandum

To: Chloe Suzanne Graham   **Sex**: F   **DOB**: 6 Nov ----   **Acct. No.**: 190

From: Yancy Rhodes, MD, Endocrinology

RE: Non-fasting thyroid stimulating hormone (TSH) test results.

Date: 23 June ----

This memo contains your non-fasting thyroid test results drawn on 20 June ---- at the Diagnostic
Clinic at the request of Dr. Murray Travis of OB/GYN. Results are within normal limits.

		Normal Range
TSH, 3rd generation	2.46 mIU/L	0.40–4.50 mIU/L

Electronically signed by Yancy Rhodes, MD, on 23 June---- at 1530 hours.

YR:xx

Performing laboratory: Quest Diagnostics at 4770 Regent Blvd in Nashville, TN
Laboratory Medical Director: Helene S. Bergstrom, MD

Memorandum 2 – Military Style Date and Time

The Nashville Diagnostic Clinic
12221 N. Cleary Expressway
Nashville, TN 37758
Phone 615.901.1111

Memorandum

To: All Patients of Dennis Gordon, MD, Neurology

From: Larry Lukin, Office Administrator

Date: 1 December ----

Effective 31 December ----, Dr. Dennis Gordon is retiring from private practice, leaving The Nashville Diagnostic Clinic as a practicing physician after 18 years of dedicated service. The physicians and staff of NDC wish Dr. Gordon all the best in his future endeavors. We invite his patients to join us here at the clinic in a Holiday Farewell on 30 December from 1400 to 1800 hours.

As a patient of the clinic, your continued care in a familiar environment is of great importance to us. We can assure you that your health care will be appropriately served by another physician within the clinic. Drs. Wanda Dale, Cooper Timmons, Dallas Juneau, and Holly Russo are all compassionate, caring physicians who are here to serve your neurology and neurosurgery needs.

If needed, the staff can assist you in having your records transferred to another physician.

If you wish to learn more about Drs. Dale, Timmons, Juneau, or Russo, please visit our website at www.ndc.com or join us here on the afternoon of 30 Dec. Please let me know personally if you have any questions or concerns. I look forward to seeing you at our Holiday Farewell.

LL:xx

Part B: Proofreading Exercises Index

Introduction

The 12 proofreading exercises provided in Part B contain errors in spelling, grammar, punctuation, style, and format. The AHDI *Book of Style, 3rd Edition*, is the authors' main style guide, but the other reference books listed in our bibliography have also been used. These exercises can be used as the basis of a discussion on "what is an error?"

As you proofread the exercises presented in Part B, identify the errors according to your teacher's instructions. The number of errors that you should find in each document is given at the top of each exercise. (These exercises are double spaced for ease in finding and marking errors.)

Exercise#	Patient Name	Type of Proofreading Exercise
PR#1	Vivian Salters	Esophageal Motility Study
PR#2	Angela Highland	Orthopedic Consultation
PR#3	Julia Zanzibar	Orthopedic Consultation
PR#4	Linda C. Dominguez	History and Physical Examination
PR#5	Eugenia Piedmont	Orthopedic Consultation
PR#6	Hal Peterson Myers	Orthopedic Consultation
PR#7	Ellen Rappaport	Family Practice SOAP Note
PR#8	Ellen Rappaport	OB/GYN Office Visit
PR#9	Noelle Trudeau	Preoperative Evaluation
PR#10	James Knolls	Orthopedic Consultation
PR#11	Dominica Trainor	Orthopedic Clinical Note
PR#12	Ronald DeVittori	Diagnostic Imaging Services

Part B: Proofreading Exercises

Proofreading Exercise 1: Find 15 errors in the following report.

Greater Nashville Gastroenterology Associates, P.A.
1200 Superior Street NW
Nashville, TN 37189
Phone 615.555.2600

ESOPHAGEAL MOTILITY STUDY

Patient Name: SALTERS, Vivian   **Referring Physician**: Greg Farrow, FNP

Date of Study: March 7, ----   **Age/Sex**: F/43   **DOB**: 7/23/----

PROCEDURE IN DETALE

The patient was prepped and draped in the usual sterile manor. Anesthesia was administered by Miller

Travis, CRNA.

The esophageal motility study was done in the usual manner using the Beckman manometer. Using the

slow pull-through technique, the lower esophageal sphincter pressure was measured. The mean was 15

mmHg, location at 40 cm, and there was normal relaxation. Using both wet and dry swallows the peristaltic

waves were measured. In the midesophagus, the mean pressure was 41 mmHg, duration of 5 seconds, and in

the distal esophagus, 38 mmHg with a duration of 6 seconds. The upper esophageal sphincter pressure was

measured and was 55 mmHg in the anterior and posterior leads and 34 mmHg in the lateral lead. These were

all with in normal limits.

The motility appeared normal even during the episode of chest pane that the patient experienced in the

Bernstein test. 1 episode was noted on the tracing of some simultaneous waves; however, no repetitive

waves were noted.

(Continued)

ESOPHAGEAL MOTILITY STUDY

Patient Name: Salters, Vivian   Referring Physician: Greg Farrow, FNP

Date of Procedure: March 7, ----   Page 2

IMPRESSIVE: Positive Bernstein test w/normal esophageal motility study except for a few simultaneous

waves.

_____

Doris Robertson, MD, Gastroenterology

DR:xx

D: 3/07/----

T: 3/70/----

C: Greg Farrow, RN

Proofreading Exercise 2: Find 23 errors in the following report.

Merwin B. Moore Memorial Clinic
6249 Broad Street
Lebanon, TN 37106
Phone 615.555.2500

ORTHOPEDIC CONSULTATION

Patient Name: Angela Highland   **Referring Physician**: Charles W. Scott MD

Date of Consultation: 8/12/----   **Sex/Age**: F/38   **DOB**: 1/16/----

CHIEF COMPLAINT: A 38-year-old Black woman referred by Dr. Scott for complaints of pane in the left caff, along with complaints of cramping and discomfort in her hands.

HISTORY OF PRESENT ILLNESS: The patient reports that she was at home holding her 3 month old baby and was kind of dancing around when she misstepped and felt a pooping sensation in her calf. Afterwards she had continuous pain in the calf and difficulty walking. She went to Forrest General Emergency Room, where she was evaluated. She had an x-ray done, which was negative. She then saw her primary care physician, Dr. Scott, from where she was referred to me for orthopedic consultation. She reports that she still has a little discomfort in her calf. She has been walking with crutches and can not ambulate fully. She also reports that she has been experiencing some cramping in her hands. This occurs bilaterally. She complains of discomfort intermittently with activity during the day, but will oftentimes wade up at night with her hands either numb or cramping. She does report a history of a radioulnar synostosis in her left upper extremity.

(Continued)

ORTHOPEDIC CONSULTATION

Patient Name: Angela Highland

Referring Physician: Charles W. Scott, M.D.

Date of Consultation: 8/12/----

Page 2

PAST MEDICAL HISTORY: Past medical history as above; otherwise, noncontributory.

PAST SURGICAL HISTORY: Hammertoe surgery.

ALLERGIES: Penicillin, which causes a rash.

SOCIAL HISTORY: She is married. She is employed as a bookkeeper for the city fo Nashville. No use of tobacco or illicit drugs; social EtOH only.

PHYSICAL EXAMINATION: The patient is a well developed, well nourished black woman who appears her stated age. She is in no acute distress. Exam is limited to the MS system.

Evaluation of the bilateral upper extremities reveals a mild angular deformity in the left forearm with an increased radial bow. There is no passive or active pronation or supination, although the patient can functionally substitute for pronation by abducting her arm and for supination by adducting her arm. There is a mild positive Phalen's test bilaterally, greater on the left than on the right. There is a negative Tinel sign bilaterally. There is no atrophy of the thenar eminence. The fingers are warm with instant capillary refill. Sensory is intact. The radial pulse is +2 and equal.

Evaluation of the left calf reveals mild edema in the body of the gastrocsoleus medially. There is tenderness in the muscle belly in the midportion on the medial head. There is no tenderness over the Achilles' tendon. There is no pain with resisted inversion of the ankle. There is mild discomfort with extension of the knee with the ankle dorsiflexed.

(Continued)

ORTHOPEDIC CONSULTATION

Patient Name: Highland, Angela   Referring Physician: Charles W. Scott, MD

Date of Consultation: 8/12/----   Page 3

DIAGNOSTIC IMPRESSION:

1. Strain of the gastrocsoleus, left lower extremity, moderately symptomatic.

2. Bilateral carpal tunnel syndrome, mild.

RECOMMENDATIONS: We discussed the diagnoses, prognoses, and treatment options. I recommend expectant

management of the left gastroc strain. The patient was instructed to apply ice, stretch gently, and begin partial

weightbearing. She is to increase weightbearing as tolerated. If her symptoms do not resolve in 2 to 3 weeks,

return for reevaluation.

We also discussed the putative carpal tunnel syndrome in her bilateral upper extremities. I recommend that the

patient undergo a coarse of night bracing. I showed her the type of braces we employ for this. She has a deductible

for braces and did not want to purchase them here. She will look for the appropriate type brace at a pharmacy or an

equipment store. Patient will follow up with me on a prn basis if her symptoms do not resolve with the night

bracing.

Thank you, Charles, for allowing me to share in the care of this pheasant patient. I will keep you informed of her

progress and any further diagnostic or therapeutic recommendations.

_____

Olivia Glover, M.D., Orthopedics

OG:xx

D: 8/12/----

T: 8/12/----

C: Charles W. Scott, MD, OB/GYN

Proofreading Exercise 3: Find 17 errors in the following report.

James C. Thompson Memorial Clinic
#1 Lincoln Circle
Paris, TN 37904
Phone 731.555.3700

ORTHOPEDIC CONSULTATION

Patient Name: Julia Zanzibar   **PCP**: Antonia Connerly, MD

Date of Consultation: 9/10/----   **Sex/Age**: 7/F   **DOB**: 7/17/----

CHIEF COMPLAINT: The patient is a 7 year old White female referred by Dr. Connerly. She presents for followup examination regarding the complaint of left distal radius fracture. The patient is s/p closed reduction and long arm cast application, which was performed in the e.r. room 2 1/2 weeks ago. The patient and her mother, who accompanies her today, reports that she is doing well with no pain or discomfort.

PHYSICAL EXAMINATION: Patient has a well applied long arm cast in place. The skin is warm and dry at the margins of the cast. After removal of the cast, there is no evidence of deformity. The skin is warm and dry. The swelling has resolved in the extremity. The fingers are warm with instant capillary refill. There is mild tenderness to palpitation over the distal radius at the fracture cite.

RADIOGRAPHIC EVALUATION: Two views of the left wrist taken to day demonstrates a fracture of the left distal radius with stable alignment.

DIAGNOSTIC IMPRESSION: Left distal radius fracture, stable.

(Continued)

ORTHOPEDIC CONSULTATION

Patient Name: Julia Zanzibar

Page 2

PCP: Antonia Connerly, MD

Date of Consult: 9/10/----

RECOMMENDATIONS: My recommendation is the application of a short arm cast today. The patient's mother requested the use of a Gore-Tex Procel liner. The patient will be seen back in 3 weeks, at which time we will remove the short arm cast and obtain x rays out of cast, anticipating union of the fracture.

After receiving informed verbal consent the orthopedic technician applied a short arm cast with Gore-Tex Procel liner to the right upper extremity. The procedure was accomplished with no complications.

_____

Olivia Glover, MD

Orthopedics

OG:xx

D: 9/10/----

T: 9/10/----

C: Antonia Connerly, MD, Pediatrician

Proofreading Exercise 4: Find 46 errors in the following report.

Forrest General Medical Center
1038 Superior Street NW
Nashville, TN 37189
Phone 615.555.5000

History & Physical Examination

Patient Name: Linda C. Dominguez   **Admitting Physician**: David Loyola, MD

Date of Admission: 6/6/----   **Sex/Age**: F/65   **DOB**: 8/23/----

CHEF COMPLAINT: Chest pain, body aches.

HISTORY OF PRESENTS ILLNESS

Patient is a 65 year-old Hispanic Female with PMH significant for hypothyroidism, CAD status post CABG-1

disease, and mitral valve replacement with mechanical valve 4 months ago. Patient also has a history of

hypertrophic obstructive cardiomyopathy dyslipidemia, hypertension, and hypothyroidism. She presented to the

ER with the complaints of chest pain, pain in the long bones of the legs, and pain in the arms.

The patient initially stated that she has had chest pain since after the above surgery when she developed the flu and

coughed alot. She thinks that her wound has not healed well and she continues to have the chest pain. She stated

that since yesterday she has had this substernal chest pain with pain in both shoulders, pain in the arms and legs,

and pain in the long bones of the lower extremities.

(Continued)

History and Physical Examination

Patient Name: Linda C. Dominguez   Admitting Physician: David Loyola, MD

Date of Admission: 6/6/----   Page 2

The patient is stating that she has seen Dr. Rhodes, endocrinologist and has attributed these pains, which are chronic, to hypocalcemia. She was put on ergocalciferol 50000 units each week. The patient also has had some low grade fever and increased cough, so yesterday she saw an ENT, Dr. King, who ordered a head CT. Patient was told that her left sinus is totally occluded, she was put on omnicef. The patient comes into the ER now complaining of this chest pain. The patient has had this chest pain before, however, she said that since yesterday it is more severe. It is substernal and does not radiate, although the patient complains of pain in both shoulder blades. The pain in the shoulder blades plus the leg pains are of a more chronic nature

The patient denies any nausea or shortness of breath associated with the chest pain. The ER physician is asking the hospitalist service to admit this patient for chest pain rule out. As I mentioned above, the patient had a C.A.B.G. plus mitral valve replacement 4 months ago. She is on Pradaxa because of the mitral valve replacement with a mechanical valve.

PAST MEDICAL HISTORY:

Significant for CAD status post C.A.B.G. status post mitral valve replacement, history of hypertension, hypothyroidism, and dyslipidemia. The patient also has a history of paroxysmal atrial fibrillation since the surgery.

HOME MEDICATIONS:

Levothyroxine 50 mc g daily, Lopressor 50 mg bid, Pradaxa 150 mg bid, Fexofenadine, Paxil 30 mg daily, Betapace 80 mg bid, Oxazepam 50 mg daily, Lovastatin 40 mg at night, Ergocalciferol 50,000 units per week. The patient also has been put on Omnicef secondary to a sinus problem. Multivitamins.

(Continued)

History and Physical Examination

Patient Name: Linda C. Dominguez   Admitting Physician: David Loyola, MD

Date of Admission: 6/6/----   Page 3

PAST SURGICAL HISTORY:

The patient has had nasal septal surgery, had a pacemaker 5 years ago, has had a hysterectomy, a lumpectomy in the left breast, has had Nissan fundoplication, and has had a C.A.B.G. and mitral valve replacement with mechanical valve.

ALLERGIES: The patient is allergic to sulfa, Cipro, and nitrofurantoin.

SOCIAL HISTORY:

A widow. She does not smoke, drink, or use elicit drugs.

FAMILY HISTORY:

Positive for cardiovascular disease in parent's and deceased husband; 5 children are L&W.

REVIEW OF SYSTEMS:

The patient denies any headache, visual changes, or dysphasia. Positive for occasional GERD. Positive for chest pain, as described. Denies shortness of breath and nausea. Has complaints of leg pains, pain in the long bones of the leg, and also arm and shoulder pain. Has had low-grade fever. Denies a history of diabetes. Has hypothyroidism. She is unaware if she is anemic or not.

PHYSICAL EXAMINATION:

GENERAL: The patient is alert, oriented, and in some pain.

VITAL SIGNS: Blood pressure 129 over 50, pulse 67, respirations 18, temperature 99.9.

HEENT: Head is normocephalic, atraumatic. PERRLA, EOMI. Anicteric sclerae. Oral mucosa is moist and pink. No exudates.

NECK: Supple. No JVD. No lymphadenopathy. No thyromegaly.   (Continued)

History and Physical Examination

Patient Name: Linda C. Dominguez   Admitting Physician: David Loyola, MD

Date of Admission: 6/6/----   Page 4

CARDIOVASCULAR: Regular rhythm. S1, S2. I appreciate no murmur or gallops.

LUNGS: Decreased breath sounds at basis. Otherwise, clear to auscultation bilaterally. No rales, no wheeze, no rhonchi.

ABDOMEN: Soft, nontender. Bowel sounds present. No HSM.

EXTREMITIES: No edema. No cyanosis. Pedal pulses present bilaterally.

NEURO: Cranial nerves II-XII intact. The patient moves all extremities. Nonfocal.

SKIN: Warm and dry. No skin ulcerations or abrasions of upper or lower extremities.

LABORATORY DATA: Sodium 142, potassium 4.4, bicarb 29, chloride 104, BUN and creatinine 15 and 0.6, glucose 98. CK is 156, MB fraction 3.7, troponin 0.03. H&H are 13 and 41.2, white cells 14.4, platelets 202. PT and INR 33.6 and 2.7, respecfully. Influenza A and B are negative.

ASSESSMENT/PLAN: A 65-year-old Hispanic female with multiple medical problems, here secondary to body aches and chest pain.

1. Body aches: A chronic problem for this patient, it has lingered for sometime. As I mentioned, the patient has seen Dr. Rhodes, who has put her on a calcium supplement. For now, I will treat her with supportive care and pain medication.

2. Chest pain: Very atypical for a cardiac patient. However we will rule the patient out for acute coronary syndrome by serial CK's, EKG's. Continue with Lopressor. The patient is on Pradaxa.

3. History of paroxysmal atrial fibrillation, status post pacemaker. Patient is on Betapace, which we will continue. I will check the TSH and also Magnesium level.

4. Hypothyroidism: Continue with Synthroid. Check TSH in the morning.

5. Dyslipidemia: Continue with Lovastatin. Check lipid profile in the morning.

(Continued)

History and Physical Examination

Patient Name: Linda C. Dominguez   Admitting Physician: David Loyola, MD

Date of Admission: 6/6/----   Page 5

6. Leukocytosis: A head CT was ordered yesterday; however, it has not been read by Radiology yet. The

patient is stating that they told her that her left sinus is occluded. I will start her on IV antibiotics; some

penicillin; Zosyn antibiotic, since the patient is allergic to Cipro; and the patient can be discharged home

tomorrow on the same Omnicef that she came in on. I will give the patient some saline nasal

decongestant.

7. Prophylaxis with Protonix. We are going to modify our medical management depending on the patients'

outcome and her response to treatment.

8. Get an opinion from Radiology on the head CT from 5 June prior to discharge.

9. Followup with her PCP, Dr. Lucinda Patrick, within a week of discharge.

_____

David Loyola, MD, Hospitalist

DL:xx

D: 6/5/----

T: 6/6/----

C: Lucinda Patrick, MD, Internal Medicine

        Yancy Rhodes, MD, Endocrinology

Proofreading Exercise 5: Find 18 errors in the following report.

Merwin B. Moore Memorial Clinic
6249 Broad Street
Lebanon, TN 37106
Phone 615.555.2500

ORTHOPEDIC CONSULTATION

Patient Name: Eugenia Piedmont   **PCP**: Anderson Phipps, MD

Date of Consultation: 16 Oct   **Sex/Age**: F/63   **DOB**: 03/23/----

CHIEF COMPLAINT: Left shoulder pain

HISTORY OF PRESENT ILLNESS: Dr. Phipps referred this 63-year-old woman, who presents with a 2-month history of left shoulder pain. There is no specific injury or trauma that she can identify other then possibly reaching back in her car with her left arm. She experiences pain, has difficulty sleeping on her left side, and has pain with certain lifting and reaching type motions, particularly at her left side. She is seen in orthopedic consultation.

PAST MEDICAL/SURGICAL HISTORY: Otherwise unremarkable. She is in good health.

MEDICATIONS: Multivitamins only.

ALLERGIES: No known drug allergies.

SOCIAL HISTORY: The patient denies alcohol, tobacco, and illicit drugs used.

FAMILY HISTORY: Noncontributory.

(Continued)

ORTHOPEDIC CONSULTATION

Patient Name: Eugenia Piedmont   PCP: Anderson Phipps, MD

Date of Consultation: 16 Oct----   Page 2

PHYSICAL EXAMINATION: On examination of her left shoulder she has full ROM with forward flexion. Pain is produced with abduction above 90 degrees. She has symmetric internal rotation. Strength of the rotator cuff is 5-/5 for superspinatus and external rotation and 5/5 for internal rotation. There is a 1+ click noted with ROM of the left shoulder.

X-RAYS, left shoulder, reveals a subacromial osteophyte present at the level of the AC joint.

IMPRESSION: Subacromial impingement as well as rotator cuff tendinitis.

RECOMMENDATIONS: Patient will be given a subacromial corticosteroid injection. She was informed that it does take 2 to 3 weeks to become fully affective. She was instructed on strengthening exercises, with the use of Thera-Band, and is referred to physical therapy.

PROCEDURE: The patient's left shoulder was prepped with Betadine. Skin was anesthetized with 1% Lidocaine plain. The subacromial space was then infiltrated with 1 ml of Betamethasone with 4 ml of 1% Lidocaine plain. Patient tolerated the procedure well. We plan to see her back in the office p.r.n. If she fails to improve, contract me right away.

Olivia Glover, MD, Orthopedic Surgery

OG:xx

DD: 10/16/----

DT: 10/17/----

cc: Lamduan "La" Howard, RPT

          Anderson Phipps, MD, Family Medicine/Geriatrics

Proofreading Exercise 6: Find 22 errors in the following report.

Forrest General Medical Center
1038 Superior Street NW
Nashville, TN 37189
Phone 615.555.5000

ORTHOPEDIC CONSULTATION

Patient Name: Hal Peterson Myers   **Physician Referring**: Stephen Grimm, DC

Date of Consultation: 07/01/----   **Sex/Age**: M/21   **DOB**: 02/04/----

REASON FOR REFERRAL: The patient is seen in the office today in orthopedic consultation, for his cervical

and lumbar regions.

HISTORY OF PRESENT ILLNESS: The patient is a 21-year-old white male student who was a seat belted

driver involved in a MVA on May 29, ----. The patient was traveling South on a 2 lane road when a vehicle 2 cars

in front of him stopped to make a left turn. The vehicle in front of him stopped abruptly. The patient swerved to

the left to avoid striking the rear of the vehicle in front. The vehicle behind him swerved as well, not knowing

what was in front of him, striking the rear of the patients' vehicle and pushing the patients' vehicle into the first car

that was making the left turn, thereby the patient received 2 impacts. He denies any loss of consciousness although

he was dazed at the time of the impact. He later developed pain, tightness, and stiffness within his neck and

subsequently pain in his lower back. He was taken by Fire Rescue to Forrest General medical center, where he was

evaluated. Subsequently patient was seen by Stephen Grimm, DC, a few days following the accident from whom

he received therapy until approximately 1 week ago.

(Continued)

ORTHOPEDIC CONSULTATION

Patient Name: Hal Peterson Myers   Physician Referring: Stephen Grimm, DC

Date of Consultation: 07/01/----   Page 2

At present, patient continues to have tightness and stiffness within his neck and low back, with his neck being the more symptomatic of the 2 locations. He has difficulty with bending, and has persistent tightness and achiness.

The patient had been involved in a previous motor vehicle accident approximately 2 years ago with no resulting injuries. He has no previous history of neck or back pain.

PAST MEDICAL HISTORY: The past medical history is otherwise unremarkable. He is in good health.

PAST SURGICAL HISTORY: Tonsils removed as a child; otherwise, unremarkable.

MEDICATIONS: The Patient takes only vitamins.

ALLERGIES: No known allergies.

SOCIAL HISTORY: The patient denies x3.

FAMILY HISTORY: Noncontributory. Parents and 2 siblings are L & W.

PHYSICAL EXAMINATION is limited to the musculoskeletal system. On physical examination, of his cervical spine, he has a mild-to-moderate increased in muscle tone noted across the superior border of the trapezoidal muscles on the right greater then left. This does extend more proximally to the base of the occiput and distally into the interscapular region.

(Continued)

ORTHOPEDIC CONSULTATION

Patient Name: Hal Peterson Myers

Date of Consultation: 07/01/----

Physician Referring: Stephen Grimm, DC

Page 3

He has a limited range of motion with extension. He has 5/5 strength for biceps, triceps, wrist flexion and

extension, EPL, APB, and first DI.

Examination of the lumbar spine reveals mild increase in muscle tone noted in the longissimus muscles on both

the right and left sides from the lower thoracic region to the lumbosacral junction. He has a full range of motion

with forward flexion, extension, side bend to the right and the left, and rotation to the right and left. Motor strength

is 5/5 for hip flexors, abductors, adductors, quadriceps, hamstrings, tibialis anterior, and gastrocsoleus. Sensation

to light touch is intact.

MRI EVALUATION: Review of MRI report of the cervical spine reveals loss of the normal lordosis of the

cervical spine. There is no reported evidence of disc herniation.

IMPRESSION

1. Cervical strain.

2. Lumbar strain.

RECOMMENDATIONS/DISCUSSION: This male patient who is 21-years-old and has had no previous history

of neck or back pain now has persistent symptomatology in both of these locations following the accident of May

29, ----. It is felt with a reasonable degree of medical probability that Mr. Myers' present symptoms are the direct

result of the above stated accident and have resulted in a permanent impairment. Using the Guides to the

Evaluation of Permanent Impairment published by the American Medical Association, it is felt that the patient has

an approximately 6% to 7 percent whole-person permanent impairment.

(Continued)

ORTHOPEDIC CONSULTATION

Patient Name: Hal Peterson Myers

Physician Referring: Stephen Grimm, DC

Date of Consultation: 07/01/----

Page 4

The patient is encouraged to continue on home exercises for stretching and strengthening. He does have the potential for flair ups in the future, which may require additional physical therapy, chiropractic treatment, anti-inflammatories, and/or muscle relaxers. We plan to see Mr. Myers back in the office in 6 months for a follow-up visit.

Thank you for this kind referral Dr. Grimm. I will keep you posted on any diagnostic or therapeutic modalities deemed necessary in the future. I see no need for surgery at this time.

_____

Olivia Glover, MD, Orthopedics

OG:xx

DD: 7/1/----

DT: 7/2/----

cc: Stephen Grimm, DC

         Lamduan "La" Howard, RPT

Proofreading Exercise 7: Find 20 errors in the following report.

Carl E. Loftin Memorial Clinic
9465 Enterprise Circle
Cookeville, TN 37269
Phone 931.555.4900

FAMILY PRACTICE SOAP NOTE

Patient Name: Ellen Rappaport   **PCP**: Anderson Phipps, MD

Date of Visit: 11/15/   **Sex/Age**: F/62   **DOB**: 06/13/----

SUBJECTIVE: The patient comes in today for a multitude of problems. I will go over them as best I can with as much thoroughness as I can.

1. In today for flu shot. Flu vaccine will be given. Only allergies are to Adrenalin, Demerol, contrast dye, Lortab.

2. Hypertension. Blood pressure has been stable, 120 to 130/80, although today it is 140/88. Will make no changes on her medicine. Currently, she is taking multiple meds for her blood pressure with good control.

3. Hyperlipidemia has been under excellent control on Lipitor. Will check lab today, but do not anticipate any changes.

4. It is time to check all of her lab, we will do lipids. Liver enzymes done 6 months ago. Will also do hemoglobin $A1_C$ for glucose intolerance. That has been gone over with patient as well.

5. Hypothyroidism has been followed by Endocrinology.

6. She had some microscopic hematuria and were recently worked up by Dr. Kelly, with a normal renal ultrasound. The patient also had an IVP and cystoscopy with bilateral retrogrades. That evidently was okay as done by Urology. She had normal bilateral retrograde pyelograms, not an IVP.

7. Patient is up-to-date on her GYN exams. Had a colonoscopy done within the last 6 months as well.

8. She comes in today for a new problem of pain in the back, going around to her sciatic area, somewhat down her leg. The main thing she has is right lower quadrant pain and right groin pain, which is a little

(Continued)

confusing since she points to the right lower quadrant and groin area where it hurts. She does not

remember injuring herself. It hurts sometimes but it just hurts to press on the area. It is noteworthy she

has just been seen by Urology and undergone retrograde pyelograms and cystoscopy. She has had GYN

checkups, and she is actually absent her uterus, having had a hysterectomy in her 40's. She had

cystoscopy done recently. Has had no x-rays done of her hip or her GI tract that I know of. She has had

no change in bowel habits, no fevers, no chills.

OBJECTIVE

VITAL SIGNS: Weight 187 pounds. Height 5'2". Blood pressure 160/90. Pulse is 72. She is afebrile.

GENERAL: Alert, cooperative, white female in today for a multitude of problems, which have been listed below.

NECK: Supple.

LUNGS: Clear.

CV: Regular rate with out murmur.

ABDOMEN: Soft, some tenderness in the right lower quadrant to deep direct pressure, particularly in the right

groin area. I do not detect a hernia. I am unsure if their is scar tissue or adhesions in the abdomen.

MS: Right hip has a full range of motion with very little pain. Very little pain in her back or going down the

sciatic region that I can ascertain, although that is where she points to. Says the pain goes from the right anterior

aspect of her right hip into her back.

EXTREMITIES: No cyanosis, clubbing, or edema.

BACK: Full range of motion with very little pain.

(Continued)

Family Practice SOAP Note   PCP: Anderson Phipps, MD

Patient Name: Ellen Rappaport   Page 3

Date of Visit: 11/15/----

ASSESSMENT

1.   New onset pain in the right lower quadrant for 3 weeks and goes into the back in the sciatic area and

     somewhat down her leg. Normal ultrasound of the kidneys. Normal cystoscopy. Normal retrograde

     pyelogram.

2.   Hyperlipidemia, stable.

3.   Hypertension, fair control.

4.   Flu vaccine today.

5.   History of hematuria worked up by Urology with normal bilateral retrograde pyelograms, normal renal

     ultrasound done.

6.   Glucose intolerance, presently stable.

PLAN

1.   Lab work to be done tomorrow.

2.   Today will do an x-ray of the right hip to make sure we are not dealing with some generalized arteritis in

     the hip referring the pain. Could be groin strain or muscular problem causing it. Will also do a CT of the

     lower abdomen, pelvis and hip itself along with an MRI of the back, which is referring the pain down her

     leg.

3.   The impression as the cause of her right lower quadrant pain is not known as she was tender in the grown

     area to pressure. Also, the pain went through to her back; so I'm not sure if this is arthritic, groin strain,

     muscular, or if it is related to the GI tract. I doubt this is urologic, only guess adhesions could do this but

(Continued)

Family Practice SOAP Note   PCP: Anderson Phipps, MD

Patient Name: Ellen Rappaport   Page 4

Date of Visit: 11/15/----

     where her pain is, is a little hard to ascertain. All the workup is ordered. She is allergic to contrast dye.

4.   Flu vaccine given today. Lab work pending.

_____

Greg Farrow, FNP, for

Anderson Phipps, MD

Family Medicine/Geriatrics

GF:xx

D: 11/15/----

T: 11/16/----

C: Dana Kelly, MD Urology

Proofreading Exercise 8: Find 13 errors in the following report.

Carl E. Loftin Memorial Clinic
9465 Enterprise Circle
Cookeville, TN 37269
Phone 931.555.4900

OB/GYN OFFICE VISIT

Patient Name: Ellen Rappaport   **PCP**: Anderson Phipps, MD

Date of Visit: 11/17/----   **Sex/Age**. F/62   **DOB**: 06/13/----

SUBJECTIVE: The patient is here, mainly for consultation. She started having some hip pain recently saw Dr. Phipps and he ordered a battery of lab tests and some x-rays. She has not even seen the x-rays yet. She just wanted to make sure there was not something going on in her pelvic.

I actually was able to pull up the x-rays of her hip. She had a normal hip x-ray but she has what looks like 2 level disease at the lumbosacral area on her spine. This may be the cause of her pain.

She is still scheduled for CT of the abdomen and pelvis then for an MRI of her back. I think probably this is going to be musculoskeletal or neurologic in nature. She just wanted to make sure that she did not need to do anything more from a GYN standpoint.

OBJECTIVE: Vitals include age 62, weight 183 pounds, BP 153/72 mmHg.

(Continued)

OB/GYN Office Visit

Patient Name: Ellen Rappaport   PCP: Anderson Phipps, MD

Date of Visit: 11/17/----   Page 2

PLAN: Once Ellen gets the CT she is going to call me. I will review those results, and make sure that it looks like she is fine as far as GYN issues in the pelvis. Then she must followup with Dr. Phipps accordingly.

Thanks for this consult—I'll keep you informed of the results.

————————————

Dr. Charles W. Scott, MD

Obstetrics/Gynecology

CWS:xx

D: 11/17/----

T: 11/17/----

Proofreading Exercise 9: Find 15 errors in the following report.

James C. Thompson Memorial Clinic
#1 Lincoln Circle
Paris, TN 37904
Phone 731.555.3700

PREOPERATIVE EVALUATION

Patient Name: Noelle Trudeau   **PCP**: Sandra Peebles, MD

Date of Evaluation: 04/25/----   **Sex/Age**: F/35   **DOB**: 11/28/----

CHIEF COMPLAINT: The patient is seen in the office today for preoperative evaluation of her right shoulder.

HISTORY OF PRESENT ILLNESS: This French female referred by Dr. Peebles is 35 years old. She is being evaluated for a diagnostic and operative arthroscopy with arthroscopic SLAP repair and subacromial decompression and acromioplasty. She continues to complain of marked pain within her shoulder difficulty with lifting and reaching type motions and a heaviness and achiness to her shoulder.

PAST HISTORY: Patient's Past Medical History is reviewed and found to be noncontributory.

SOCIAL HISTORY: Married, with 2 children living and well. No EtOH or illicit drugs. She does smoke 10 cigarettes a day, and has done so for several years. Her husband travels internationally.

MEDICATIONS: Birth control pills, aspirin, and multivitamins.

ALLERGIES: NKDA.

(Continued)

PREOPERATIVE EVALUATION

Patient Name: Noelle Trudeau   PCP: Sandra Peebles, MD

Date of Evaluation: 04/25/----   Page 2

PHYSICAL EXAMINATION: Vital signs are WNL. The patient's head is normocephalic, atraumatic.

Extraocular movements are intact. Oral cavity is noncontributory. Neck is suppel without lymphadenopathy.

Lungs are clear to auscultation bilaterally. Heart has a regular rate and rhythm without murmur. Abdomen is

benign. Genitalia exam is deferred. Gate normal. Psychiatric: Good attitude toward the upcoming procedure.

Examination of the right shoulder reveals a painful range of motion to the right shoulder above 90 degrees of

forward flexion and abduction above 90 degrees. Strength of the rotator cuff is 5-/5 for supraspinatus and external

rotation and 5/5 for internal rotation. There is a 1+ click noted with range of motion to the shoulder.

IMPRESSION: Right shoulder SLAP lesion as well as impingement syndrome.

RECOMMENDATION: My recommendations is that the patient be admitted to Forrest General early

tomorrow morning and taken to the operating room to undergo a diagnostic and operative arthroscopy under general

anesthesia. This operative procedure will most likely consist of arthroscopic SLAP repair subacromial

decompression and acromioplasty.

The patient and her husband were counseled as to the nature of the surgery as well as the associated risks including, but

not limited to: infection, bleeding, nerve damage, stiffness, persistence of pain, loss of motion, and recurrence

of pain. The patient understands these risks and they have elected to proceed with the proposed procedure.

(Continued)

PREOPERATIVE EVALUATION

Patient Name: Noelle Trudeau   PCP: Sandra Peebles, MD

Date of Evaluation: 04/25/----   Page 3

Preop instruction sheet given to patient. She stopped her Aspirin 2 days ago and will be n.p.o. after midnight.

An appointment was made to see Noelle in the office 48 hours after surgery. They are to notify either me or Dr.

Glover prior to this appointment if the patient has any bleeding, swelling, fever, or any other problems or concerns

postop.

Emily Adkins, MD, Surgical Resident for

Olivia Glover, MD, Orthopedic Surgery

EA:xx

DD: 03/25/----

DT: 03/25/----

C: Sandra Peebles, Internal Medicine

Proofreading Exercise 10: Find 18 errors in the following report.

James C. Thompson Memorial Clinic
#1 Lincoln Circle
Paris, TN 37904
Phone 731.555.3700

ORTHOPEDIC CONSULTATION

Patient Name: James Knolls   **Referring Physician**: Connerly, Antonia MD

Date of Consultation: 12/13/----   **Sex/Age**: M/16   **DOB**: 2/18/----

CHIEF COMPLAINT: Referred by Dr. Antonia Connerly the patient is a 16-year-old black male who presents for orthopedic evaluation regarding a complaint of left knee discomfort.

HISTORY OF PRESENT ILLNESS: The patient reports that he injured his left knee about a week ago. He reports that on Sat he began experiencing pain in his left knee. He initially stated that he did not recall anything causing the pain. However, later he and his father stated that he went ice-skating the day before and he did have an episode where someone pushed him or bumped him, and he fell to the ground; he may have injured his left knee in doing so. He reports that yesterday he tried to run and had some pain in his right calf when he was running around the tract. He is still experiencing some discomfort in his left knee, but it is not severe. He reports that last week he did go to a walk in clinic and then went to the emergency room at Forrest General Medical Center for evaluation. He was given a knee immobilizer, which did not fit satisfactorily, and he hasn't been using this. He has been using crutches intermittently. He presents now for orthopedic consultation.

PAST MEDICAL HISTORY: Significant for childhood asthma.

(Continued)

ORTHOPEDIC CONSULTATON

Patient Name: James Knolls   Referring Physician: Antonia Connerly, MD

Date of Consultation: 12/13/----   Page 2

PAST SURGICAL HISTORY: Tube tympanostomy and adenoidectomy.

SOCIAL HISTORY: He is in high school and lives locally with his father, grandmother, and 3 siblings. No use of

tobacco, ethanol, or illicit drugs.

PHYSICAL EXAMINATION: The patient is a well-developed, well-nourished, black teenaged male who

appears his stated age. He is in no acute distress. His gait is grossly tandem, nonantalgic. Exam is limited to the

musculoskeletal system.

Evaluation of the bilateral lower extremities reveal no angular or rotational deformity. There is a grossly normal

appearance of the left and right knees.

There is no tenderness to palpation over the right calf either anteriorly or posteriorly. There is no pain with range

of motion of the right knee and no pain with range of motion of the right angle.

Evaluation of the left knee reveals mild tenderness to palpitation over the inferior poll of the patella or the superior

aspect of the patellar tendon. There is 5-/5 strength on knee extension. There is mild discomfort with flexion to

endpoint. The skin is warm and dry. There is a negative effusion. The calf is soft and supple. The patient is able to

extend and flex the knee actively and against resistance.

RADIOGRAPHIC EVALUATION: Three views of the left knee taken today demonstrates normal appearance of

the patella and normal appearance of the articular components of the left knee.

DIAGNOSTIC IMPRESSION: Left knee pain, probable patellar tendon strainer.

(Continued)

ORTHOPEDIC CONSULTATON

Patient Name: James Knolls   Referring Physician: Antonia Connerly, MD

Date of Consultation: 12/13/----   Page 3

RECOMMENDATIONS: I discussed with the patient his diagnosis, prognosis, and treatment options. I

recommend the use of Aleve, 2 tablets twice a day. I recommend application of ice for 30 minutes, 3 to 4 times a

day. He should avoid running, jumping, or strenuous activity until his pain resolves. He may then resume activities

as tolerated in a grated fashion.

I advised James not to ice skate or jump until his pain fully resolves. I discussed this with the patient's Father as

well. If his symptoms have not resolved in 2 to 3 weeks patient is to return for reevaluation at that time.

Thank you Dr. Connerly for allowing me to share in the care of this interesting patient. I will be happy to provide

further diagnostic and therapeutic modalities, as required.

_____

David Lanewala, MD

Orthopedic Surgery

DL:xx

D: 12/13/----

T: 12/13/----

C: Antonia Connerly, MD, Pediatrics

Proofreading Exercise 11: Find 15 errors in the following report.

James C. Thompson Memorial Clinic
#1 Lincoln Circle
Paris, TN 37904
Phone 731.555.3700

ORTHOPEDIC CLINIC NOTE

Patient Name: Dominica Trainor   **PCP:** N/A

Date of Visit. 10/61/----   **Sex/Age:** F/49   **DOB:** 01/30/----

CHIEF COMPLAINT: The patient is seen in the Clinic today for evaluation of her right foot.

HISTORY OF PRESENT ILLNESS: The patient is a 49-year-old Haitian woman who presents with an approximately 2 to 3 week history of pain in the planter aspect of her right foot. She has made some gradual improvement over the past week. However, she still has discomfort, primarily over the posteromedial aspect of the heal.

PHYSICAL EXAMINATION: Patient has point tenderness directly over the medial aspect of her heel. She is able to dorsiflex and planterflex the ankle and invert and evert, which is pain-free. She is neurovascularly intact distally. Her calf is supple, and she has a mildly tight arc. She ambulates without antalgia.

X-RAYS: X-rays reveal a minimal osteophyte present on the planter aspect of her heel.

(Continued)

ORTHOPEDIC CLINIC NOTE

Patient Name: Dominica Trainor

Date of Visit: 10/16/----

Page 2

IMPRESSION: Mild planter fasciitis.

RECOMMENDATIONS: The patient was instructed on stretching exercises. She was instructed on icing down the heel and using a tennis ball and/or a frozen bottle of water on the bottom aspect of the heel, rolling it on the undersurface of her heel. She should avoid high heeled shoes at this time; instead, she is to wear running shoes or sports shoes that fit good.

We plan to see Dominica back in the office on an as needed basis. If she fails to improve she should contact the Clinic for an appointment for further evaluation and consideration of treatment.

_____

Olivia Glover, MD

Orthopedics Surgery

OG:xx

DD: 10/16/----

DT: 10/17/----

Proofreading Exercise 12: Find 15 errors in the following report.

Forrest General Medical Center
1038 Superior Street NW
Nashville, TN 37189
Phone 615.555.5000

Diagnostic Imaging Services

Patient Name: Ronald DeVittori   **Referred by**: Holly Russo, MD

Date of Procedure: 7/28/----   **Sex/Age**: M/59   **DOB**: 11/25/----

Name of Procedure: MRI, lumbar spine.

CLINICAL HISTORY: Back pain in a 59-year-old Canadian Male.

TECHNIQUE: Multisequence T1 and T2 weighted images were obtained. Images were obtained in the neutral seated position.

FINDINGS: The conus medullaris appear normal. There is a 25 degree levoscoliosis with the apex at L2-3. There is decreased intervertebral disk space height and signal at L2-3, L3-4, and L4-5 suggestive of disk desiccation. The lordotic curvature of the lumbar spine is preserve. No evidence of abnormal solid or cystic lesions are identified. No prevertebral or paravertebral masses or fluid collections is seen, and there is no evidence for abnormal marrow-replacing lesion. Segmental analysis of the lumbar spine is listed below.

(Continued)

Name of Procedure: MRI, lumbar spine

Patient Name: Ronald DeVittori   Referring by: Holly Russo, MD

Date of Procedure: 7/28/----   Page 2

At L1-2 there is an anterior disk herniation. No central canal stenosis. No neural foraminal stenosis.

At L2-3 there is a circumferential disk bulge causing impression on the anterior thecal sac. No central canal stenosis. No neural foraminal stenosis.

At L3-4 there is an anterior disk herniation superimposed on a circumferential disk bulge plus bilateral facet hypertrophic changes causing mild central canal stenosis measuring .9 cm. Mild right neural foraminal stenosis and moderate left neural foraminal stenosis is noted.

At L4-5 there is a circumferential disk bulge with bilateral facet hypertrophic changes causing impression on the anterior thecal sac . No central canal stenosis. No neural foraminal stenosis.

At L5-S1 there is a left lateral disk herniation superimposed on a circumferential disk bulge causing impressive on the anterior thecal sac. No central canal stenosis. Mild right neural foraminal stenosis is noted. No left neural foraminal stenosis.

IMPRESSION

1.   A 25-degree levoscoliosis with the apex at L2-3.

2.   Disk desiccation at L2-3, L3-4, and L4-5.

3.   At L1-2 there is an anterior disk herniation.

4.   At L2-3 a circumferential disk bulge is causing impression on the anterior thecal sac.

5.   At L3-4 there is an anterior disk herniation superimposed on a circumferential disk bulge and bilateral facet hypertrophic changes causing mild central canal stenosis, mild right neural foraminal stenosis, and moderate left neural foraminal stenosis.

(Continued)

Name of Procedure: MRI, lumbar spine

Patient Name: Ronald DeVittori   Referring by: Holly Russo, MD

Date of Procedure: 7/28/----   Page 3

6.   At L4-5 there is a circumferential disk bulge with bilateral facet hypertrophic changed

       causing impression on the anterior thecal sac.

7.   At L5-S1 left lateral disk herniation is superimposed on a circumferential disk bulge

       causing impression on the anterior thecal sac and right neural foraminal stenotic.

Thank you for your kind reference.

_____

Charles Tew, MD

Certified Neuroradiologist

CT:xx

DD: 7/28/----

DT: 7/28/----

C: Holly Russo, MD, Neurosurgery

CHAPTER 20

PROFESSIONALISM/ ETHICS

Introduction

The information presented in this chapter will provide the healthcare documentation specialist (HDS) with valuable information relative to professionalism and ethics in their chosen profession. Included are tips on pursuing a career as an HDS, interviewing, creating an effective résumé, samples of employment letters, and information about "scribes" in the medical profession. Computer etiquette, speech recognition/voice recognition, medical editing, quality assurance, and the need for acute-care healthcare documentation specialists are also included in this chapter. *NB*: Career-enhancing information can be found in *Getting Your Foot in the Door: Two Years' Experience Not Required,* which is a resource published by AHDI for new HDS graduates.

Critical Thinking Exercise

?

You are teaching a healthcare documentation specialist class, and one of the students asks if it is ever okay to transcribe without using ear phones, e.g., using their speakers playing out loud. How do you reply to this student?

Tips for Job Searching and Interviewing as a Healthcare Documentation Specialist

These tips and resources will help enhance your knowledge of the industry and better prepare you for working in the healthcare documentation profession.

- Become credentialed. Check out the Association for Healthcare Documentation Integrity web site at http://www.ahdionline.org for information about the field of healthcare documentation plus AHDI as the professional association for healthcare documentation specialists and credentialing. Becoming credentialed as a registered healthcare documentation specialist (RHDS) or a certified healthcare documentation specialist (CHDS) shows professionalism and respect for your chosen career field and is an external indicator to others of your commitment to the profession and to continuing education. Membership and participation in AHDI will allow you to meet, network with, and make friends with other professionals in the field, learn the latest industry news and trends, and maybe provide job opportunities you otherwise would not have known about. Network! AHDI has local, state, and regional components throughout the United States and Canada. Visit the AHDI web site to learn where the nearest AHDI component is and how you can get involved.

- Update your résumé. (Read "Tips on Creating an Effective Résumé," p. 297.) You can also go to the AHDI web site and type "How to Write a Resume" in the search box. You'll fine articles that will offer suggestions for creating an effective résumé. (See p. 299 for a sample.)

- Make business cards—a true mark of professionalism. Design and print your own business cards or order them from any number of local or online printing companies. Shop around and look at samples. A simple but clever business card will surely catch people's eyes and hold you memorable in their minds. Find a mentor. Some students are fortunate to have the opportunity of an internship or externship with a medical transcription service organization (MTSO) prior to graduation in order to gain hands-on experience. Others begin their careers as an apprentice with an independent contractor, a person with an at-home business, or MTSO who is willing to help them get started. For the independent contractor or MTSO, hiring a beginning HDS is both costly and time consuming. New HDSs should be prepared to commit to the job and to learn all they can about creating, transcribing, and editing medical documents as well as how to run a business. New employees can also learn a great deal by working in-house, by having access to patient charts, by seeing how office personnel work together, and by learning how healthcare documentation fits into the larger scheme of things.

- Explore myriad employment avenues. With copies of your résumé and business cards in hand, go to medical office buildings, including labs and radiology offices, and ask to speak to the office manager. Make an appointment, if necessary. Also search job sites on the Internet and network with others in the industry to find out which companies are hiring. When you do get an interview, remember to research the company and learn all you can about it so that you can customize your interview answers as to why you want to work for that specific company. An employer is more likely to hire someone who has taken the initiative to learn about their company and who also shows enthusiasm and genuine interest in working for their company.

- Build your network. Wherever you apply, be sure to pick up that company's business card and keep notes about who you spoke with, if they are currently hiring or not, whether or not you got an interview, the number of years of experience required, and any other helpful details.

- At the interview they are going to want to know what you can offer THEM. Do not be demanding. Instead, be prepared to match your skills to their needs. Make sure they know all your best qualities, how you will fit into their business, and how your expertise will help to make them more successful. Ask that they keep your résumé and business card on file for future reference.

- Offer to be backup for the office, covering healthcare documentation and/or editing for weekends, holidays, sick leave, and/or vacation time. Offer to help clear up their backlog of work. Getting something to list on your résumé is the most important thing right now.

- When leaving the interview, be gracious, smile, thank the office manager, the receptionist, etc., even if they have said "no" to you. Every interview is a learning experience. ALWAYS write a short, positive thank-you note to your interviewer in your own handwriting. See example on page 302.

- Think positively. This whole process is a learning experience. Keep notes so you can evaluate your experience later. Who knows, this may be the first day of the REST OF YOUR LIFE!

Dos and Don'ts Checklist

Being interviewed can be a nerve-wracking process. To help set your mind at ease and be better prepared for your interview, follow the recommendations below provided by experienced interviewers and be sure to make a positive first impression. *NB:* A large percent of the healthcare documentation workforce works from a remote location, e.g., home office. Be prepared to interview by phone or online via Skype or some other technical venue.

- DO shake hands with a firm grip, use good eye contact, and smile.

- DO use courteous greetings and polite small talk (stay away from controversial topics such as politics or religion).

- DO dress professionally and groom neatly: clean, pressed clothes, shined shoes (no flip-flops, facial piercings, tattoos showing, or low-seated pants.)

- DO NOT chew gum.

- DO keep your cell phone or other electronics on vibrate or turned off.

- DO ensure your voice mail phone message is clear and friendly. For example, "I'm away from the phone. Please leave your name and number so I can return your call."

- DO NOT bring family members, including children, or friends to your interview. If a family member or friend gave you a ride to your interview, ask them to stay in the car or wait in a nearby restaurant.

- DO research the company with which you are interviewing. Know pertinent details such as how long they have been in business, whether they have a national presence, etc., which may come up during the interview.

- DO ask questions—make sure they are pertinent to the job for which you are applying. For

example, how many HDSs do they employ, do they reimburse or compensate the cost of credentialing exams or continuing education credits, what is the supervisory structure, do they use quality assurance (QA) personnel and give feedback on errors found?

- DO prepare a brief introductory speech about yourself—who you are, what your background is, what you are looking for, and why you are perfect for this job—two to three minutes tops.

- DO follow up the interview with a personal thank-you note. (See sample on page 302.)

- DO contact the interviewer about three days after the interview to let him know how much you appreciate the meeting, how much you would like to work at the company, etc. Be ready for followup questions and a potential second interview. A second interview may be with someone else—someone higher up in the company—so stay prepared.

Here is a site for more information on interviewing: http://www.helpguide.org/life/interviewing_techniques_tips_getting_job.htm

Tips for Creating an Effective Résumé

Your résumé is often the first opportunity a potential employer has to learn about you. It presents a snapshot of your work experience and education. It is a timeline intended to catch an employer's eye and show what you can do for the company; therefore, it should stand apart from other résumés the employer might have received. While the document gives a picture of you, it should be short and to the point.

In creating a résumé, here are some pointers:

Begin with your *personal contact information*: Insert your complete legal name, address, phone numbers, fax number, and email address as the heading for the page.

Next list your *employment objective:* This statement should be concise but reflect thought. It should include more than just what you <u>want</u>; it should include what you can <u>offer</u>. Use different objective statements for different jobs. You can have more than one résumé.

In the next section, describe your *educational background,** with the most recent educational experience listed first, like the certificate you may have just earned.

---

*These educational background and work experience sections can be reversed depending on what information is most pertinent to the job for which you are applying.

Any extra classes you completed should be listed, too; for example, anatomy and physiology, coding and billing, etc.

List your work experience, with the most recent job first. For each job, list the dates employed (month and year), employer's name, job title, supervisor, contact number, and your primary responsibilities. When you list your duties, use action verbs; for example, "Answered phone, exercised patients' limbs, and bathed patients." Also, be sure that the statements are parallel in grammatical structure.

Because this section of the résumé is a timeline, if there was a time you were not working, indicate what you were doing, i.e., out of town assisting a relative, touring Europe, recovering from surgery, etc. Include any part-time or summer jobs or volunteer projects that show you are responsible, dependable, and would be an asset.

List any experience you had with any medical transcription platforms such as DocuScribe or DocuManage.

If you worked two jobs at one time, be sure to include the days of the week or the shifts so that it is easy to see how they meshed together. For example, maybe you do one thing during the week and something else on weekends. You might have a full-time day job with a part-time evening job. However, if your part-time job is not pertinent to either your experience or the career field in which you are interested, you can leave it out.

In the next section, include areas of interest, hobbies, school or community activities, and participation in service organizations. Include special skills, such as being bilingual, knowing sign language, knowing CPR, etc.

A comment about references should be the last section of the résumé. You can simply say "Available upon request." Information relative to references should be listed on a separate page and carried to the interview—it is given to the interviewer only upon request.

Ask someone else to proofread your résumé for accuracy. A huge part of being an HDS is accuracy, so make sure it is reflected in your résumé.

Remember, this is the only picture of you that the prospective employer has. The ideal résumé is one page long, but two pages can be acceptable.

REMEMBER: Your résumé must stand out from the crowd! Employers throw résumés with typos into the trash!

Scribes in the Medical Profession

As the documentation of medical records moves from paper-based to electronic, some hospitals and medical facilities are beginning to utilize scribes to input information as physicians gather it. The scribe accompanies the doctor during examination of patients and documents findings, labs or diagnostics ordered, prescriptions needed, treatment plan, and other items noted by the physician. Once the scribe has completed documenting the record, the physician checks the accuracy of the information, makes any necessary additions or corrections, and signs off on it.

Many of the scribes are nursing and pre-med students who need to make extra money. Facilities are finding that the use of scribes can allow physicians to see more patients and increase efficiency in the billing process, and thereby increase revenue for the facility. However, they do see turnover with nursing and pre-med students as graduation occurs.

Healthcare documentation specialists would be perfect as scribes. Not only are they specifically trained for documentation, but this is their chosen career field—there would be much less turnover using an HDS as a scribe.

Computer Etiquette

Never forward random emails to people on your contact list. It makes you look unprofessional at best, ultimately hurting your career; at worst, it can cause people to block your correspondence.

It is not appropriate to send emails with subject matter that includes jokes, reports of viruses (most are fake), anything political, anything of an adult nature, and anything that could be found offensive to work colleagues, your boss, or clients. These types of things are never appropriate for mass sharing. Never use a company's email account to send them to personal contacts either. People can mark such emails as spam, which could result in your company's email server being put on a black list as a spammer.

A few things are appropriate to forward; for example, the latest industry news is relevant to a list of people to whom it will matter. These shared tidbits are important for keeping current in your career. Forward select association news to those whom you know would be interested. Forward positive information regarding your company. Everyone likes to see their company gain positive exposure. Essentially, forward purposeful news that is relevant to the receivers. Keep in mind, however, that some people will not be interested in even this type of forwarding. Include a brief note in your email explaining why you forwarded the email (e.g., continuing education opportunity, important drug updates included, new terms list, etc.), and include an invitation for the recipient to be removed from your "forwarded emails" list if they so desire. Respect their request by remembering to remove them from the list of people to whom you forward emails.

(Sample Résumé)

Diane Smith
73009 Mockingbird Road
Nashville, TN 37557
615.445.5501 (cell)
dsmithrn@comcast.net

OBJECTIVE   To work as a human resources manager in a multi-physician clinic

EDUCATION   Florida State University, Tallahassee, FL: BS in Nursing with minor in Human Resources Management, Aug 1995

Miami-Dade Community College, Miami, FL: AA degree in Anatomy & Physiology, May 1993

EXPERIENCE

Dec 2007 to Present   **The Nashville Diagnostic Clinic**

Title: RN

<u>Duties</u>: Assist physicians with patient care, help in minor surgical procedures, keep instruments sterile, help in dictation of reports, maintain employees' HIPAA and CPR status, and other office duties as required.

Supervisor: Fred Anderson, MD, Phone: 615.901.1111 ext 35

Dec 1998 to Nov 2007   **James C. Thompson Memorial Clinic**

Title: Human Resource Assistant

<u>Duties</u>: Assisted HR director with day-to-day activities of the department, communicated with personnel relative to individual employment issues, and conducted new employee orientation/training.

Supervisor: Travis L. Longino, Phone: 731.555.3700 ext 90

Aug 1995 to Dec 1998   **Forrest General Medical Center**

Title: RN

<u>Duties</u>: Assisted with hospital patient care; supervised surgical floor nursing duties, worked various shifts, maintained employees' HIPAA and CPR status, organized nursing shifts, and filled in when necessary.

Supervisor: Tyron Nguyen, RN, Phone: 615.555.5000 ext 72

Diane Smith   Page 2

HONORS   **Florida State University**

                          Outstanding senior nursing major, president of Student Nursing Association, and vice
                          president of Student Human Resources Association

                          Miami-Dade Community College

                          Beta Club, student government association, and yearbook staff

REFERENCES AVAILABLE UPON REQUEST

(*NB*: References should be typed on a separate page and taken to the interview. Provide each reference's full legal
name, position, address, phone number, and email address.)

EXAMPLE

Mr. Travis L. Longino, Director
Human Resources Department
James C. Thompson Memorial Clinic
#1 Lincoln Circle
Paris, TN 37904
Phone: 731.555.3700 ext 90
tlongino@comcast.net

Sample Cover Letter (to accompany résumé)

Diane Smith, RN
73009 Mockingbird Road
Nashville, TN 37758
615.445.5501 (cell)
<u>dsmithrn@comcast.net</u>

July 2, ----

Fred Anderson, MD
The Nashville Diagnostic Clinic
12221 N. Cleary Expressway
Nashville, TN 37758

Dear Dr. Anderson:

Ms. Nadine Longfield, a nurse employed at the clinic, referred me for a job as manager of Human Resources at The Nashville Diagnostic Clinic. I have several years' experience working as a clinic nurse, including working in human resources, which should qualify me for this job.

Please review the enclosed résumé for additional information about my education and related work experience. I am available for an interview at your convenience.

Thank you for your consideration.

(handwritten signature here)

Enclosure

(Sample Thank-You Letter)

Diane Smith, RN
73009 Mockingbird Road
Nashville, TN 37758
615.445.5501 (cell)
dsmithrn@comcast.net

July 28, ----

Fred Anderson, MD
The Nashville Diagnostic Clinic
12221 N. Cleary Expressway
Nashville, TN 37758

Dear Dr. Anderson:

I would like to express my thanks for the time you spent with me yesterday for both the interview and the tour of your facilities. It is clear that you have devoted yourself to providing the best in clinical and diagnostic care for your patients.

I look forward to hearing from you in the near future.

Most sincerely,

(add handwritten signature here)

NB: The thank-you letter is part of the etiquette used when looking for a job. After you have obtained a job, certain points of etiquette should be followed as well. See Computer Etiquette below.

If you are going to forward something that is relevant, such as industry news, be sure to clean up the email. When you click *forward*, remove all the forwarding addresses. Send it to yourself and use BCC for any copies. In the body of the email, remove all of the past headers. Make the email look clean and professional, not left as something that you just carelessly clicked *Forward* and sent.

If you keep all of this in mind, resisting that urge to forward unnecessary or junk email, you will maintain friends, not enemies, keep your professional reputation intact, and be on your way to a bright career. If distributing important workplace-appropriate information is a passion of yours, speak with your boss about starting a company-wide, office, or departmental newsletter that could be sent out regularly with input from the entire staff.

Speech/Voice Recognition and Medical Editing

Referred to as "speech rec" and "voice rec," these are virtually the same thing.

Speech/voice recognition is the process of capturing the spoken word as an input to a computer program, with the goal of creating faster and more efficient documentation. In the healthcare domain, speech recognition can be implemented in the front-end or back-end of the medical documentation process. Front-end speech recognition is where the provider dictates into a speech-recognition engine, the recognized words are displayed as they are spoken, and the dictator is responsible for editing and signing off on his own document(s).

Back-end or deferred speech recognition is where the provider dictates into a digital dictation system, the voice is processed through a speech-recognition engine, and the recognized draft document is routed along with the original voice file to the healthcare documentation specialist (HDS). In this case, the HDS is acting as a medical editor to complete (or finalize) the report. Deferred speech recognition is widely used in medicine currently.

Medical editing of dictated medical records is an extension of the act of transcribing the original documents from a blank screen. The HDS, acting as medical editor, listens to the dictation and edits what has been recorded via the speech recognition engine. Special programs and keyboard applications are used in this process to help the HDS follow the dictation through the text. Medical editors must employ vigilant attention and focus while editing as the eyes, ears, and brain work together to help ensure accuracy of the record. This is a bit of a different skill set from that used in traditional medical transcription in which the HDS is producing transcribed text based on what is heard versus the brain processing and matching what the eyes see on the screen with what the ears hear during medical editing. Once the document has been corrected with regard to accurate terminology and spelling, grammar, and necessary clarifications of the record, it is sent to the originating provider for signature.

Quality Assurance (QA)

QA provides a bridge between the healthcare documentation specialists, the supervisors, and the dictating physicians. QA specialists proofread the completed work, research errors, correct them, and give feedback to each HDS. In this way, individual employees are helped in their learning process of specialized medical terminology and the individual dictators' styles. Management, in turn, is helped in their process of employee evaluation. When employees come up for review, the QA documentation allows the employer to see what errors have been made and how each HDS is learning and growing in the job.

QA feedback can be accomplished as monthly developmental meetings or individually. This feedback, especially when done one-on-one, is important for the HDS to keep up with changes in drugs, terms, procedures, etc. Feedback works best when done often (e.g., daily, weekly, monthly, or quarterly), but this would depend upon the size of the company and how it is organized. Other factors that would be taken into consideration would be how experienced the HDS is and how long they have been with the company. Less experienced HDSs and new employees will need QA performed more often to ensure their work meets quality standards and that they are following site-specific information appropriately. Many companies will have new employees on 100% QA review for a certain period of time to evaluate their work (e.g., two weeks). Likewise, experienced HDSs generally do not need QA performed as often, though quality checks should still be performed on a routine basis.

Quality assurance departments are not present in every company, but for companies that do provide QA review and feedback, there are definite advantages (1) to the dictating physicians in the way of correctly transcribed medical records, (2) to the supervisors in the way of increased efficiency, (3) to the healthcare documentation specialists in the way of continuing education, and (4) to management in the way of informed employees and a smoothly running operation.

Is Healthcare Documentation Going Away?

All kinds of people—from vendors and healthcare professionals to healthcare documentation specialists themselves—have been saying for years that the HDS profession is going away. However, hospitals and MTSOs are looking for full-time **acute-care healthcare**

documentation specialists in every nook and cranny. An author of this text knows a person who left the industry many years ago and later received a call regarding a résumé she had sent in more than five years ago. That is how desperate some companies are for an acute-care HDS, dredging their entire past databases.

Schools that teach healthcare documentation often have requests for more than 100 acute-care-trained HDSs a year. Production companies want to hire acute-care HDSs as well. Résumés have been requested everywhere imaginable—through résumé sites, through email blasts, forums, social media, etc. The vast majority of responses are from people who have experience only in clinic work.

What students may not fully realize is that **CLINIC WORK** in healthcare documentation is not always a viable long-term plan. The work is relatively simple and is the first to go offshore or to 100% speech recognition. **ACUTE CARE** healthcare documentation, however, is an acceptable standard for long-term success; and it remains in high demand. Those who went the route of clinical work are now looking to step up their skill set so they will be viable long-term healthcare documentation specialists in the acute-care arena.

While the myth of jobs being scarce likely will continue, those with acute-care training will continue to enjoy their security and in-demand status as more and more clinic work HDSs realize that they need additional training to remain viable in a fast-moving industry. No, healthcare documentation is definitely not going away; but those who enjoy this career field must upgrade their skills via continuing education to stay ahead of the game.

Other potential areas of employment for acute-care healthcare documentation specialists include legal transcription, scribes, quality-assurance professionals, instructors, trainers/facilitators, patient advocacy, authors, and editors.

Sims, Lea. *The Book of Style for Medical Transcription*, 3rd ed. Modesto: AHDI, 2008.

Dorland. *Dorland's Illustrated Medical Dictionary*, 32nd ed. Philadelphia: Elsevier Saunders, 2011.

Rice, Jane. *Medical Terminology: A Word Building Approach*, 7th ed. New York: Pearson, 2012.

Pitman, Sally. *Radiology Imaging: Words and Phrases*, 2nd ed. Modesto: Health Professions Institute, 2005.

Stedman's Medical Dictionary, 28th ed. Baltimore: Lippincott Williams & Wilkins, 2006.

Stedman's Orthopedic & Rehab Words, 6th ed. Baltimore: Lippincott Williams & Wilkins, 2009.

Stedman's Medical Dictionary for the Health Professions and Nursing, 5th ed. Baltimore: Lippincott Williams & Wilkins, 2005.

Tessier, Claudia. *The Surgical Word Book*, 3rd ed. St. Louis: Elsevier Saunders, 2004.

Postal Addressing Standards, Publication 28. United States Postal Service, 2000, *www.ftb.ca.gov/aboutFTB/Projects/ITSP/USPS*_Publication_28.pdf.

Davis, Neil. *Medical Abbreviations: 32,000 Conveniences at the Expense of Communication and Safety*, 15th ed. Westminster: Davis, 2010.

Lance, Leonard. *Quick Look Drug Book*. Hagerstown: Lippincott Williams & Wilkins, 2011.

Turley, Susan. *Medical Language*, 2nd ed. Upper Saddle River: Prentice Hall, 2011.

Diehl, Marcy. *Medical Transcription Techniques and Procedures*, 7th ed. Philadelphia: Elsevier Saunders, 2012.

Drake, Ellen. *Sloane's Medical Word Book*, 5th ed. St. Louis: Saunders Company, 2011.

Drake, Ellen & Drake, Randy. *Saunders Pharmaceutical Word Book*. St. Louis: Saunders, 2012.

The Merck Manual, 18th ed. Whitehouse Station: Merck Sharp & Dohme Corp., 2006.

Merriam-Webster. *Merriam-Webster's Collegiate Dictionary*, 11th ed. Springfield: Merriam-Webster, Inc., Springfield, 2003.

Lippincott, Williams, & Wilkins publishes medical reference books in the following specialties:
   Stedman's OB/GYN and Pediatric Words
   Stedman's Cardiovascular & Pulmonary Words With Respiratory Words
   Stedman's Oncology Words Includes Hematology, HIV & AIDS
   Stedman's Pathology & Laboratory Medicine Words Includes Histology
   Stedman's GI & GU Words
   Stedman's Plastic Surgery, ENT & Dentistry Words
   Stedman's Radiology Words Includes Nuclear Medicine and Other Imaging
   Stedman's Neurology & Neurosurgery Words
   Stedman's Endocrinology Words
   Stedman's Surgery Words Includes Anatomy, Anesthesia & Pain Management
   Stedman's Organisms & Infectious Disease Words

General online resources consulted:

http://www.webmd.com/

http://www.nlm.nih.gov/

http://www.cdc.gov/

http://www.mayoclinic.com

http://www.mtdesk.com

http://www.cancer.gov

http://www.ninds.nih.gov/

http://www.medicaltranscription.com/

http://www.surgery.com/

http://www.jointcommission.org

Note: All sites listed in individual chapters in the text were consulted as well.

Contents

List of Dictating Healthcare Professionals' names (including specialties and accents)

Last Name	First Name	Specialty	Accent
Adkins, MD	Emily	Surgical Resident	Southern state
Alloy, MD	Stella J.	Anesthesiology	*
Altman, MD	Robert	Pulmonary Surgery/ Respiratory Medicine	Scotland
Bay, MD	Jackie	Hospitalist (Internal Medicine)	Boston
Bruckman, DO	Grayson	Radiology	British
Connerly, MD	Antonia	Pediatrics	NY
Dale, MD	Wanda P.	Neurology	NY
Davis, CRNA	Diane	Anesthesiology	*
Farrow, FNP	Greg	Family Nurse Practitioner	NY
Ferrell, MD	Antoine	Pathology	French
Glover, MD	Olivia	Orthopedic Surgery	NY
Gonzales, PhD	Cynthia G.	Psychology/Social Services	*
Grimm, DC	Stephen	Chiropractic	*
Guajardo, MD	Rachel	Psychiatry	*
Hampton, MD	Faye	Rheumatology	Long Island
Holcomb, MD	Daniel	Ophthalmology	Irish
Howard, RPT	Lamduan "La"	Physical Therapy	*
Hutto, MD	Jennifer	Cardiac Surgery	Dutch
Jackson, MD	Toni	Cardiology	NY
Kelly, MD	Dana (Female)	Urology	Northeastern
King, MD	Miranda	ENT	*
Lanewala, MD	David	Orthopedic Surgery	Indian/Pakistani
Light, RN	Theresa	Surgical Nurse	*
Lindsey, PA-C	Ray Jo	Physician Assistant, Certified	*
Logan, MD	Stacey Lee (Female)	Infectious Disease	Boston
Long, MD	Julia	Neonatology	Russian
Moffett, MD	Michel (Male)	ENT/Oral Surgery	French
Mosel, MD	Grace	Hospitalist (Internal Medicine)	Long Island
Nguyen, RN	Tyron	Surgical Nurse	*
Oswalt, MD	Savant (Male)	Hematology/Oncology	Indian/Pakistani
Palmer, PA-C	Bobby J.	Physician Assistant, Certified	*
Patrick, MD	Lucinda	Internal Medicine	Dutch
Peebles, MD	Sandra	Internal Medicine	Chicago
Phipps, MD	Anderson	Family Medicine/Geriatrics	Southern state

q̃

Pruitt, MD	Catherine	Radiation Oncology	NY
Quimby, MD	Judith	General Surgery	NY
Reyes, MD	Anthony	General Surgeon	British
Rhodes, MD	Yancy (Male)	Endocrinology	British
Robertson, MD	Doris	Gastroenterology	NY
Russo, MD	David	General Surgery	*
Russo, MD	Holly	Neurosurgery	Southern state
Scott, MD	Charles W.	Obstetrics/Gynecology	Irish
Sherman, MD	Jamie Z. (Female)	Pediatrics	NY
Sherwood, DPM	Donna	Podiatry	NY
Shuff, MD	Phyllis	Nephrology	Jamaican
Swafford, MD	Mark	Plastic & Reconstructive Surgery	Arabic
Tew, MD	Charles	Radiology	Chinese
Timmerman, MD	Callie	Dermatology	*
Travis, CRNA	Miller	Anesthesiology	*
Travis, MD	Murray	Obstetrics/Gynecology	Local
Trigg, MD	Dominika	Pathology	Russian
Upshaw, MD	Jody	Anesthesiology	*
Van Cleave, MD	Martin T.	Retinal Specialist	*
Warren, MD	Tonya	Hematology/Oncology	NY
Webb, MD	Zachary	Vascular Surgery	Jamaican
Wilder, MD	Connie C.	Emergency Medicine	NY
Wolfe, MD	Jeffery	Cardiac Surgery	Scotland
Wong, DDS	Sans	Dentistry	*

*No dictation

List of Confusing Terms

Many letters and words sound similar. Listen carefully, use critical thinking skills, and consider the surrounding context before choosing which word to transcribe.

abduction – the act of drawing away from (often dictated "a-b-duction")
adduction – the act of drawing toward a center (often dictated "a-d-duction")
subduction – the act of drawing downward; infraduction

aberration – deviation from the usual course or condition
abrasion – the wearing away of a substance or structure through some unusual or abnormal mechanical process

absorption – the soaking up of a substance by skin or other surface
adsorption – the adherence of a substance to a surface

acathexia – the inability to retain bodily secretions
cachexia – general ill health and malnutrition

afferent – carries impulses *toward* a center or part
efferent – carrying *away* from a central organ or part

allograft – transfer or transplants between two individuals of the same species
autograft – transfers or transplants from the same person

anuresis – retention of urine in the bladder
enuresis – urinary incontinence

aphagia – inability to swallow
aphasia – absent or impaired comprehension or communication by speech or writing—may be transient, as in acquired lesion or swelling of the brain

apophysis – outgrowth or swelling
epiphysis – a center for formation of bone substance at each extremity of long bones

areola – (n) a circular area of a different color surrounding a central point, as in the breast
areolae – plural of areola
areolar – (adj) pertaining to or containing areolae

arrhythmia – irregular heartbeat
eurhythmia – regular pulse

arteriosclerosis – a group of diseases characterized by thickening and the loss of elasticity of arterial walls
atherosclerosis – hardening of the arteries caused by the deposition of calcium and cholesterol in the arterial walls
arteriostenosis – ossification of an artery
arteriotomy – surgical opening of an artery

arteritis – inflammation of artery
arthritis – inflammation of a joint
arterial – pertaining to one or more arteries
arteriole – a small arterial branch

arthropathy – any joint disease
arthroplasty – plastic surgery of a joint

aural – pertaining to the ear
oral – pertaining to the mouth

bronchi – plural of bronchus
rhonchi – pertaining to a rattling in the throat or dry, coarse rales in the bronchial tubes

bursa – a sac or sac-like cavity filled with viscid fluid
bursae – plural of bursa

calculous – (adj) pertaining to, of the nature of, or affected with calculus
calculus – (n) a hard, pebble-like mass formed within the body, as in the gallbladder

callous – (adj) unfeeling; the adjective form of callus
callus – (n) a callosity; hard skin

cancellous – (adj) of a reticular, spongy, or lattice-like structure; said mainly of bony tissue
cancellus – (n) any structure arranged like a lattice

canker – an ulceration, primarily of the mouth and lips
chancre – the primary lesion of syphilis

cerebellum – that part of the brain behind the cerebrum
cerebrum – the main portion of the brain

cirrhosis – a progressive disease in which healthy liver tissue is replaced with scar tissue, thereby preventing the liver from functioning properly
xerosis – abnormal dryness, as of the eye, skin, or mouth
sclerosis – hardening, as hardening of a part from inflammation

cite – to quote
site – a location
sight – the function of seeing, a view, or to take aim

colectomy – excision of a portion of the colon
colpectomy – excision of the vagina

colonic – pertaining to the colon
clonic – pertaining to muscular contractions and relaxations that alternate in rapid succession

cornua (noun), corneal (adj.) – pl. of cornu, a structure resembling a horn in shape, i.e., cornua uteri

cornea (noun), corneal (adj) – the transparent structure forming the anterior part of the sclera of the eye, i.e., cornea of the eye

cystoscopy – direct visual examination of the urinary tract with a cystoscope

cystostomy – the formation of an opening into the bladder

cystotomy – surgical incision of the urinary bladder

dilation – the act of being dilated or stretched

dilatation – condition of being stretched beyond the normal dimensions

diuresis - an increased secretion of urine

uresis – the passage of urine

dysphagia – difficulty in swallowing

dysphasia – impairment of speech

dysplasia – abnormality of development

effusion – escape of a fluid into a part

affusion – pouring of water upon the body to reduce temperature

infusion – continuous introduction of solution, especially into a vein

emphysema – a pathological accumulation of air in tissues or organs, as in the lungs

empyema – accumulation of pus in a cavity

enervation – lack of nervous energy

innervation – the supply of nervous energy or of nerve stimulus sent to a part

enterocleisis – closure of a wound in the intestine

enteroclysis – the injection of a nutrient or medicinal liquid into the bowel

epididymis – the structure attached to the back of the testis

epididymitis – inflammation of the epididymis

exostosis – a bony growth that emanates from the surface of a bone

enostosis – an osseous tumor within the cavity of a bone

facial – pertaining to the face

fascial – pertaining to the fascia (a layer of fibrous tissue)

facioplasty – plastic surgery of the face

fascioplasty – plastic surgery on a fascia

fascicular – pertaining to a fascicle

vesicular – composed of or relating to small, sac-like bodies

testicular – pertaining to a testis

facies – pertaining to the anterior or ventral aspect of the head from forehead to chin

feces – the excrement discharged from the intestines

fascicle – a small bundle, like muscle or nerve fibers

vesicle – a small fluid-containing sac

fecal – pertaining to excrement discharged from the intestines

thecal – pertaining to an enclosing case or sheath

fossa – a trench or channel; a general term for a hollow or depressed area

fossae – plural of fossa

fundus – the bottom or base

fungus – a vegetable cellular organism that subsists on organic matter—a mushroom is a fungus

hemithorax – one side of the chest

hemothorax – a collection of blood in the pleural cavity

pneumothorax – accumulation of air or gas in the pleural space

hemostasis – the arrest of bleeding
homeostasis – a tendency to stability in the normal body states of an organism

hyperglycemia – abnormally increased content of sugar in the blood
hyperglycinemia – heredity disorder involving excessive glycine in the blood
hypoglycemla – abnormally low content of sugar in the blood

hypertension – persistently high arterial blood pressure
hypotension – abnormally low blood pressure

ileum – part of the small intestine (gastrointestinal system)
ilium – part of the pelvis (musculoskeletal system)
ileus – disease (obstruction of the small intestine)

ketosis – a condition characterized by an abnormally elevated concentration of ketone bodies in the body tissues and fluids
keratosis – a horny growth

loupe – a pair of glasses worn by a surgeon in ocular surgery; "loupe magnification"
loop – an instrument used to grasp and remove the lens; "lens loop"

M (header)

malleolus – a bone of the ankle
malleus – a bone of the ear

mammaplasty <u>or</u> **mammoplasty** – plastic reconstruction of the breast
mammillaplasty – plastic surgery of the nipple and areola

metacarpal – relating to the hand
metatarsal – relating to the foot, between the instep and the toes

mucosa – **(n)** a mucous membrane
mucosal – **(adj)** pertaining to the mucous membrane

mucous – **(adj)** pertaining to or resembling mucus
mucus – **(n)** secretion or slime of the mucous membrane

myelitis – inflammation of the spinal cord
myositis – inflammation of a voluntary muscle

naris – the nostril; one side of the nasal opening
nares – plural of naris; both nasal openings

nephritis – inflammation of a kidney
neuritis – inflammation of a nerve

nuchal – the back, nape, or scruff of the neck
knuckle – the dorsal aspect of any phalangeal joint

ostial – between two distinct cavities within the body
osteal – bony

palate – the partition separating the nasal and oral cavities
palliate – to reduce the severity of

palpation – the act of feeling with the hand
palpitation – unduly rapid action of the heart

para – combining form meaning beside, near, past, beyond, the opposite, abnormal
peri – prefix meaning around or about

pericardial – **(adj)** pertaining to the membrane surrounding the heart and great vessels
pericardium – **(n)** the membrane surrounding the heart

perineal – pertaining to the perineum or genital region

peritoneal – pertaining to the peritoneum, the membrane lining the abdominal wall

peroneal – pertaining to the fibula or the outer side of the leg

peritoneum – the serous membrane lining the abdominopelvic walls

perineum – the pelvic floor and the associated structures occupying the pelvic outlet

plain x-ray – no contrast media was used; a noncontrast film

plane x-ray – a tomogram

pleural space – space between the parietal and visceral layers of the pleura

plural space – more than one space

precordial – pertaining to the region over the heart and lower part of the thorax

precordium – the region of the thorax immediately over the heart

psittacosis – an infectious disease of parrots and other birds that may be transmitted to humans

psychosis – a general term for any major mental disorder of organic or emotional origin

sycosis – a disease marked by inflammation of the hair follicles

radical – directed to the cause; directed to the root or source of a morbid process

radicle – any one of the smallest branches of a vessel or nerve

reflux – a backward flow

reflex – an involuntary response to a stimulus

scirrhous – **(adj)** pertaining to a cancer that is stony hard to the touch; scirrhous carcinoma

scirrhus – **(n)** hard, a hard tumor

serious – said or done in earnest; sincere

supination – the act of rotating the arm so that the palm of the hand is forward or upward

suppuration – the formation or discharge of pus

tendinous – resembling a tendon

tendinitis – inflammation of a tendon or tendons

ureter – tube through which urine travels to the bladder—we have a left and a right ureter

urethra – a membranous canal through which urine travels from the bladder to the surface—we have one urethra

ureteral – pertaining to the ureters

urethral – pertaining to the urethra

vena cava – one of two venae cavae, superior or inferior

venae cavae – the two largest veins in the body

vesical – pertaining to the urinary bladder

vesicle – any small bladder or sac containing liquid

villous – **(adj)** shaggy with soft hairs; covered with villi

villus – **(n)** a small vascular process or protrusion

viral – pertaining to a virus

virile – possessing masculine traits

List of Medical Instruments (partial list)

A

Abadie clamp
ACMI gastroscope
Adair-Allis tissue forceps
Adson forceps
Adson-Brown forceps
Allport-Babcock mastoid
   retractor
argon laser

B

Babcock forceps
Backhaus dilator
Backhaus towel clamps
Bacon rongeur
Bailey-Gibbon rib contractor
Bainbridge goiter clamp
Bakes common duct
   dilator
Balfour retractor
Ballenger-Lillie mastoid bur
Ballenger tonsil forceps
Bard-Parker blade
Barraquer iris forceps
Beck-Schenck tonsil snare
Beckman goiter retractor
Bellucci scissors
Benedict gastroscope
Bennett retractor
Berens lens expressor
Berens mastectomy
   retractor
Bernstein gastroscope
Bethune rib shears
Beyer rongeur forceps
Blanchard hemorrhoid
   forceps
Blohmka tonsil hemostat
Boettcher antrum trocar
Bonney dissecting forceps
Boucheron ear speculum
Bovie unit
Bozeman forceps
Braasch bulb ureteral
   catheter
Bronson-Turtz iris retractor

Brown-Buerger cystoscope
Burford rib spreader

C

Cameron flexible gastroscope
Caparosa burs
Carmel clamps
Castroviejo-Arruga forceps
Cavanaugh-Wells tonsil suturing
   forceps
Chevalier Jackson gastroscope
Church scissors
Cicherelli rongeur/forceps
Clark common duct dilator
Cloward instrument
Collin forceps
Cottle-Neivert retractor
C-P suction (Chaffin-Pratt)
Crile hemostatic forceps
Crutchfield tongs
Cushing retractor
Cushing vein retractor

D

Dandy forceps
Davidson electric bur
Davis-Crowe mouth gag
Deaver retractor
Debakey-Cooley retractor
deCourcy goiter clamp
DeMartel-Wolfson forceps
Depuy-Weiss tonsil needle
Deschamps ligature needles
Desjardin gallstone forceps
Desmarres lid elevator
Deutschman cataract knife
DeVilbiss cranial rongeur
DeWecker eye scissors
Dormia basket
Doubilet sphincterotome
Doyen intestinal occlusion
   clamp
Doyen raspatory
Doyen retractor
Duckbill rongeur

Duffield scissors
Dunning periosteal elevator
Duval-Allis forceps

E

Eder gastroscope
Elliott forceps
Ellsner gastroscope
Elschnig cataract knife
Emerson suction

F

Farabeuf periosteal elevator
Faulkner antrum gouge
Fehland clamps
Fein antrum trocar
Fenger forceps
Ferguson needle
Ferris-Robb tonsil knife
Finochietto rib spreader
Foley catheter
Frankfeldt grasping forceps
Frazier retractor
Freer elevator
French catheter
Fritsch retractor
Furniss-Clute clamp

G

Gavin-Miller forceps
Gelepi retractor
Gerzog mallet
Gifford curette
Gigli saw
Gill scissors
Gomco clamp
Gomco suction tube
Goodell dilator
Goodhill tonsil forceps
Graham scalene elevator
Grover meniscotome
Gruenwald rongeur
Guyton-Park lid speculum

Hajek elevator/mallet
Hall air drill
Hank dilator
Harrison-Shea curet
Hartmann forceps
Heaney forceps
Heerman chisel
Hegar dilator
Hemovac drain
Herrick clamp
Heyman-Paparella angular scissors
Hibbs retractor
Hibbs-Spratt curette
Hirschowitz gastroduodenal
    fiberscope
Holter valve
Hotz ear probe
House-Dieter Malleus nipper
House myringotomy knife
Housset-Debray gastroscope

Jaboulay button
Jackson laryngoscope
Janeway gastroscope
Jansen forceps
Jesberg scope
Jewett osteotomy plate
Johns Hopkins forceps
Joker dissector
Judd-DeMartel forceps

Kahler forceps
Keeler pantoscope
Kehr T-tube
Kelly forceps
Kelly-Murphy forceps
Kelman forceps
Kerrison rongeur/forceps
Key periosteal elevator
Kifa skin clip
Kirschner wire
Klebanoff gallstone scoop
Knapp cataract knife

Kocher clamp
Krukenberg pigment spindle
Krwawicz cataract extractor

Lahey forceps
Lambotte osteotome
Lane forceps
Langenbeck retractor
LeFort catheter
Lempert knife
Luer bone rongeur
Luer-Korte scoop
Luer-Whiting rongeur forceps

MacDonald dissector
Mahoney speculum
Malecot catheter
Mathieu retractor
Mayo scissors
McCaskey curette
McGuire scissors
McIndoe scissors
McIvor gag
Mentor wet field coagulator
Metzembaum scissors
Meyerding finger retractor
Michel clips
Moersch esophagoscope
Mollison mastoid retractor
Molt mouth gag
Morris retractor
mosquito forceps
Moynihan artery forceps
Mueller mastoid curette

Nesbit resectoscope

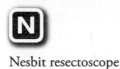

O'Brien forceps
Ochsner forceps

Olivecrona rongeur/forceps
Ollier rake retractor
O'Sullivan-O'Connor retractor

Parker-Heath cautery
Parker ribbon retractor
Payr clamps
Pean forceps
Penrose drain
Pezzer catheter
Potts-Smith forceps

R

Rampley sponge holding
    forceps
Rapaport common duct
    dilators
Reich-Nechtow forceps
Reiner rongeur
Rigby self-retaining
    retractor
Rizzuti iris retractor
Roux retractor
Rubinstein cryoprobe
Ruskin mastoid rongeur

S

Sam Roberts head rest
Sarot needle holder
Satinsky clamp
Sauerbruch box rib
    rongeur
scalpel
Schiotz tenometer
Schnidt forceps
Schroeder forceps
Schuknecht knife
Sengstaken balloon
Senn retractor
Shallcross forceps
Shambaugh irrigator
Shea curette
Shoemaker thyroid
    scissors
Siker laryngoscope

Sims probe
Storz-Beck tonsil snare
Sump drain

Thorek scissors
Timberlake obturator

VanBuren urethral sounds
Varco forceps

Volkmann rake retractor
von Graefe cataract knife
von Petz clamp

Wagner antrum punch
Wangensteen clamp
Weiner-Pierce antrum trocar
Weitlaner retractor
Weitlaner self-retaining retractor
Wellaminski antrum perforator
Westcott scissors
Winsbury-White deep retractor
Woodson plastic instrument

Yankauer antrum punch
Yankauer suction tube

Zeiss operating microscope
Ziegler knife
Zipser clamp

Supportive Resources for Equipment

Stedman's Medical & Surgical Equipment Words, 4th ed. Baltimore: Lippincott Williams & Wilkins, 2004.

The Surgical Word Book by Claudia Tessier, 3rd ed. St. Louis, MO: Elsevier Saunders, 2004.

http://www.sklarcorp.com/   Search for "resources"; click on Skylar Surgical Instruments—Surgical Resources.

http://www.surgical911.com   Click on links of interest; this site has an extensive list of instruments.

Types of Sutures and Suture Materials (partial list)

a
Acier stainless steel
Acufex bioabsorbable
  Suretac
Acumed suture anchor
Ailee
Anspach suture anchor
ArthroSew suturing
  system
Atralease
atraumatic

b
bioabsorbable
BioSorb
Biosyn

Bondek absorbable
Bralon braided nylon
bridle
buried
buried-knot

c
chromic catgut
coaptation
colposuspension
Connell
continuous
Cushing
Cutalon
cutaneous

d
Dacron
Dafilon
Dagrofil
Deklene II
Deknatel
Dermalene
Dermalon
Dexon

e
Ethicon
Ethiflex
Ethilon
Ethistrip skin closures
everting

f
figure-of-8
Flexon

g
Giampapa
Grams nonabsorbable

h
Halsted
hemostatic

i
Investa

k
Kelly plication

l
Lembert
limbal
Linatrix
Littre
lock-stitch vertical
   mattress
Lukens PGA

m
mattress
Maunsell
Maxon
Mersilene
Mersilk black silk
Micrins microsurgical
MicroMite anchor
Miralene
Mitek
Mitek Mini GII
Monocryl
monofilament
Monosyn
multifilament

n
Novafil
Nurolon

p
Palfyn
Panacryl
PDS
PeBA
Petit
PGA
plication
Polydek
polyethylene
Polysorb
Prolene
Pronova
pursestring

r
Ramdohr
Rapide
Reddick-Saye
retention
right-angle

Ritisch
running lock

s
Safil
Serralene
Serralnyl
Serralsilk
Silkam
silk-braided
Sofsilk
Softcat
stainless steel
Statak
Steelex
steel mesh
stick tie
subcuticular
superior rectus
Supramid
Suretac
Surgilon
Sutralon
SutraSilk
Suture Clinch

Suture Lok
Sutured-Clip
Sutureloop
Synthofil

t
Tevdek
through-and-through
tongue-in-groove
traction
Tycron or Ti-Cron

u
Ultrasorb
undyed

v
Vascufil
Vicryl
Vicryl Rapide
visceroparietal

y
Y-sutures

z
Zimmer Statak

Types of Anesthetic Agents (partial list)

Anestacon
Brevital
Carbocaine
cocaine
Demerol
Ethrane
fentanyl
Fluothane

Forane
halothane
ketamine
   hydrochloride
lidocaine
Marcaine hydrochloride
morphine
Nembutal

Nescacaine
Nisentil
nitrous oxide
Novocain
Nupercaine
   hydrochloride
Pontocaine
procaine hydrochloride

sodium pentothal
sufentanil
tetracaine
   hydrochloride
thiopental sodium
topical cocaine
Valium
Xylocaine

Supportive Web Site for Anesthesia

http://www.nlm.nih.gov/medlineplus/   Click on "Health Topics"; search for "anesthesia" and select links of interest.

Types of Dressings (partial list)

ABD pad
Adaptic
Aeroplast
Desault bandage,
    ligature
Esmarch bandage,
    tourniquet

Kerlix gauze
Kling bandage, dressing
Kos-House
Owen cloth
Robert-Jones compression
    bandage
Sayre bandage

scultetus binder
Semken dressing
spica cast
stent surgical
    dressing
Steri-Drape
    (3-M drape)

Steri-Strip skin closure
Steri-tape
Telfa
Unna paste boot
Vaseline wick dressing
Velpeau bandage
Xeroform gauze dressing

Types of Surgical Incisions (partial list)

ab-externo
Auvray
buttonhole
Cherney
circumferential
collar
coronal
crosshatch
cruciate
curvilinear
Deaver

Dührssen
elliptical
endaural
Fowler
gridiron
hockey-stick
infraumbilical
intracapsular
Kehr
Kocher
Küstner

Langenbeck
lateral flank
lateral rectus
Mackenrodt
McBurney
median
midline
muscle splitting
paramedian
Parker
Pfannenstiel

racquet or racket
rectus muscle splitting
Rockey-Davis
Schuchardt
suprapubic
transverse
Vischer lumboiliac
Z-flap
Z-shaped

Types of Operative Positions (partial list)

decubitus
dorsal recumbent or
    dorsorecumbent
jackknife

knee-chest
Kraske
lateral

lithotomy
Proetz
prone

Sims
supine
Trendelenburg

Joint Commission Official "Do Not Use" List[1]

Do Not Use	Potential Problem	Use Instead
U, u (unit)	Mistaken for "0" (zero), the number "4" (four) or "cc"	Write "unit"
IU (International Unit)	Mistaken for IV (intravenous) or the number 10 (ten)	Write "International Unit"
Q.D., QD, q.d., qd (daily)	Mistaken for each other	Write "daily"
Q.O.D., QOD, q.o.d, qod (every other day)	Period after the Q mistaken for "I" and the "O" mistaken for "I"	Write "every other day"
Trailing zero (X.0 mg)*	Decimal point is missed	Write X mg
Lack of leading zero (.X mg)		Write 0.X mg
MS	Can mean morphine sulfate or magnesium sulfate	Write "morphine sulfate" / Write "magnesium sulfate"
MSO_4 and $MgSO_4$	Confused for one another	

[1]Applies to all orders and all medication-related documentation that is handwritten (including free-text computer entry) or on pre-printed forms.

*Exception: A "trailing zero" may be used only where required to demonstrate the level of precision of the value being reported, such as for laboratory results, imaging studies that report size of lesions, or catheter/tube sizes. It may not be used in medication orders or other medication-related documentation.

Additional Abbreviations, Acronyms and Symbols
(For possible future inclusion in the Official "Do Not Use" List)

Do Not Use	Potential Problem	Use Instead
> (greater than) < (less than)	Misinterpreted as the number "7" (seven) or the letter "L" Confused for one another	Write "greater than" Write "less than"
Abbreviations for drug names	Misinterpreted due to similar abbreviations for multiple drugs	Write drug names in full
Apothecary units	Unfamiliar to many practitioners Confused with metric units	Use metric units
@	Mistaken for the number "2" (two)	Write "at"
cc	Mistaken for U (units) when poorly written	Write "mL" or "ml" or "milliliters" ("mL" is preferred)
µg	Mistaken for mg (milligrams) resulting in one thousand-fold overdose	Write "mcg" or "micrograms"

Two-Letter Postal Codes from United States Postal Service

According to USPS Publication 28, PE.USPS.GOV, pp 63–64.

Use the abbreviations below when addressing mail. Using the two-letter state abbreviations makes it possible to enter the city, state, and five-digit ZIP Code (or ZIP+4 code) on the last line of the address within 29 positions when necessary: 13 positions for city, one space between city and state abbreviation, two positions for the state, two spaces (preferred) between the state and ZIP Code, and 10 positions for the ZIP+4 code.

State/Possession	Abbreviation	State/Possession	Abbreviation
Alabama	AL	Nevada	NV
Alaska	AK	New Hampshire	NH
American Samoa	AS	New Jersey	NJ
Arizona	AZ	New Mexico	NM
Arkansas	AR	New York	NY
California	CA	North Carolina	NC
Colorado	CO	North Dakota	ND
Connecticut	CT	Northern Mariana Islands	MP
Delaware	DE	Ohio	OH
District of Columbia	DC	Oklahoma	OK
Federated States of		Oregon	OR
Micronesia	FM	Palau	PW
Florida	FL	Pennsylvania	PA
Georgia	GA	Puerto Rico	PR
Guam	GU	Rhode Island	RI
Hawaii	HI	South Carolina	SC
Idaho	ID	South Dakota	SD
Illinois	IL	Tennessee	TN
Indiana	IN	Texas	TX
Iowa	IA	Utah	UT
Kansas	KS	Vermont	VT
Kentucky	KY	Virgin Islands	VI
Louisiana	LA	Virginia	VA
Maine	ME	Washington	WA
Marshall Islands	MH	West Virginia	WV
Maryland	MD	Wisconsin	WI
Massachusetts	MA	Wyoming	WY
Michigan	MI		
Minnesota	MN	Military "State"	
Mississippi	MS	Armed Forces Europe, The	
Missouri	MO	Middle East, & Canada	AE
Montana	MT	Armed Forces Pacific	AP
Nebraska	NE	Armed Forces Americas	
		(except Canada)	AA

Text Expanders

Text expanders allow a healthcare documentation specialist (HDS) to increase productivity by minimizing key strokes. A typical expander works by recognizing short forms that are developed for words, then expanding them into the long form. Many suggest using the first three letters of a word plus the last letter as the short form; for example, "abdl" for abdominal. Every time this shortcut is used, you would save about four letters. Some use "pt" for patient, "hy" for history, "rx" for prescription, and so on. Just these few simple shortcuts can save many keystrokes over time.

An HDS can and should develop a personal list of shortcuts, which is much better than simply importing lists from others. The goal is to use shortcuts that you know and will use versus looking simply to build a large database.

People usually begin by using Microsoft Word's autocorrect feature to define some basic shortcuts. This may work well in the beginning; it becomes burdensome, however, to add new forms quickly, backup, and take the shortcuts with you.

Using a commercial expander program* allows an HDS to develop, edit, import, and export shortcuts quickly. It also allows shortcuts to be saved on a thumb drive for when travel is a necessity. Text expander programs work with any Windows program seamlessly. These programs quickly pay for themselves in time and strokes saved.

*SpeedType, PhraseExpress, and InstantText are just a few of the commercial expander programs available on Google or Amazon or can be purchased retail.

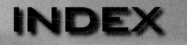

INDEX